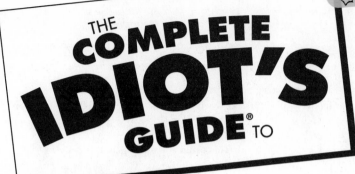

THE COMPLETE **IDIOT'S** GUIDE® TO

Total Nutrition

Fourth Edition

by Joy Bauer, M.S., R.D., C.D.N.

ALPHA

A member of Penguin Group (USA) Inc.

This book is dedicated to my husband, Ian, my daughters, Jesse and Ayden Jane, and my son, Cole, who are always there to make me smile.

ALPHA BOOKS

Published by the Penguin Group

Penguin Group (USA) Inc., 375 Hudson Street, New York, New York 10014, U.S.A.

Penguin Group (Canada), 10 Alcorn Avenue, Toronto, Ontario, Canada M4V 3B2 (a division of Pearson Penguin Canada Inc.)

Penguin Books Ltd, 80 Strand, London WC2R 0RL, England

Penguin Ireland, 25 St Stephen's Green, Dublin 2, Ireland (a division of Penguin Books Ltd)

Penguin Group (Australia), 250 Camberwell Road, Camberwell, Victoria 3124, Australia (a division of Pearson Australia Group Pty Ltd)

Penguin Books India Pvt Ltd, 11 Community Centre, Panchsheel Park, New Delhi—110 017, India

Penguin Group (NZ), cnr Airborne and Rosedale Roads, Albany, Auckland 1310, New Zealand (a division of Pearson New Zealand Ltd)

Penguin Books (South Africa) (Pty) Ltd, 24 Sturdee Avenue, Rosebank, Johannesburg 2196, South Africa

Penguin Books Ltd, Registered Offices: 80 Strand, London WC2R 0RL, England

Copyright © 2005 by Joy Bauer

International Standard Book Number: 1-59-257439-4
Library of Congress Catalog Card Number: 2005929455

08   07   06   8   7   6   5   4

Interpretation of the printing code: The rightmost number of the first series of numbers is the year of the book's printing; the rightmost number of the second series of numbers is the number of the book's printing. For example, a printing code of 05-1 shows that the first printing occurred in 2005.

Printed in the United States of America

Note: This publication contains the opinions and ideas of its author. It is intended to provide helpful and informative material on the subject matter covered. It is sold with the understanding that the author and publisher are not engaged in rendering professional services in the book. If the reader requires personal assistance or advice, a competent professional should be consulted.

The author and publisher specifically disclaim any responsibility for any liability, loss, or risk, personal or otherwise, which is incurred as a consequence, directly or indirectly, of the use and application of any of the contents of this book.

Most Alpha books are available at special quantity discounts for bulk purchases for sales promotions, premiums, fundraising, or educational use. Special books, or book excerpts, can also be created to fit specific needs.

For details, write: Special Markets, Alpha Books, 375 Hudson Street, New York, NY 10014.

Publisher: *Marie Butler-Knight*
Editorial Director: *Mike Sanders*
Senior Managing Editor: *Jennifer Bowles*
Acquisitions Editor: *Tom Stevens*
Development Editor: *Michael Hall*
Production Editor: *Janette Lynn*

Copy Editor: *Ross Patty*
Illustrator: *Richard King*
Cover/Book Designer: *Trina Wurst*
Indexer: *Brad Herriman*
Layout: *Ayanna Lacey*
Proofreading: *Donna Martin*

Contents at a Glance

Contents

Appendixes

Foreword

In a very real way, knowing too much about nutrition can be a curse. Even though I adore my job as health director of *SELF* magazine, I long for the days when I could eat a meal thinking more about how hungry I was and what sounded good than the fiber, fat, and carb content of every forkful.

Nowadays that's nearly impossible, and not just for those of us who are tummy-deep in every new finding about how nutrition affects your health. Thanks to the barrage of information—some accurate, some erroneous, most designed to get you to buy a specific product—it's hard to know what your body needs.

Think back to the last time you picked up a menu. Your thought process probably went something like this: "I'd like a sandwich, but what kind? Let's see ... can't have salami because of the saturated fat. Can't have the ham because of the nitrites. What about turkey? Hate it without cheese, but too much of that will give you a heart attack ... it's high in cholesterol. Okay, so no cheese—ooh, and no mayo—but maybe plain turkey. But no bread ... carbs are bad, right? No, wait, now I've heard they're good, as long as they're whole grain. Is rye a whole grain? I wonder how much fiber is in rye bread ... any antioxidants?" You get the idea.

Enter Joy Bauer and *The Complete Idiot's Guide to Total Nutrition*. By the way, you're not a complete idiot—you're just understandably confused. Working with Joy at *SELF*, where she's a columnist and a contributing editor, I've come to rely on her not just for her ability to cut through the conflicting headlines so I might bring our readers the straight dope, but for her commonsense approach to eating well.

That's because to Joy, "well" doesn't only mean healthfully. She is aware that food—whether you're trying to lose weight, keep a disease in check, or just eat for maximum energy—must be satisfying to the soul as well as to the body. She knows that the best diet is one that you'll stick to. She also has built-in bull radar, which detects overblown and misleading claims and marketing. All of these elements of Joy's philosophy leave her advice—and this book—fad-free.

When I had my first working lunch with Joy, I loaded my tray with salad, vegetables, grilled chicken—what I thought would impress her as informed dietary choices. For my drink, I picked water. I don't remember what she had. After eating food I don't recall even tasting, I ogled a fellow diner's enormous chocolate cupcake. "You should have one," Joy said. "As long as you don't eat the whole thing and don't have one every day, there's no reason a cupcake can't be a treat."

In truth, if she hadn't been around, I probably would have gotten one in the first place, scarfed it down, and then felt guilty about it. But Joy's way of thinking about how a cupcake can fit into a realistic eating plan—how devil's food cake is not, in fact, the devil—made it seem less forbidden. I got the cupcake, and found that a third of it was enough to satisfy me, so I didn't feel deprived.

In short, nowhere in *The Complete Idiot's Guide to Total Nutrition* will you find finger-wagging, tongue-clucking, or moralistic judgment about how you eat.

What you will find is clear, bottom-line information about what to eat and how much, served up with humor and style and empathy for how difficult it can be to make good choices in today's food environment. Keep it nearby and refer to it whenever you want to be sure you're doing the best thing for your body.

—Stephanie Dolgoff, health director, *SELF* magazine.

Introduction

If you're confused by the enormous amount of nutrition information that bombards us on a daily basis, this book is for you! It's an up-to-date, comprehensive guide to eating smart and becoming fit that is both trustworthy, and—most importantly—reader-friendly. It's the product of *years* of personal and professional experience working with people who want to slim down, bulk up, maintain good health, combat diseases, or just plain look and feel great.

How to Use This Book

To make the reading easier for you, I've divided these pages into six areas of interest:

Part 1, "Time for a Nutrition Tune-Up," is all about the fundamentals of food. This section dissects the dietary guidelines and offers simple strategies to help you incorporate the five basic food groups into your life. You'll also get the inside scoop on simple and complex carbohydrates, the power of protein, and the relationship between excess fat intake and heart disease. Finally, you'll learn the facts about fiber, salt, and those vital vitamins and minerals your body requires.

Part 2, "Making Savvy Food Choices," shows you that dining healthfully does not mean giving up the pleasure of eating. In this section, you'll learn how to become a Sherlock Holmes in your local grocery store—capable of decoding the nutrition information on product labels and making more-informed food choices. You'll take a "virtual" tour through a supermarket and load your cart with healthy foods to stock in your kitchen. You'll also find many easy-to-make, low-fat recipes, as well as the best bets in ethnic and fast-food restaurants for when you just don't want to cook. Lastly, you'll learn strategies for creating holiday menus that don't forfeit taste *or* tradition.

Part 3, "The ABCs of Exercise," provides the tools and inspiration to get you moving and *keep* you moving. That's right—a crash course on becoming physically fit. You'll hear the lowdown on strengthening your heart and lungs through aerobic exercise, and get tips on how to buff your bodacious bod through appropriate weight training and conditioning. You'll learn the importance of warming up, cooling down, and stretching your body, *plus* get the education you need to enter a gym with confidence. There's also a comprehensive guide to sports nutrition that will help you learn how to fuel your body for both casual exercise and competitive sport.

Part 4, "Beyond the Basics: Nutrition for Special Needs," discusses how good nutrition can help prevent or slow the progress of various diseases and conditions—from cancer, diabetes, and heart disease to gastrointestinal ailments, migraines, and

PMS. There's also a section on food allergies and intolerances, and one on the various types of vegetarian diets. You'll also find a comprehensive guide to herbal remedies for things like depression, insomnia, arthritis, cancer, liver and heart disease, respiratory ailments, and benign prostatic hyperplasia.

Part 5, "Pregnancy and Parenting," provides essential information that will help you manage your growing baby's nutritional needs. You'll learn how much weight you should gain, the right foods to eat, and which foods to avoid. This section also includes recipes for healthy after-school snacks, strategic ways to disguise vegetables and help your kids eat healthier, and tips to encourage more physical activity.

Part 6, "Weight Management 101," provides you with a sensible plan of attack—whether you want to lose weight, gain weight, or just stop obsessing about food. For those of you who want to trim *down*, check out my "Bubble" weight-loss plan. And for those of you who want to bulk *up*, there are tons of calorie-cramming strategies and food supplements to help you achieve your goals. Finally, you'll find a section on life-threatening eating disorders that includes resources to help you find balance when food and exercise go beyond health and get way out of control.

Extras

To help you get the most out of this book, I've sprinkled it with the following helpful information boxes.

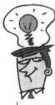

Food for Thought

Follow these tips on eating and exercising to make everyday nutrition and fitness fun.

Nutri-Speak

This box provides definitions of food and exercise jargon.

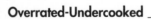

Overrated-Undercooked

You should keep these warnings in mind when eating or exercising.

Q & A

The questions we all want to ask and their answers.

Acknowledgments

Many thanks to the tremendous number of people who helped pull this book together. First, let me extend my eternal gratitude to my nutrition team at Joy Bauer Nutrition: Lisa Mandelbaum-Brown, M.S., R.D.; Jennifer Medina, M.S., R.D., C.D.E.; Laura Pumillo, M.A., R.D.; Maria Baldo, M.S., R.D., C.D.E.; Elyssa Hurlbut, M.S., R.D.; Nicole DiLorenzo, M.S., R.D.; Erica Ilton, M.S., R.D.; Suzanne Magnotta M.S., R.D.; and Rebecca Gainen, M.S., R.D.

A special thanks to Erica Ilton for her unstoppable brilliance—this fourth edition shines because of her research and editorial expertise. Thanks to Jennifer Medina for providing her invaluable knowledge on diabetes mellitus and as always, thanks to Rosemary Black, a talented writer who is there whenever I call.

Many thanks to Mitch Douglas for making this book happen over and over again. Tremendous thanks to Tom Stevens, Michael Hall, Jan Lynn, and Ross Patty for perfecting this fourth edition—and Mike Sanders, Ginny Bess, and Katherin Bidwell for their dedication on the previous editions.

Sincere thanks to Geralyn Coopersmith and Evan Spinks, two outstanding fitness consultants who shared their sense of humor and invaluable information. Thanks to Suki Hertz, a talented chef who provided great ideas and creative recipes in the holiday chapter. And thanks to Karen Robinowitz, a great writer and an exceptional person. I am also grateful to Frances Aaron, Michael Simon, Grace Leder, Meg Fein, Dany Levy, Candy Gulko, and Jane Stern for contributing their input and recipes.

On a personal note, I would like to extend a sincere thanks to my incredible parents, Ellen and Artie Schloss, who have always taught me that *anything* and *everything* is possible! My Grandma Martha, for constantly cheering me on (I miss you!). "The gang": Debra, Steve, Ben, Noah, Becca, Pam, Dan, Charlie, Glenn, Elena, Harley, Jason, Mia, Nancy, Jon, Camrin, Karen, Lisi, Kael, Harvey, and Jenny. To Shannon Green for being the wonderful person she is. My super in-laws, Carol and Vic, along with Grandma Mary and Grandpa Nat for their support and encouragement. And, most of all, my partners in crime, Ian, Jesse, Cole, and Ayden Jane!

Special Thanks to the Nutrition Revision Consultant

The Complete Idiot's Guide to Total Nutrition, Fourth Edition was reviewed by an expert who double-checked the accuracy of what you'll learn here, to help us ensure that this book gives you everything you need to know about nutrition. Special thanks are extended to Erica Ilton, R.D.

Trademarks

All terms mentioned in this book that are known to be or are suspected of being trademarks or service marks have been appropriately capitalized. Alpha Books and Penguin Group (USA) Inc. cannot attest to the accuracy of this information. Use of a term in this book should not be regarded as affecting the validity of any trademark or service mark.

Part 1

Time for a Nutrition Tune-Up

After reading and listening to conflicting food advice from friends, relatives, store clerks, websites, and even hairdressers, it's no wonder people are more confused than ever about what they should be eating!

The first part of this book proves that eating healthfully does *not* have to be complicated or restrictive. Quite the contrary—food is one of life's great pleasures, and everyone deserves a good meal that nourishes both body and soul. This section unravels the most recent dietary guidelines, and gives the inside scoop on carbohydrates, protein, fat, fiber, and salt. After grasping these food fundamentals, you'll be ready to read further and learn the specifics about total nutritional health.

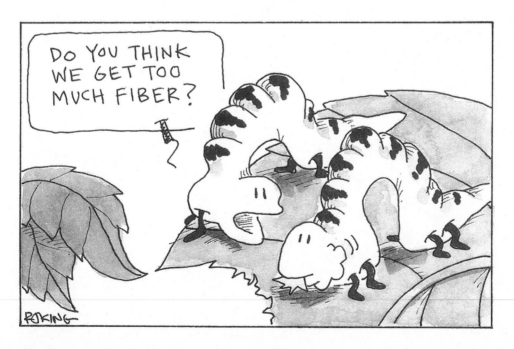

The Dietary Guidelines

In This Chapter

- Unraveling the Dietary Guidelines
- Balancing your food groups
- Where do calories fit in?
- The keys to successful eating
- Scheduling time to fuel your body

After thumbing through hundreds of complicated nutrition articles and magazine ads, catching random food advice from friends and relatives, and listening wearily to endless infomercials promising an instant bodacious bod, you're probably more confused than ever about what you should be eating.

So what exactly should you be eating? Believe it or not, healthy eating doesn't mean driving miles to some obscure health food store in search of organic produce. It also doesn't mean eating bean sprouts sprinkled with wheat germ for dinner (mm, mm). All you have to do is check out the *Dietary Guidelines for Americans*—a state-of-the-art "roadmap" to eating healthfully.

Food for Thought

Nutrients that have been shown to be lacking in the average American diet are fiber, calcium, potassium, magnesium, beta carotene, vitamin C, and vitamin E. Chapters 6, 7, and 8 of this book will give you lots of ideas about how to increase your intake of these vital nutrients without loading up on saturated and trans fats, cholesterol, salt, sugar, and alcohol.

Food for Thought

Chapter 27 will tell you everything you need to know about how to lose weight in a healthy manner. You'll find information about why crash diets don't work, how to calculate your ideal body weight, how to design a well-balanced eating plan for weight loss, and how to maintain your newly trim physique.

Unraveling the Dietary Guidelines

The Dietary Guidelines are aimed at helping people choose a diet and exercise plan that will reduce their risk for major chronic diseases.

The guidelines are a joint production of the U.S. Department of Agriculture (USDA) and the U.S. Department of Health and Human Services (HHS) and are revised every five years so as to keep up with the latest scientific evidence. The first edition came out in 1980 and the most recent one was released in 2005. The current edition features *nine* basic guidelines that focus on weight control, exercise, and getting the most nutritional bang for your caloric buck—all things that nutritionists have been preaching for ages!

1. **Eat nutrient-dense foods within caloric needs.** Eat a variety of nutrient-dense foods and limit your intake of saturated and trans fats, added sugars, cholesterol, salt, and alcohol.

2. **Maintain a healthy weight.** Maintain a healthy body weight by balancing calories *in* (from food) and calories *out* (from physical activity).

3. **Be physically active on most days.** Regular exercise is an important factor in keeping your weight in check and your body *and* mind in great shape.

    To help prevent chronic diseases, try to exercise for at least 30 minutes on most days.

    To help prevent weight gain, aim for about 60 minutes of exercise on most days.

    To maintain weight loss, shoot for 60 to 90 minutes of exercise on most days.

4. **Encourage certain food groups.** Vegetables, fruits, whole grains, and low-fat dairy RULE!

   Make a point of having dark green, orange, and starchy vegetables—as well as legumes—several times a week.

   Make most of your grains *whole* grains (try for at least 3 servings per day).

   Consume 3 cups of fat-free milk, low-fat milk, or equivalent milk products per day.

5. **Choose the right fats.** Keep your *total* fat intake around 20 to 35 percent of daily calories, and go for mainly polyunsaturated and monounsaturated fats—the kind found in fish, nuts, and vegetable oils.

   Keep trans fat consumption as low as possible, consume less than 10 percent of calories from saturated fat, and aim for a cholesterol intake of less than 300 mg per day.

   When selecting meat, poultry, and milk products, choose lean, low-fat, or fat-free types.

6. **Choose healthy carbohydrates.** Choose fiber-rich fruits, vegetables, and whole grains often and try to avoid packaged products that contain lots of added sugars.

7. **Get less sodium and more potassium.** Choose and prepare foods with little salt, while consuming *lots* of potassium-rich foods. Your daily sodium intake should be less than 2,300 mg—that's approximately *1 teaspoon* of table salt.

Food for Thought _____

Chapter 10 gives you the low-down on the healthiest choices in the vegetable, fruit, grain, and dairy departments of your local supermarket.

Chapter 4 is all about good fats (monounsaturated), bad fats (saturated), and truly *ugly* fats (trans).

Chapter 2 cuts through the hype and gives you the real scoop on carbohydrates.

Chapter 5 focuses on salt, and Chapter 20 lists tons of potassium-rich foods.

Chapter 18 outlines safe food practices for the general population, as well as for individuals with compromised immune systems.

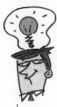

Food for Thought _____

Women: "Moderation" is defined as *up to* one 12-ounce beer, one 5- to 6-ounce glass of wine, or 1¼ ounces of distilled spirits per day.

Men: "Moderation" is defined as *up to* two 12-ounce beers, two 5- to 6-ounce glasses of wine, or 3 ounces of distilled spirits per day.

8. **Limit alcoholic beverages.** If you choose to drink alcohol, do so sensibly and in moderation.

9. **Keep your food safe.** Avoid food-borne illness—especially if you are pregnant or have a compromised immune system.

Balancing Your Food Groups

The Dietary Guidelines emphasize the importance of eating from the five main food groups. They also allow for a limited amount of fats, oils, and "discretionary calories."

Discretionary calories are the calories from fat or sugar that remain after you've eaten the correct number of servings from the basic food groups. For example, if you drink full-fat milk instead of fat-free or low-fat milk (or fruit canned in syrup instead of fresh fruit), then you have used up some of your discretionary calories. I think it's easiest to think of discretionary calories with my 90/10 rule of thumb: if you eat a healthy diet approximately 90 percent of the time, then you should be able to have some "fun foods" 10 percent of the time. Of course, this is not exact math, but a food strategy that's helpful for maintaining a healthy lifestyle. Some of my favorite treats are a small cone of frozen yogurt (about 200 calories), a small bag of soy crisps (140 calories), and an ounce of dark chocolate (about 150 calories).

The following chart shows how many servings from each group you should choose for your particular caloric needs (more about how to determine *your* caloric level later in this chapter).

Calorie Level	1,000	1,200	1,400	1,600	1,800	2,000	2,200	2,400	2,600	2,800	3,000	3,200
Vegetables	2 srv	3 srv	3 srv	4 srv	5 srv	5 srv	6 srv	6 srv	7 srv	7 srv	8 srv	8 srv
Fruits	2 srv	2 srv	3 srv	3 srv	3 srv	4 srv	4 srv	4 srv	4 srv	5 srv	5 srv	5 srv
Grains	3 oz-eq	4 oz-eq	5 oz-eq	5 oz-eq	6 oz-eq	6 oz-eq	7 oz-eq	8 oz-eq	9 oz-eq	10 oz-eq	10 oz-eq	10 oz-eq
Whole Grains	1.5	2	2.5	3	3	3	3.5	4	4.5	5	5	5
Other Grains	1.5	2	2.5	3	3	3	3.5	4	4.5	5	5	5
Lean Meat & Beans	2 oz-eq	3 oz-eq	4 oz-eq	5 oz-eq	5 oz-eq	5.5 oz-eq	6 oz-eq	6.5 oz-eq	6.5 oz-eq	7 oz-eq	7 oz-eq	7 oz-eq
Milk	2	2	2	3	3	3	3	3	3	3	3	3
Oils	15g	17g	17g	22g	24g	27g	29g	31g	34g	36g	44g	51g
Discretionary Calorie Allowance	165	171	171	132	195	267	298	362	410	426	512	648

Source: Appendix A-2 USDA Food Guide from The Dietary Guidelines For Americans, 2005

The serving sizes for the basic food groups are as follows:

1. **Vegetables:** Vegetables are packed with vitamins and minerals and are super-low in calories and fat. Try to eat several servings of dark green and orange vegetables—like spinach, kale, sweet potatoes, and carrots—per week.

   One serving =

   $1/2$ cup raw or cooked vegetables

   1 cup leafy salad greens

   6 ounces vegetable juice

2. **Fruits:** Fruit is a terrific source of vitamins and minerals—especially vitamins A and C. Choose whole fruit over juice whenever possible for the fiber boost.

   One serving =

   1 medium piece of fruit

   $1/2$ cup fresh, frozen, or canned fruit

   6 ounces fruit juice

   $1/4$ cup dried fruit

3. **Grains:** Grains and grain products (especially ones made from whole grains) provide fiber, vitamins, and minerals. They're also our prime source of energy. Try some of the more "exotic" grains—like quinoa, amaranth, spelt, and kamut—the next time you want a change from rice.

   One serving (1-ounce equivalent) =

   $1/2$ cup cooked grains, pasta, or cereal

   1 ounce dry grains, pasta, or ready-to-eat cereal

   1 slice bread, $1/2$ small bagel, or $1/2$ large pita

4. **Lean meat and beans:** Along with supplying substantial amounts of protein, this group contains B-vitamins, iron, and zinc.

   One serving (1-ounce equivalent) =

   1 ounce cooked lean meat, poultry, or fish

   1 egg

   $1/4$ cup cooked dry beans or tofu

1 tablespoon peanut butter

$^1/_2$ ounce nuts or seeds

5. **Milk:** This food group is rich in bone-building calcium. If you can't eat milk or milk products, Chapter 8 will help you find other sources of calcium.

   One serving =

   1 cup milk or yogurt

   $1^1/_2$ ounces natural cheese or 2 ounces processed cheese

5. **Oils:** Fats and oils are not officially billed as a food group, but they're still important components of a healthy diet. They are our sole source of essential fatty acids; they help us absorb vitamins A, D, E, and K; and they serve as building blocks for cell membranes. Check out Chapter 4 for advice on which fats to choose, and which to lose.

Food for Thought

The Dietary Guidelines list servings from this group in grams (g). You should know that 14 g of oil or fat is approximately 3 teaspoons. So, for example, if you consume 2,000 calories per day, your fat allotment is 27 g, or about 6 teaspoons.

Food for Thought

The USDA's new food pyramid can be found at www.mypyramid.gov.

Where Do Calories Fit In?

All the foods we eat contain *calories*—some more than others. In order to maintain a healthy weight and to have enough energy to power you through the day, you should try to take in only the amount of calories your body needs—no more, no less (I know—easier said than done!).

Nutri-Speak

A **calorie** is the amount of energy that food provides. The number of calories is determined by burning food in a device called a calorimeter and measuring the amount of heat produced. One calorie is equal to the amount of energy needed to raise the temperature of one liter of water one degree Celsius. Carbohydrates and protein contain 4 calories per gram, fat contains 9 calories per gram, and alcohol has 7 calories per gram.

How Many Calories Are Right for You?

How do you find the perfect balance between calories in and calories out? Not by nitpicking over calorie counting, that's for sure! You *should* pay attention to what and how much you eat, but not to the point that you carry a calculator and whip it out after each bite of food.

To get a *rough* idea of how many calories you should be taking in, look at the following chart. This chart only offers three general caloric ranges, so keep in mind that your personal daily requirements might fall somewhere between two that are listed. Remember, everyone is different. Caloric intake will vary depending upon your age, sex, size, genetics, and level of activity.

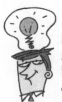

Nutri-Speak

Sedentary folks generally have desk jobs, watch a lot of TV, and tend to sit around most of the time. **Active** folks are constantly on the go. They do a lot of walking, take the stairs, play sports, or regularly work out.

General Daily Calorie Requirements

1,600 calories	Number of calories needed for many sedentary women and some older adults.
2,200 calories	Number of calories needed for most children, teenage girls, active women, and many sedentary men. Women who are pregnant and breastfeeding may need somewhat more.
2,800 calories	Number of calories needed for teenage boys, many active men, and some *very* active women.

Source: USDA 1992

Food for Thought

Live by a 90/10 food strategy; 90 percent healthy foods and 10 percent fun foods!

The Keys to Successful Eating: Variety and Moderation

I know this sounds like the kind of advice your mom or grandmother would give, but it really *is* a major part of eating healthfully. When you eat a *variety* of healthy foods in *moderate* amounts from all the food groups, you're bound to get the vitamins, minerals, and other nutrients your body needs. Moderation also allows for occasional indulgences that make eating more fun and even help prevent all-out pig-outs that lead to weight gain. Instead of denying yourself that piece of chocolate cake you're craving, why not enjoy a small piece once in a while?

Scheduling Time for Breakfast, Lunch, and Dinner

What kind of an eating schedule are you on? Do you make time in your day for breakfast, lunch, and dinner; or do you run on empty until dinner and then pig out from starvation? Everyone has his own eating regimen—some better than others. You should be fueling your body *throughout* the day when you need the energy.

Breakfast with a Bang

You've heard it a million times: *Breakfast is important!*

Think of your body as a car: it needs fuel to run properly. When you wake up from a good night's sleep, your body has been fasting for about eight hours (if you're lucky enough to get that much sleep). "Break-fast" in the morning helps kick your body into gear by supplying it with energy. Eating a smart breakfast can also help regulate your appetite throughout the day so you don't overdo it at lunch and dinner.

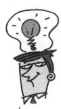

Food for Thought

Numerous studies have proven that breakfast eaters are more likely to be productive and attentive in the morning than non–breakfast eaters.

Source: U.S. Departments of Agriculture and Health and Human Services.

Fueling Your Body All Day

Remember, breakfast alone just won't cut it. Your body needs to be constantly energized throughout the day to help keep you going. You don't necessarily have to eat the standard three square meals. In fact, some prefer six mini-meals. Do whatever works best for your schedule and eating style, but be sure that your daily food intake resembles the Dietary Guidelines.

The Least You Need to Know

- Make sure to eat a variety of foods from the five food groups. Become familiar with the *Dietary Guidelines*, which provide an eating style that supports proper nutrition.

- Don't get caught up with counting calories; it can drive you crazy! Simply focus on eating healthy foods in moderation.

- Get out of your food rut and be adventurous. Try new and exciting foods, recipes, and restaurants.

- Schedule time to fuel your body *throughout* the day. Food can help keep you alert, energetic, and focused.

Chapter 2

A Close-Up on Carbohydrates

In This Chapter

- ◆ What's a carbohydrate?
- ◆ Simple carbs versus complex carbs
- ◆ How many carbohydrates should you eat?
- ◆ Do starchy carbs make you fat?
- ◆ The Glycemic Index and the Glycemic Load
- ◆ To artificially sweeten or not

All the foods you eat are composed of three macro-nutrients known as carbohydrate, protein, and fat. Some foods consist primarily of only one macro-nutrient (in other words, bread is mainly carbohydrate, turkey meat is protein, and butter is fat), whereas other foods contain combinations of all three (for example, pizza, sandwiches, and burritos).

Your body needs all three of these macro-nutrients to function properly, but *not* in equal amounts. Most nutrition professionals recommend that carbs make up a minimum of 40 percent of your diet. Despite all the backlash against them in recent years, carbs are *still* our prime source of energy and (if you choose the right ones) a great source of vitamins, minerals, and fiber.

This chapter covers the "real deal" on carbs, from simple to complex.

What Exactly Is a Carbohydrate?

Technically speaking, a carbohydrate is a compound made up of carbon, hydrogen, and oxygen. The most basic carbohydrates are called simple sugars and include honey, jams, jellies, syrup, table sugar, candies, soft drinks, fruits, and fruit juices. Glucose (also called dextrose) is a common simple sugar found in fruits, honey, and vegetables. It is also the substance measured in blood. (In other words, blood sugar equals blood glucose.) As you can see from the following figure, they are relatively small compounds. When several of these simple sugars are linked together, they form more complicated molecules known as complex carbohydrates.

Complex carbohydrates that come from plants are called starch and are found in quality foods such as grains, vegetables, breads, seeds, *legumes*, and beans. Whether it's a handful of jelly beans or freshly sliced whole grain bread, it's all carbohydrate!

Nutri-Speak _____

Legumes are vegetables in the bean and pea family that are rich in complex carbohydrates, protein, and fiber. They supply iron, zinc, magnesium, phosphorous, potassium, and several B-vitamins, including folic acid. Because these provide both complex carbs and protein, they fit in the meat and beans group *and* the vegetable group. Legumes include black beans, pinto beans, kidney beans, lima beans, navy beans, soybeans, black-eyed peas, chickpeas (garbanzos), split peas, lentils, and nuts and seeds, which are higher in fat.

Simple sugar.

Sweet Satisfaction: The Lowdown on Simple Sugars

So your favorite sugary sweets are classified as carbohydrates—and you're supposed to eat a lot of carbohydrates—*so it's okay to load up on gummy bears and licorice, right?*

Not a chance. Here's why: the *quality* of your carbohydrates matters tremendously. Simple sugars such as candy, sodas, and sugary sweeteners found in cakes and cookies offer little in the form of nutrition except providing your body with energy and calories. These foods are literally "empty calories"—calories with no nutritional value. In moderation, simple sugars are perfectly fine (and, I admit, yummy), but people who consistently load up on the sweet stuff often find themselves too full for, or uninterested in, the healthy foods their bodies require. The end result is too much sugar and not enough nutrition.

Does sugary candy promote dental cavities?

Actually, all foods that contain carbohydrates (rice, pasta, potato, cakes, cookies, and, yes, candy) can mix with the bacteria in plaque and increase your risk for tooth decay. Sadly, nutrient-dense raisins are amongst the worst offenders. But don't panic. By brushing a few times each day, flossing daily, and swishing water around in your mouth after eating, you can fight off the drill.

Where Do Fruits and Fruit Juices Fit In?

There are some exceptions to the "no sugar" rule. For example, fruits and fruit juices contain fructose (a natural simple sugar) and provide several vitamins and minerals. Eating fresh fruit or drinking 100 percent fruit juice is far from pumping "empty calories" into your system. When you can, choose whole fruit over fruit juice: you get the same nutrients, as well as more complex carbohydrates and fiber. You'll read more about this in Chapter 6.

As you can see in the following table, juice and cola both contain simple sugars, but juice provides a lot more nutrition.

8 oz. of orange juice	8 oz. of cola
110 calories	100 calories
26 grams carbohydrate	26 grams carbohydrate
25 grams sugar	26 grams sugar
120% daily vitamin C	0% daily vitamin C
12% daily potassium	0% daily potassium
20% daily folic acid	0% daily folic acid

All About Complex Carbohydrates

Now that you know what you shouldn't load up on, let's take a look at the foods you should eat. By now, you should be clued-in to which foods are rich in *complex carbohydrates* (pasta, grains, breads, cereal, legumes, and vegetables). Although they're actually made from hundreds—or even thousands—of simple sugars linked together, they react quite differently inside your body. After you ingest a complex carbohydrate (or starch), several enzymes break it down into its simplest form, called glucose.

Nutri-Speak

Simple carbohydrates (simple sugars) are molecules of single sugar units or pairs of small sugar units bonded together. **Complex carbohydrates (complex sugars)** are compounds of long strands of many simple sugars linked together.

Glucose is the simple sugar that your body recognizes and absorbs. All types of carbohydrate (simple and complex) must be broken down and converted into glucose before your body can absorb and use it for energy.

If all carbs wind up as glucose, why can't we just eat simple sugars? I've already touched on the first reason. Many simple sugars are nutrition zeroes, whereas complex carbs often provide phytochemicals, vitamins, minerals, and even fiber, depending on the food.

In fact, your *best* complex carbs include vegetables and whole grains (not the white, refined stuff). Check out this comparison: a large baked sweet potato (high-quality, complex carb) versus a 20-ounce bottle of cola (simple carb). Although both provide about 280 calories, that's where the similarity ends. The sweet potato supplies potassium, magnesium, vitamin A, folic acid, vitamin C, and significant fiber, along with several other vitamins and minerals. And the cola—you probably guessed—*provides zilch*. Just plain sugar (18.5 straight teaspoons!). What's more, the sweet potato provides you with a fuller and more satisfied feeling. As you can see, eating complex carbs certainly does make a difference, even though it all ends up as glucose.

Another reason to choose complex carbohydrates is that the glucose created during digestion gets released into your blood more slowly. Simple carbohydrates are already broken down—they go straight into the blood, resulting in what is unofficially known as the "sugar rush"—whereas complex carbohydrates are larger molecules that must be broken down. As your body processes complex carbs, small glucose molecules are released into the blood over an extended period of time. This helps to regulate blood-sugar levels, especially in people who may have problems with their blood sugars (for example, people with *hyperglycemia*, *hypoglycemia*, or *diabetes mellitus*).

For the best regulation of problematic blood-sugar levels, choose carbohydrates that supply soluble fiber, including oatmeal, apples, sweet potatoes, beans, artichokes, grapefruits, squash, peas, brussels sprouts, and oranges.

Nutri-Speak

Hyperglycemia is a condition resulting in abnormally high blood-glucose (blood-sugar) concentration. *Hyper* means "too much," *glyce* means "glucose," and *emia* means "in the blood." **Hypoglycemia** is characterized by abnormally low blood sugar. Here, *hypo* means "too little." **Diabetes mellitus** is a disorder of blood-sugar regulation usually caused by the body's inability to either produce enough insulin or use it effectively.

How Much Carbohydrate Should You Eat?

As mentioned earlier, no less than 40 percent of your diet should consist of carbohydrates, specifically, complex carbohydrates. Most athletes and growing children and adolescents will need far more carbs than this, though. But no matter how high or low you go—always make the bulk of your carbs healthy ones.

Food for Thought

Some excellent sources of carbohydrates include fruits, vegetables, legumes, brown rice, barley, oatmeal, whole grain bread, whole wheat tortillas, high-fiber cereal, and high-fiber crackers.

Do Starchy Carbs Make You Fat?

In this era of trendy low-carb and no-carb diets, this may be the best thing you've heard in a while: carbohydrates will *not* make you fat! Consistently overeating *calories* will make you fat—and those calories may come from protein, fat, and/or carbohydrate. Always remember that appropriate amounts of high-quality carbohydrates will prolong your energy and improve your health.

Why all the confusion? For starters, some people confuse weight gain from fat with weight gain from carbohydrates. One gram of fat has more than double the amount of calories as one gram of carbohydrate. What some people don't realize is that fat usually accompanies carbohydrates at a meal. For instance, people remember that they had pasta for dinner but forget that the pasta was swimming in oil, butter, cheese, or Alfredo sauce. Clearly, the culprit for weight gain was the fat (butter, oil, and so on), not the carbohydrate (pasta).

Another example is many a New Yorker's favorite staple—the bagel. Alone, a bagel is a straightforward, complex carbohydrate. Add all that butter or cream cheese, and you'll wind up with a lot more calories and fat than you bargained for. The next time you question whether pasta or other carbs make you fat, reevaluate. It's likely the fat that is making you fat.

Expand your grain vocabulary:

- **Quinoa (pronounced "keen-wah").** A native South American grain, quinoa is high in protein, calcium, and iron and good in puddings, soup, and stir-fry.

- **Barley.** Good in soups, stews, side dishes, puddings, and cereals, barley is found in grocery stores and available as "pot" or "scotch barley."

- **Millet.** Good as a side dish or stuffing for poultry and high in phosphorus and B-vitamins, millet is available in health food stores.

- **Wild rice.** High in protein and a good source of B-vitamins, this pseudograin is really a grass seed.

- **Amaranth.** High in protein, iron, and calcium, amaranth is from South America and available in health food stores and some upscale grocery stores. It serves as a good side dish or cereal.

- **Wheat berries.** Found in most grocery stores and health food stores, wheat berries serve as a good high-fiber cereal or substitute for rice.

On the other hand, Americans tend to overeat everything, and we *love* the starchy carbs! Do you ever eat a bagel for breakfast, sandwich on a hero roll for lunch, jumbo bag of pretzels for a snack, large bowl of pasta with a few slices of bread for dinner, and a granola bar before bed? Although low in fat, your diet is heavy in carbohydrate calories. And unless you're incredibly active, there is a great chance you'll gain weight because you've taken in more calories than your body can efficiently burn.

What's more, numerous studies have confirmed that portions have dramatically increased over the years, and it's no surprise that muffins, bagels, and pasta entrees are high on the list. A deli bagel can weigh in at 5 ounces—that's the equivalent of 5 slices of bread or 400 calories. A typical pasta entree is 5 to 6 servings (based on 1/2 cup standard serving size), and provides 600 calories before you even consider the sauce.

Remember, to maintain an ideal weight, you need that balance of "calories in, calories out." It doesn't matter if those extra calories come from carbohydrates, protein, or fat: *Excessive calories will be stored by your body as fat.* When it comes to carbohydrates, choose wisely and eat appropriate portions.

The Glycemic Index and the Glycemic Load

The Glycemic Index and the Glycemic Load are gaining acceptance by many health professionals as a way for people to incorporate healthier carbohydrates into their diets.

The *Glycemic Index* is a measure of how quickly a particular carbohydrate-rich food is turned into blood sugar (glucose). Why is this important? Because every time you eat a carb-rich food, your blood sugar goes up and a hormone produced in the pancreas called *insulin* has to bring it down. Too many high blood sugar spikes lead to an overproduction of insulin, which can cause hunger (and subsequent weight gain), cardiovascular disease, and diabetes. One way to keep your blood sugar level steady is to choose carbs that do not create such big spikes in blood sugar, in other words—ones that are low on the Glycemic Index.

Having said all that, there *are* problems with the Glycemic Index. Namely, it doesn't take into account how *much* of a particular food you're eating *or* how healthy that food is.

It just standardizes all foods to a 50-gram carbohydrate content. Now, while 50 grams *is* the amount of carbs in a typical 3-ounce bagel, to get that many carbs from carrots you'd have to eat about 4 cups worth! A more typical serving of carrots is $^1/_2$ cup, and that amount contains only about 6 grams of carbohydrate.

Food for Thought

Fat, fiber, and the way a food is prepared affect its Glycemic Index ranking. For instance, fat tends to slow down sugar absorption, which makes many unhealthy high saturated fat foods—like Snickers Bars—get a relatively low ranking. Fiber also slows down sugar absorption, but this is a *good* way to put on the brakes!

Food for Thought

For the most comprehensive Glycemic Index/Load on the web, check out http://diabetes. about. com/library/mendosagi/ ngilists.htm.

This is where the *Glycemic Load* comes into play. To calculate the Glycemic Load of a typical serving of food, you just multiply the grams of carbohydrate in the serving size you're eating by the food's Glycemic Index percentage.

For example, the Glycemic Load for $1/2$ cup of carrots is:

.47 (47%) × 6 = 2.8

So you can see that with a Glycemic Load of only 2.8, carrots don't deserve the bad rap they've been getting after all!

Glycemic Index Range

Low	55 or less
Medium	56–69
High	70 and higher

Glycemic Load Range

Low	10 or less
Medium	11–19
High	20 or more

To Artificially Sweeten or Not

People often have to use artificial sweeteners because of a medical condition. For example, sugar substitutes can be great for diabetics, who can't tolerate *real* sugar because their bodies can't produce the hormone insulin. Insulin delivers the sugar from our blood to our cells, where we utilize it as energy. When your body doesn't have enough insulin, sugar builds up in the blood and doesn't get into the cells. This condition is known as high blood sugar and can be extremely dangerous for people with diabetes. Because sugar substitutes do not contain any glucose (and therefore do not require insulin), they can be effective sweeteners for people with diabetes.

A more popular reason for using artificial sweeteners is saving calories. However, this notion might not be as effective as you think. Although it is true that diet soft drinks and other artificially sweetened foods can save you a lot of sugar calories, several studies have shown that people who "save calories" with these diet foods usually wind up eating those saved calories somewhere else. Pretty ironic, huh? Did you know that a real sugar packet (that's 1 teaspoon) has only 16 calories? You can easily burn that off walking an extra flight of stairs. It's certainly something to think about the next time you grab artificial sweetener.

Artificial sweeteners have always been the subject of much controversy. Before you tear open your gazillionth nonsugar packet, read the following and learn the facts.

Saccharin

One of the first sugar substitutes to receive U.S. Food and Drug Administration (FDA) approval was saccharin (Sweet & Low), and it continues to be popular. Although several studies suggest that saccharin in large quantities can cause cancer (specifically bladder tumors) in laboratory rats, no harmful effects have been shown in humans.

Aspartame

Another popular artificial sweetener is aspartame, better known as NutraSweet or Equal. Aspartame consists of two protein fragments (phenylalanine and aspartic acid) and has had FDA approval since 1981. It is presently found in more than 5,000 differ-ent products, and there is no evidence of any harmful effects from its use. However, because aspartame does contain phenylalanine, individuals with the metabolic disor-der PKU (an inherited disease in which the body cannot dispose of excess phenylala-nine) should consult their physicians before using this sweetener.

Stevia

A little more obscure, but gaining popularity, is the sweetener called Stevia. Stevia (STEE-vee-uh) is a South American shrub whose leaves have been used as a sweet-ener for centuries by native peoples in Paraguay and Brazil. *Stevioside*, the main in-gredient, is virtually calorie-free and hundreds of times sweeter than table sugar. Although not commonly used in the United States, Canada, or European countries, this sweetener is quite accepted in Japan and has been used by manufacturers since the early 1970s.

To date, the FDA has not approved Stevia simply because there is not enough data to conclude its safety. In fact, one study suggested that large amounts of Stevia can cause reproductive problems in both men and women. There's also a slight question about the potential for cancer. Clearly, more information needs to be gathered, but until then, if you use Stevia, do so in small to moderate amounts.

Sucralose

Another recent artificial sweetener to come into the market is called Splenda (sucralose). Splenda was discovered in 1976 and is made by replacing three hydrogen-oxygen groups on the sugar (sucrose) molecule with three tightly bound chlorine atoms. Because sucralose is not broken down, the sweetener has no calories, and the body does not recognize it as a carbohydrate. Approximately 600 times sweeter than sugar, Splenda is exceptionally stable and can withstand long shelf-life and hot cooking temperatures. Furthermore, sucralose received FDA approval in April 1998 for use in 15 food and beverage categories, the broadest initial approval ever given to a no-calorie sweetener.

Splenda Brand Sweetener (sucralose) has been subjected to one of the most extensive and thorough safety testing programs ever conducted on a new food additive. Over 50 regulatory agencies worldwide have permitted the use of Splenda Brand Sweetener, including the FDA, the Joint FAO/WHO Expert Committee on Food Additives (JECFA), the Health Protection Branch of Health and Welfare Canada, and Australia's National Food Authority.

Neotame

The newest sweetener to recently gain FDA approval is Neotame. Depending upon its food application, Neotame is approximately 7,000+ times sweeter than sugar, and may be used in most cooking applications. Neotame is a free-flowing, water-soluble powder, and has undergone more than 113 animal studies. To date, the FDA concludes that this sweetener is safe for human consumption. Stay tuned for further information.

The bottom line is that artificial sweeteners can safely be part of a well-balanced diet. Just don't get so carried away that you view sugar as the enemy. Remember, the dietary guidelines suggest eating real sugar in moderation, not avoiding it altogether.

The Least You Need to Know

- ◆ No less than 40 percent of your total food for the day should come from carbohydrates (mostly high-quality, complex carbohydrates). Carbohydrate-rich foods include fruit, vegetables, legumes, whole grain bread, high-fiber cereal, brown rice, pasta, and all other grain products.

◆ Limit your intake of candy, cola, and other sugary sweets. Although they are carbohydrates, simple sugars provide you with nothing more than "simply sugar."

◆ Fruit and fruit juices are the exception to the "simple sugar" rule. Although considered simple carbohydrates, they provide a variety of important nutrients. That said, go easy on the juice!

◆ Carbs aren't fattening; however, almost anything you consistently overeat will put on the pounds—including carbohydrates.

◆ The Glycemic Load may help you choose healthier carbs, but you don't really need it to tell you that vegetables, beans, and whole grains are better for you than cookies, cakes, and candy.

◆ In moderation, artificial sweeteners can be an effective sugar substitute for people with diabetes mellitus and part of a well-balanced diet for the general population. The choice between sugar and sugar substitutes is yours.

3

The Profile on Protein

In This Chapter

- ◆ The importance of protein
- ◆ Amino acids—the building blocks
- ◆ Animal protein versus vegetable protein
- ◆ Combining incomplete proteins
- ◆ Your personal requirements
- ◆ The facts, the fallacies

It's time to learn the many powers of protein—one incredibly versatile molecule. Almost everyone seems to have a basic idea of which foods are rich in protein, but do you actually know your personal requirements or understand why protein is important and how it works? Stay tuned: this chapter presents the facts.

What's So Important About Protein?

First, protein is not just in food; it's floating around all over your body. Did you know that your bones, organs, tendons, ligaments, muscles, cartilage, hair, nails, teeth, and skin are all made up of protein? That's just the beginning. *Working proteins* are busy performing specific tasks in your body. These include …

- **Enzymes.** Proteins that facilitate and accelerate chemical reactions. They are also known as protein catalysts. Each enzyme has a specific function to perform in the body.

- **Antibodies.** Proteins that help fight illness and disease. They are found in red blood cells.

- **Hemoglobin.** Proteins that transport oxygen all over the body.

- **Hormones (most).** Proteins that regulate many body functions. Hormones signal enzymes to do their job, such as equalizing blood-sugar levels, insulin levels, and growth.

- **Growth and maintenance proteins.** Proteins that serve as building materials for the growth and repair of body tissues.

The list is endless. But I promise not to take you back to high school biology.

A Brief Return to Chemistry 101

Protein consists of carbon, hydrogen, oxygen, and nitrogen. The addition of nitrogen gives protein its unique distinction from carbohydrate and fat, along with establishing the signature name, amino acid. Much like simple sugars, which link together to form a complex carbohydrate (see Chapter 2), amino acids are the building blocks for the more complicated protein molecule.

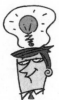

Food for Thought

Protein was named over 150 years ago after the Greek word *proteios*, meaning "of prime importance."

Nutri-Speak

Proteins are compounds made of carbon, hydrogen, oxygen, and nitrogen and arranged as strands of amino acids.

Amino Acids: The Building Blocks of Protein

There are a total of 20 different amino acids, and depending upon the sequence in which they appear, a specific job or function is carried out in your body. Think of amino acids as similar to the alphabet—26 letters that can be arranged in a million different ways. These arranged letters create words, which then translate into an entire language. The arrangement of amino acids is your body's "protein language," which dictates the exact tasks that need to be carried out. Therefore, *proteins* that make up your enzymes will have one sequence, whereas those that form your muscles will have a completely different one.

Your Bod: The Amino Acid Recycling Bin

Your body continually gets the amino acids it needs from its own amino-acid pool and from a diet that meets your daily protein requirements. After you eat a food that contains protein, your body goes to work, breaking it down into the various amino acids. (Different foods yield different amino acids.) When the protein is completely dissected, your body absorbs the amino acids (resulting from your digested food) and rebuilds them into the sequence that you need for a specific body task. Your body is sort of like a recycling bin.

Let's take this amino acid talk a bit further. Out of 20 amino acids, 11 can actually be manufactured within your body. However, that means nine cannot be manufactured. You cannot function without each and every amino acid. It is "essential" that you get these nine from outside food sources. Therefore, they are appropriately called *essential amino acids*.

Nutri-Speak

Amino (*a-MEEN-o*) **acids** are the building blocks for protein that are necessary for every bodily function.

Essential Amino Acids	Nonessential Amino Acids
Histidine	Glycine
Isoleucine	Glutamic acid
Leucine	Arginine
Lysine	Aspartic acid
Methionine	Proline
Phenylalanine	Alanine
Threonine	Serine
Tryptophan	Tyrosine
Valine	Cysteine
	Asparagine
	Glutamine

Animal Protein Versus Vegetable Protein

In general, animal proteins (meat, fish, poultry, milk, cheese, and eggs) are considered good sources of *complete proteins*. Complete proteins contain ample amounts of all essential amino acids.

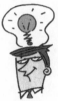

Food for Thought

Gelatin is the only animal protein that is not considered a complete protein.

Nutri-Speak

Complementary proteins are two incomplete proteins in a food that, when combined, compensate for one another's shortfalls.

On the other hand, vegetable proteins (grains, legumes, nuts, seeds, and other vegetables) are *incomplete proteins* because they are missing, or do not have enough of, one or more of the essential amino acids. That's not such a big deal. You already know that grains and legumes are rich in complex carbohydrate and fiber. Now you learn that they can be an excellent source of protein as well; it just takes a little bit of work and know-how. By combining foods from two or more of the following columns—voilà—you create a self-made complete protein. You see, the foods in one column may be missing amino acids that are present in the foods listed in another column. When eaten in combination at the same meal (or separately throughout the day), your body receives all nine essential amino acids.

You can combine the following vegetable proteins to make complete proteins.

Sources of Complementary Proteins

Grains	Legumes	Nuts/Seeds
Barley	Beans	Sesame seeds
Bulgur	Lentils	Sunflower seeds
Cornmeal	Dried peas	Walnuts
Oats	Peanuts	Cashews
Buckwheat	Chickpeas	Pumpkin seeds
Rice	Soy products	Other nuts
Pasta		
Rye		
Wheat		

Combinations to Create Complete Proteins

Combine Grains and Legumes	Combine Grains and Nuts/Seeds	Combine Legumes and Nuts/Seeds
Peanut butter on whole-wheat bread	Whole-wheat bun with sesame seeds	Hummus (chickpeas and sesame paste)

Also, by adding small amounts of animal protein (meat, eggs, milk, or cheese) to any of the groups, you create a complete protein. Here are some examples:

- Oatmeal with milk
- Macaroni and cheese
- Casserole with a small amount of meat
- Salad with beans and a hard-cooked egg
- Yogurt with granola
- Bean and cheese burrito

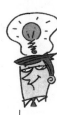

Food for Thought

Hey, did you know that the mineral iron is best absorbed from the following animal proteins: liver, beef, pork, lamb, chicken, and turkey.

Your Personal Protein Requirements

This chart presents the Recommended Dietary Allowances (RDAs) of protein for a variety of age categories:

Infants	Up to 5 months	13 grams
	5 months–1 year	14 grams
Children	1–3 years	16 grams
	4–6 years	24 grams
	7–10 years	28 grams
Males	11–14 years	45 grams
	15–18 years	59 grams
	19–24 years	58 grams
	25+ years	63 grams
Females	11–14 years	46 grams
	15–18 years	44 grams
	19–24 years	46 grams
	25+ years	50 grams

continues

Pregnant		60 grams
Lactating	first 6 months	65 grams
	second 6 months	62 grams

However, this chart does not take into account your size—and larger people tend to have greater protein requirements. The following calculation is a more popular method for calculating daily protein amongst most health professionals:

Your weight in pounds multiplied by .36 to .50 = Daily protein requirement (in grams)

Avid exercisers and athletes require even more. Check out Chapter 16 for more information.

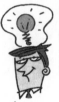

Food for Thought

Keep in mind that pregnant or lactating women have increased protein requirements. Pregnant women need an additional 10 grams of protein a day, whereas breast-feeding women need 12 to 15 extra grams a day for the first six months.

Protein for the Day in a Blink of an Eye

The previous chart gave you a number; let's see how quickly 63 grams can translate into food. The following chart lists the protein content of commonly eaten foods.

Protein Content of Common Foods

Animal Proteins	Grams of Protein	Vegetable Proteins	Grams of Protein
Steak, sirloin	26	Peanuts (1 oz.)	7
Ground meat	20	Walnuts (1 oz.)	4
Hamburger	14	Peanut butter (2 TB.)	8
Bologna	10	Sesame seeds (1 oz.)	5
Hot dog	10	Sunflower seeds (1 oz.)	6
Venison	26	Flaxseeds (1 oz.)	6
Buffalo	13	Tofu (6 oz.)	12
Bacon (1 slice)	21	Soybeans ($1/2$ cup)	11
Ham	2	Soy milk (1 cup)	7
Turkey breast	26	Kidney beans ($1/2$ cup)	8
Roast beef	21	Lentils ($1/2$ cup)	9

Animal Proteins	Grams of Protein	Vegetable Proteins	Grams of Protein
Chicken, light	26	Chickpeas ($^1/_2$ cup)	10
Salmon	18	Split peas ($^1/_2$ cup)	8
Scallops	14	Tofu (5 oz.)	10
Oysters (2 oz.)	8	Oatmeal (1 cup)	6
Crab	13	Pasta (1 cup)	7
Cottage cheese ($^1/_2$ cup)	14	Brown rice (1 cup)	5
Cheddar cheese (1 oz.)	7	White rice (1 cup)	3
American cheese (1 oz.)	6	Whole-wheat bread	5
String cheese (1 oz.)	6		
Mozzarella (1 oz.)	7		
Goat cheese (1 oz.)	6		
Jarlsberg cheese (1 oz.)	7		
Blue cheese (1 oz.)	6		
Whole milk (1 cup)	8		
Skim milk (1 cup)	8		
Low-fat plain yogurt (1 cup)	10		
Low-fat fruit yogurt (1 cup)	10		
Frozen yogurt ($^1/_2$ cup)	3		
Egg (1)	6		

All are 3-ounce servings (approximately the size of a deck of cards) unless otherwise indicated.
Source: 1996 First Databank.

You can imagine how quickly these numbers add up, especially because most people tend to eat much more than a 3-ounce serving in one shot.

Let's take a look at a typical day:

Breakfast:
2 scrambled eggs
3 strips of bacon
2 slices of toast with margarine
Glass of milk

Lunch:
A big fat tuna salad sandwich (6 oz.)
2 slices of bread
Apple

Dinner:
Steak (6 oz.)
Some veggies and rice

Total protein = 137 grams (yikes!)

As mentioned earlier, people in industrialized countries don't have a problem meeting their protein requirements. In fact, as you can see, it's easy to *exceed* the amount you need because our society tends to focus on meat, fish, eggs, seafood, or dairy with almost every meal.

Should You Worry About Overeating Protein?

Well, maybe. The problem is that your body only uses what it needs. And the rest? Well, some protein may be used for energy, but most is just a lot of extra calories and usually not just protein calories. Many of these high-protein foods are also packaged with fat; therefore, excess calories, which can translate into weight gain, can be a major concern. Furthermore, filling up on enormous portions of animal protein might crowd out grains, fruits, and veggies, which would create "macro-nutrient chaos."

Go ahead and determine your personal protein needs, and then adjust your meals accordingly. You might want to prepare smaller pieces of animal protein (about 3 ounces) and load a variety of veggies and grains onto your plate.

Food for Thought

Your leanest protein sources include turkey breasts, skinless chicken breasts, egg whites, lean red meats, low-fat yogurt, skim or 1-percent milk, low-fat cheese, beans and lentils, all seafood and fish, split peas, chickpeas, and tofu.

Also, watch out for "high-protein" diets, which promise quick weight loss by encouraging large amounts of protein while severely limiting carbohydrate intake (no bread, potatoes, rice, pasta, cereal, and so on). You might lose weight, but not from any magical combination of "high protein/low carbohydrates." One reason may be loss of water because the breakdown of excessive protein causes frequent urination. Another explanation may be that your total calories usually decrease when you're limited to high-protein foods. How much plain protein can you really eat?

Furthermore, these high-protein/low-carb eating plans can be unhealthy (unless you are clinically diagnosed with hyperinsulinemia by your physician). Your body cannot burn fat efficiently without adequate carbohydrates. As a result, you produce compounds called ketones, which can accumulate in the blood and leave you feeling dizzy, nauseous, fatigued, and headachy—and give you incredibly bad breath. What's more, excessive protein can also put an added strain on your kidneys. It's pretty ironic when the goal of losing weight should be to improve your health, not make it worse.

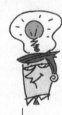

Food for Thought

Recent studies have shown that folks at risk for kidney stones would benefit from following a diet that was low to moderate in protein.

Does Excessive Protein Build Larger Muscles?

Okay, let's set the record straight. It's true that protein is needed for the development of muscle, but it's not true that "extra" protein will build bigger biceps. Body builders and other athletes do need more protein than the RDA. However, this increase is already accounted for in the typical American diet. As mentioned earlier, we cannot store excess protein. Therefore, all those extra protein calories (and the fat that came along with them) will most likely wind up on your … well, let's just say I'm not talking about your quads!

In addition, anyone eating excessive protein will urinate more frequently because the breakdown of protein produces an increase in *urea*, a waste product in urine. You can imagine the inconvenience of running to the bathroom every 10 minutes, let alone your risk of becoming dehydrated. Furthermore, body builders who take tremendous amounts of protein tend to skimp on carbohydrates—the key energy-providing ingredient for an optimal workout.

The Scoop on Amino-Acid Supplements

Amino-acid supplements are unnecessary. Your body only needs a certain amount of each amino acid, and most of us receive far more than this amount from the food we eat (both animal and vegetable protein). Although the amount that you need is vital, there is nothing miraculous about megadosing. In fact, overkill can be expensive and inefficient. Think about it: for next to nothing, you can prepare a piece of grilled chicken instead of spending more than double that for one of those "amino acid" shakes.

The Least You Need to Know

- A total of 20 different amino acids act as building blocks for the more complicated protein molecules. Nine of these amino acids must be obtained from outside food sources and are called "essential amino acids."

- Animal proteins are considered "complete proteins" because they contain ample amounts of all nine essential amino acids. Vegetable proteins are "incomplete proteins" because they are missing one or more of the essential amino acids. By combining two or more incomplete vegetable proteins during the day, you can create a complete protein with all nine essential amino acids.

- Some people have a tendency to go protein-overboard, which can also mean more fat and calories because foods high in protein may also be high in fat.

- Excessive protein and amino-acid supplements do not build larger muscles. In fact, these myths can lead to a host of problems, including dehydration and increased fat intake.

Chapter 4

Chewing the Fat

In This Chapter

- ◆ Various types of fat
- ◆ The heart disease connection
- ◆ Your cholesterol numbers and what they mean
- ◆ Gaining weight from excessive fat
- ◆ Living a low-fat lifestyle

Unless you've been living on another planet, you've heard that too much fat can create a lot of problems. Ironically, despite the "fat warnings" that bombard us every day, we remain an overweight society that eats far too much. It's one thing to *know* what to eat, but it's a whole different ballgame to actually commit to eating healthy and follow through with it.

Let's not forget the flip side: low-fat does not mean no-fat. Some people take this new "low-fat religion" to radical extremes. "I'll have a broiled fish, dry, no oil; salad with mustard on the side, no dressing; steamed veggies, nothing on them; and a baked potato, plain." You might as well remove your taste buds before digging into that meal! Come on, food is supposed to be enjoyable, right?

This chapter shows that excessive fat can lead to a host of problems, including weight gain and disease. However, it will also emphasize to all the "fat-phobics" out there that *some* fat is actually good for you, and with some hard work and realistic planning, everyone can find his or her happy medium.

Why Fat Is Fabulous

Before we begin a fat-bashing session, let's look at all the positives about fat:

♦ Fat provides you with a ready source of energy.

♦ Children need fat to grow properly.

♦ Fat supports the cell walls within your body.

♦ Fat enables your body to circulate, store, and absorb the *fat-soluble* vitamins A, D, E, and K. Without any fat, you would become deficient.

♦ Fat supplies essential fatty acids that your body can't make and must therefore get from foods.

♦ Fat helps promote healthy skin and hair.

♦ Fat makes food taste better by adding flavor, texture, and aroma.

Nutri-Speak

Fat-soluble nutrients dissolve in fat. Some essential nutrients such as the vitamins A, D, E, and K require fat for circulation and absorption.

♦ Fat provides a layer of insulation just beneath the skin. People who are extremely thin are often cold because they lack this layer of subcutaneous fat. Overweight people tend to have too much of this insulation and become uncomfortably warm in hot weather.

♦ Fat surrounds your vital organs for protection and support.

Are All Fats Created Equal?

Fat comes in a variety of packages; some are more harmful than others. In addition to watching your total fat intake, you must also pay attention to the *type* of fat you take in. Let's start from the beginning and figure out what's what in the world of fat.

First, here's all of the "fat vocabulary" you will ever need to speak like an expert at your next social function:

◆ **Triglycerides.** The general term used for the main form of fat found in food. The structure of a TG (that's fat slang for triglyceride) is a *glycerol* (carbon atoms linked together) plus three fatty acids. There are several triglyceride categories, and depending upon the fatty acid composition, a TG is classified as saturated, monounsaturated, or polyunsaturated.

You may also hear about your "triglyceride level" when the doctor takes your blood. That's because TGs, like cholesterol, are a storage form of fat in your body—circulating in the bloodstream and deposited in adipose tissue (better known as flub).

◆ **Monounsaturated fats.** As mentioned earlier, the molecular composition of a triglyceride can vary. When one double carbon bond is present in the fatty acid molecule (c=c), the fat is grouped as "monounsaturated" (one spot that is *not* saturated). Olive oils, peanut oils, sesame seed oils, canola oils, and avocados are high in monounsaturated fat. According to studies, these fats may help to lower blood cholesterol. But go easy with that olive oil if your weight is an issue. This "good" fat is still loaded with fat calories.

Nutri-Speak

Omega-3 fat supplements can be a useful tool for helping to lower triglyceride levels, improving digestive disorders, and reducing the symptoms of arthritis. Speak with your physician if you think you may benefit.

Overrated-Undercooked

All types of fat when eaten in excess can cause weight gain, but overloading on saturated fat, specifically, can also put you at risk for serious health problems, including heart disease.

◆ **Polyunsaturated fats.** Another type of unsaturated fat is polyunsaturated. Where a "mono" has one double carbon bond, the "poly" fat has several (c=c=c) spots that are *not* saturated. Corn oils, cotton seed oils, safflower oils, sunflower oils, soybean oils, and mayonnaise are all predominant in polyunsaturated fat. The fat in fish is also polyunsaturated (a type called omega-3 fatty acids). Didn't think fish had any fat? Well, it does (especially mackerel, salmon, albacore tuna, and sardines), but much less than most meats. What's more, the poly-fats have also been shown to help reduce the risk of heart disease. So fish away—just don't fry it.

◆ **Saturated fats.** When triglyceride molecules contain only single carbon bonds (c-c-c, unlike the double bonds you saw in mono- and polyunsaturated), the fat is grouped as "saturated." Saturated fats are the demons of all fats because they can raise your blood cholesterol, which, in turn, can lead to heart disease. Hard to believe a simple molecular change can make such a difference, but it can, and these guys are destructive. Animal fats found in meat, poultry, and whole milk dairy products are all high in saturated fats. Although most vegetable oils are unsaturated, some "saturated" exceptions include coconut, palm, and palm kernel oils (found in cookies, crackers, nondairy creamers, and other baked products). Do your body a favor: make a concerted effort to cut back on these fats. You'll help protect yourself from heart disease, certain cancers, and other potential health problems.

◆ **Trans-fatty acids.** This type of fat is *not* naturally occurring but is created when innocent unsaturated fats undergo a manufacturing process called hydrogenation. Hydrogenation is when a liquid or semisoft fat is transformed into a more solid state. Trans-fatty acids can be harmful because they act like saturated fats inside the body and raise blood cholesterol. Why mess with a good thing and "hydrogenate?" The process can help preserve food or enable a food company to change the texture of a product. For example, margarine in the liquid form is unsaturated, but with some hydrogenation, it becomes semisoft (tub margarine). With further hydrogenation, it becomes hard (stick margarine). Unfortunately, most people prefer tub and stick over liquid margarines and end up paying the "trans-fatty" penalty. Other trans-fatty culprits include partially hydrogenated vegetable oils, commonly found in cakes, crackers, cookies, and other baked goods. If you ever read the ingredients on food products, you'll know that trans-fats are everywhere.

Starting in 2006, trans fats will be listed on food labels, making it easier for you to spot (and avoid) them. Because of this new labeling act, food manufacturers have *already* started reformulating their products to make them trans-fat free.

Is it better to use butter or margarine?

Butter is loaded with saturated fat; margarine is packed with trans-fatty acids. Which one do you choose? Although both contain artery-clogging fat, a serving of butter contains *more* artery-clogging fat than most margarines. Give your blood vessels a break and only buy soft tub margarine spreads that also say "trans free" on the label. If you're looking to save additional calories, buy reduced-fat, trans-free soft tub spreads.

Most Fats Contain Combinations of All Three Types of Fat but Are Predominantly One Type

Saturated	Monounsaturated	Polyunsaturated
Beef fat	Canola oil	Corn oil
Butter	Olive oil	Cottonseed oil
Whole milk	Peanut oil	Safflower oil
Cheese	Sesame oil	Soybean oil
Coconut oil	Most nuts	Sunflower oil
Palm oil	Avocados	Margarine (soft)
Palm kernel oil		Mayonnaise
		Fish oils
		Sesame oil
		Flaxseed oil

The Cholesterol Connection and Heart Disease

If you've ever read a nutrition label, you know that dietary fat and cholesterol make up two very different categories. In fact, they are even measured in different units; fat is shown in grams, whereas cholesterol is shown in milligrams. We've already explored the facts on fat; now it's time for cholesterol.

Cholesterol is a waxy substance that contributes to the formation of many essential compounds, including vitamin D, bile acid, estrogen, and testosterone. At this point, you might be thinking, "Hey, if this stuff does so many great things, why can't I eat as much as I want?" The problem is that your liver makes all the cholesterol you'll ever need, and the unused portion all too often gets stored as plaque in your arteries.

All animal-related foods and beverages contain cholesterol because all animals have livers. Eggs, meats, fish, cheese, milk, and poultry are all sources of cholesterol. Needless to say, a slab of liver is loaded with the stuff. What's more, plant foods do not contain cholesterol, simply because they never had a liver.

How do you lower triglycerides?
Reduce your fat intake, specifically saturated fat; cut down on simple sugars such as candy, fruit juice, and so on; avoid alcoholic beverages; and engage in regular aerobic exercise. Also, speak with your doctor about fish oil supplements.

Don't Be Fooled by Misleading Labels

When a label reads "no cholesterol," the food in question is not necessarily low in calories and fat. Here is a perfect example. I walked into a famous cookie store and noticed these incredibly decadent peanut butter cookies. Next to them was a sign proclaiming "No-Cholesterol Cookies." Well, as far as I know, a peanut has never had a liver, and therefore, peanut butter doesn't have any cholesterol. But WOW, those cookies were packed with fat; the ingredients included peanut butter, margarine, and vegetable oil. Unfortunately, the majority of people mistook these cookies for low-calorie/low-fat just because of the no-cholesterol label. The next time you grab something that reads "no-cholesterol," check out the fat content; it might not be all it's cracked up to be.

How does saturated fat work its way into the cholesterol picture? This artery-clogging culprit can also raise blood cholesterol levels. Just imagine how harmful the high-fat animal foods such as marbled red meats and whole milk dairy products can be; they contain *both* saturated fat and cholesterol.

Total Fat, Saturated Fat, and Cholesterol Content of Common Foods

Food Name	Total Portion	Saturated Fat (g)	Fat (g)	Cholesterol (mg)
Ground beef, med. fat	3 oz.	17.7	6.9	76
Ground beef, lean	3 oz.	15.7	6.2	74
Frankfurter	3 oz.	24.8	9.1	43
Bacon	2 slices	6.2	2.2	11
Pork chops	3 oz.	11.0	4.0	70
T-bone steak	3 oz.	20.0	8.0	57
Veal, leg, braised	3 oz.	4.3	2.0	115
Chicken breast, no skin	3 oz.	3.0	0.9	72
Turkey breast, no skin	3 oz.	1.0	0.2	71
Liver, braised	3 oz.	4.2	1.6	331
Pâté (foie gras)	2 TB.	11	4.0	39
Sole/flounder	3 oz.	1.3	0.3	58

Food Name	Total Portion	Saturated Fat (g)	Fat (g)	Cholesterol (mg)
Scallops	3 oz.	3.0	0.5	27
Shrimp	3 oz.	1.0	0.25	166
Oysters	2 oz.	3.0	0.0	20
Swordfish	3 oz.	4.4	1.2	43
Salmon, Atlantic	3 oz.	6.9	1.0	60
Tofu, firm	3 oz.	4.0	0.5	.0
Tofu, fried	3 oz.	17	2.5	.0
Whole egg	1	5.0	1.6	213
Egg yolk	1	5.0	1.6	213
Egg white	1	0.0	0.0	0
Whole milk	1 cup	8.1	5.1	33
Skim milk	1 cup	0.4	0.3	4
Cheddar cheese	1 oz.	9.4	6.0	30
American cheese	1 oz.	8.8	5.6	27
Mozzarella/skim milk	1 oz.	4.5	2.9	16
String cheese	1 pc	5.0	3.0	15
Ice cream	¹/₂ cup	12.0	7.0	45
Ice cream, low-fat	¹/₂ cup	2.0	1.0	5
Yogurt, low-fat fruit	8 oz.	3.0	1.5	15
Nuts	1 oz.	14.1	2.0	0
Peanut butter	2 TB.	16.0	3.3	0
Butter	1 TB.	11.4	7.1	31
Margarine	1 TB.	11.4	2.1	0
Margarine, red. fat	1 TB.	5.7	1.0	0
Olive oil	1 TB.	13.5	1.8	0
Salad dressing, Ranch	2 TB.	16.0	2.3	1.3
Salad dressing, Caesar	2 TB.	17.0	2.6	1.0
Cream cheese	2 TB.	10.0	6.3	32
Mayo, regular	1 TB.	11.0	1.6	8.0
Mayo, low-fat	1 TB.	1.0	0.0	0.0

Source: First Databank.

Your Cholesterol Report Card

Yikes! The doctor just sent you a report indicating that your blood cholesterol level is high. Are you now at risk for heart disease?

Although it's certainly not in your favor to have clogged arteries, don't give away your prized possessions yet. In fact, most people have tremendous control over lowering their numbers by limiting the fats and oils in their diet, increasing foods rich in soluble fiber, losing weight if it's warranted, and becoming more physically active.

What do those numbers on the report card mean anyway?

- **Total blood cholesterol.** This number refers to the amount of cholesterol circulating in the bloodstream and provides a direct correlation to the amount of plaque deposited in your arteries. It is a combination of both types of cholesterol—HDL (good) and LDL (bad). Total cholesterol levels less than 200mg/dL are considered desirable. To help remember which "DL" is which, just remember this: "L" in LDL stands for "lousy," and "H" in HDL stands for "helpful."

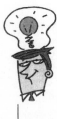

Food for Thought

Although shellfish contains a considerable amount of cholesterol, it has substantially less total fat and saturated fat than red meat and is clearly a leaner choice.

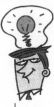

Food for Thought

Some people are born with a genetic predisposition to high cholesterol and therefore might need the assistance of cholesterol-lowering medication.

- **HDL.** The "good guys" actually help your body get rid of the cholesterol in your blood (sort of like garbage men clearing out the gar-bage). Thus, the higher your HDL–cholesterol number, the better off you are. An HDL–cholesterol of less than 40mg/dL is considered low and increases your risk for heart disease.

- **LDL.** The "bad guys" cause the cholesterol to build up in the walls of your arteries. Thus, the higher your LDL–cholesterol number, the greater your risk for heart disease. Optimal LDL–cholesterol is less than 100mg/dL.

Getting Fat from Eating Fat

The consequence from eating excessive fat is one that most of us know all too well: *weight gain.* Gram for gram, fat delivers more than twice as many calories as carbohydrates and protein. In other words, high-fat foods (such as chips, cakes, and whole milk dairy products) are more calorically dense than low-fat foods (grains, fruits, and veggies). And boy, those fat calories can add up quickly. A measly chocolate bar contains 240 calories; by contrast, so does an entire plateful of low-fat foods such as an apple, a banana, and a handful of pretzels. There is no comparison; you get a lot more quantity for the same amount of calories when you go low-fat. Sure, the candy bar might sound more appealing, but consider the other fats you may have consumed that same day: salad dressings, fried foods, whole milk dairy, and fatty meats. That's a lot of fat, which means a tremendous amount of calories.

CAUTION

Overrated-Undercooked

Even though excess calories from carbohydrates and protein can put on pounds, it's *a lot* easier to get fat from eating a lot of *fat*. One gram of fat supplies more than twice the number of calories your body gets from carbohydrates and protein:

1 gram carbohydrate = 4 calories

1 gram protein = 4 calories

1 gram fat = 9 calories

Don't get me wrong: no one should deprive himself of the things he loves. However, as with money, you must budget your fat so you don't go overboard by the end of the day. In this case, consistently going over budget won't leave you broke; it will leave you fat.

Filling up on fatty foods might also crowd out the healthy stuff that keeps us fit. Great—chubby and malnourished! Believe me, I sympathize. It's tough limiting all those delicious donuts, cakes, and gooey, chocolate treats. I'm certainly not one of those "genetic lean machines" who can eat whatever he wants and not gain an ounce. (I hate every one of them.) For most people, maintaining an ideal weight means watching total fat intake.

How Much Fat and Cholesterol Should We Eat?

The American Heart Association recommends the following:

◆ No more than 30 percent of the day's total calories should come from fat.

◆ For healthy people, saturated fat plus trans fat should not exceed 10 percent of total calories. If you have coronary heart disease, diabetes, or high LDL cholesterol, keep that number to less than 7 percent.

◆ Healthy people should limit their total daily cholesterol intake to less than 300 milligrams. For people with cardiovascular disease, keep it to less than 200 milligrams.

A Guide to Recommended Daily Fat Intake for Healthy People

Daily Calories	Fat Calories	Total Fat Grams	Saturated Fat Grams
1,200	<360	<40	<13
1,500	<450	<50	<17
1,800	<540	<60	<20
2,000	<600	<67	<22
2,500	<750	<83	<24
2,800	<840	<93	<28
3,000	<900	<100	<33

**Based on 30 percent of total calories coming from fat and 10 percent of total calories coming from saturated fat.

Some Fats Are Easier to Spot than Others

Although some fats and oils are rather obvious, others are hidden deep within our food. Take a look:

◆ **Visible fats.** Butter*, cream cheese*, lard*, sour cream*, mayonnaise, oil-based salad dressings, cream-* or cheese-based salad dressings, animal shortenings*, guacamole, cooking oils, peanut butter, and margarine.

◆ **Invisible fats.** Whole milk dairy*, high-fat meats* (including bologna, pepperoni, sausage, bacon, pastrami, spareribs, and hot dogs), donuts*, cakes*, cookies*, nuts, candy bars*, chocolate chips*, avocado, ice cream*, fried foods, pizza*, coleslaw, macaroni salad, and potato salad.

*Contains saturated fat

Food for Thought

Forty to sixty percent of all cancers may be diet-related. Evidence strongly suggests that people who eat low-fat diets have substantially less risk for certain types of cancer.

Slicing Off the Fat Without a Knife

These are tips to help you reduce the fat in your diet. Read through them and learn how to painlessly develop a low-fat lifestyle:

- Choose low-fat and nonfat dairy products whenever possible: skim or 1-percent milk, low-fat cheese and yogurts, low-fat sour creams, and reduced-fat ice cream.

- Prepare foods by roasting, baking, broiling, boiling, steaming, lightly stir-frying, or grilling.

- Use nonfat cooking sprays or nonstick pans when frying.

- Remove all skin from poultry and trim all visible fat from meats.

- Limit your intake of red meats and try to completely avoid the higher-fat selections, including salami, bologna, sausage, pepperoni, bacon, and hot dogs. Buffalo and venison may be eaten more frequently because they are very lean.

- Buy reduced-fat versions of margarine, butter, mayonnaise, and cream cheese.

- Buy low-fat salad dressings, or make your own by mixing balsamic vinegar, a lot of spices, and moderate amounts of olive oil.

- Instead of using butter and oily sauces, flavor your vegetables with herbs and seasonings. Also try lemon juice, spicy mustard, salsa, and flavored vinegars.

- Watch out for pastas swimming in oil and cream sauce. Instead, substitute marinara or other tomato-based sauces.

- Opt for egg white omelets (or egg substitutes) rather than whole eggs with yolk. If you can't live without eating whole eggs, limit yourself to three to four yolks per week.

- Pass on the ice cream, chips, and cookies. Instead, snack on pretzels, fig bars, fresh fruit, and frozen yogurt.

- Use extra-lean ground turkey breast or ground sirloin instead of ground beef in your favorite recipes.

The "Fat-Phobic" Generation

Sure, a low-fat lifestyle is the way to go, but some misinterpret this message and become utterly neurotic. Are you afraid to even touch anything that might have once possibly come in contact with fat? When ordering in a restaurant, do you create such chaos that your waiter is off and running to his or her shrink?

It might sound funny, but it's no laughing matter to be completely preoccupied with fat. Certainly, a low-fat diet is an essential part of being healthy. However, taking this concept to radical extremes can place serious restraints on social eating, let alone set you up for a serious eating disorder. If your reason is weight control, think again. Some fat is helpful, and I promise you can maintain your ideal body weight (within reason, of course) and still allow yourself to enjoy foods with fat.

In fact, joining a "fat-free cult" doesn't necessarily mean that you automatically lose weight. Quite frequently, I meet clients who cannot seem to drop an aggravating 5 or 10 pounds—even while following a strictly fat-free regimen. How can that be?

The answer is rather obvious: they simply overcompensate with the fat-free products. For the most part, the explosion of lower-fat foods on the market has been a wonderful tool, enabling people to painlessly lower their cholesterol and total fat intakes. Unfortunately for some people, the expression "low-fat" means carte blanche to eating huge amounts. Just because a product is fat-free doesn't mean it's calorie-free. As a matter of fact, many lower-fat foods can pack in just as many calories as their original fat-containing counterparts (compensating by pumping in more carbs).

Do you have a friend who will not go near a "real" chocolate-chip cookie but doesn't hesitate to inhale half a box of the fat-free version? Which is worse: the cookie with fat at 75 calories or 10 no-fat cookies at a whopping 500 calories? Remember, no matter where they come from, calories still count in the battle of the bulge.

The Least You Need to Know

- Fats perform vital roles in the body, including providing stored energy, storing and circulating fat-soluble vitamins, and providing a layer of insulation underneath the skin.

- All types of fat, when eaten in excess, can cause a variety of health problems, including weight gain.

- Saturated fat has the destructive capability to increase blood cholesterol and therefore promote heart disease.

- Live a "low-fat lifestyle" by limiting your intake of red meat, whole milk dairy, fried foods, high-fat spreads, and oily sauces. Switch to low-fat milk, yogurts, and cheese while jazzing up foods with herbs, spices, lemon juice, and Dijon mustard.

- Although low-fat and fat-free foods are great for your diet, every diet must have some sort of fat in it. A totally fat-free diet is dangerous because fat is responsible for vital body functions.

Chapter 5

Don't As-*salt* Your Body

In This Chapter

- ◆ All about salt
- ◆ Sodium and water retention
- ◆ The high blood pressure connection
- ◆ How much is recommended
- ◆ Decreasing your intake

Salt is composed of 40 percent sodium and 60 percent chloride. However, when most people speak of the problems associated with salt, they are usually referring to the part of salt called sodium. What exactly is sodium and what does it do?

Sodium is a mineral that is essential for many important functions, such as:

- ◆ Controlling the fluid balance within your body
- ◆ Transmitting electrical nerve impulses
- ◆ Contracting muscles (including your heart)
- ◆ Absorbing nutrients across cell membranes
- ◆ Maintaining your body's acid/base balance

Nutri-Speak

Hyponatremia is the excessive loss of sodium and water due to persistent vomiting, diarrhea, or profuse sweating. In this case, both water and salt must be replenished to maintain the correct balance for your body.

With such a wonderful resumé for sodium, why worry about your intake? Although sodium is essential for good health, your body requires less than $1/10$ teaspoon of salt on a daily basis. Would you believe the average American consumes 5 to 18 times more than that every day? In fact, most people could stand to substantially cut back.

Feeling a Bit Waterlogged?

Have your fingers ever been so swollen that it's literally impossible to get your rings on or off?

It's common to experience a temporary bloating or swelling after eating highly salted foods. You see, your body requires a certain balance of sodium and water at all times. Extra salt requires extra water, resulting in water retention. Where does this extra water or fluid come from? Usually your glass. Salt triggers your thirst response to balance out the sodium-water concentration. Ever wonder why you're so thirsty after munching on salty pretzels or nuts? It's no coincidence that the snacks offered in drinking establishments are covered with salt. What a strategy: the more you eat, the more you drink!

Can't Take the Pressure!

For reasons that are not completely understood, salt can play an active role in raising the blood pressure in people who are salt-sensitive.

What Exactly Is High Blood Pressure?

When your heart beats, it pumps blood into your arteries and creates a pressure within them. High blood pressure (also known as *hypertension*) occurs when too much pressure is placed on the walls of the arteries. This can occur if there is an increase in blood volume or the blood vessels themselves constrict or narrow.

People who are genetically sensitive to salt can't efficiently get rid of extra sodium through their urine. Therefore, that extra sodium hangs around, drawing in extra water, which means an increase in blood volume. This increased blood volume can then stimulate the vessels to constrict, creating increased pressure.

Imagine a garden hose with a normal flow of water running through it. No problem. Now, think about the increased pressure on the hose when you drastically turn up the amount of water rushing out. What if you were to pinch off spots of this hose, like a constricted blood vessel? A garden hose might endure the wear and tear, but your arteries can become extremely damaged by such constant pressure—so damaged that the end result might include a heart attack, stroke (a brain attack), or kidney disease.

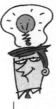

Food for Thought

Treating high blood pressure can reduce heart failure by more than 50%, strokes by 35% to 40%, and heart attacks by 20% to 25%.

Nutri-Speak

Hypertension is the medical term for sustained high blood pressure. It has nothing to do with being tense, nervous, or hyperactive.

What Causes High Blood Pressure?

According to recent statistics, one out of every four American adults—nearly 60 million people—has high blood pressure. In a small percentage of people, this increased pressure is from an underlying problem such as kidney disease or a tumor of the adrenal gland. However, in 90 to 95 percent of all cases, the cause is unclear. That's why it is known as the *silent killer*; it just creeps up without any warning. Whereas some of the contributing factors are *not* controllable, others can be quite controllable.

What's a normal blood pressure reading?

If you haven't seen your doctor in a few years, you may be in for a shock. In 2003, the definition of "normal" blood pressure (which had been 120/80) changed. Experts now recommend a systolic (that's the upper number) reading of *less than* 120 and a diastolic (the lower number) reading of *less than* 80. If your systolic pressure is between 120 and 140 and your diastolic between 80 and 90, you have "pre-hypertension." The definition of full-blown high blood pressure hasn't changed, though—it's still 140/90 or higher.

Risk factors that cannot be controlled are …

- **Age.** The older you get, the more likely you are to develop high blood pressure.

- **Race.** African Americans tend to have high blood pressure more often than whites. They also tend to develop it earlier and more severely.

- **Heredity.** High blood pressure can run in families. If you have a family history, you're twice as likely to develop it as others.

Risk factors that can be controlled are …

- **Obesity.** Being extremely overweight is clearly related to high blood pressure. In fact, nearly 60 percent of all high blood pressure cases concern overweight patients. By losing weight—even a small amount—obese individuals can significantly reduce their blood pressure.

- **Sodium consumption.** Reducing the intake of salt can lower blood pressure in people who are salt-sensitive.

- **Potassium, calcium, and magnesium consumption.** Studies have shown that eating foods rich in these minerals can play an active role in maintaining normal blood pressure.

> **How do you know if you have high blood pressure?**
>
> You don't! High blood pressure is known as the "silent killer" because it has no symptoms. In fact, many people can have hypertension for years without knowing it. By that time, their body organs may have already been damaged. Stay on top of your health and have your blood pressure checked regularly by a qualified health professional.

- **Alcohol consumption.** Regular use of alcohol can dramatically increase blood pressure in some people. Fortunately, alcohol's effect on blood pressure is completely reversible. Limit yourself to a maximum of two drinks a day.

- **Smoking.** Although the long-term effect of smoking on blood pressure is still unclear, the short-term effect is that it can raise blood pressure briefly. However, given that both smoking and high blood pressure have been linked to heart disease, smoking compounds the risk.

- **Oral contraceptives.** Women who take birth control pills may develop high blood pressure.

- **Physical inactivity.** Lack of exercise can contribute to high blood pressure. By becoming more active with moderate exercise, an inactive person can get into better shape, feel terrific, and help keep his or her blood pressure in check.

Investigating Your Blood Pressure Numbers

Your doctor measures two numbers when checking your blood pressure, systolic and diastolic. Systolic pressure is the top, larger number. This represents the amount of pressure that is in your arteries while your heart contracts (or beats). During this contraction, blood is ejected from the heart and into the blood vessels that travel throughout your body.

Diastolic pressure is the bottom, smaller number. This represents the pressure in your arteries while your heart is relaxing between beats. During this relaxation period, your heart is filling up with blood for the next squeeze. Although both numbers are critically important, your doctor might be more concerned with an elevated diastolic number because this indicates that there is increased pressure on the artery walls even when your heart is resting.

How to Lower High Blood Pressure

If your blood pressure is high, don't panic. Most people can significantly lower their numbers with know-how and determination:

- **Diet.** Follow the Dietary Approaches to Stop Hypertension (DASH) plan outlined in this chapter. Also, limit your alcohol intake, or better yet, avoid alcohol completely.

- **Weight.** Lose weight if you are overweight.

- **Exercise.** Become physically active and get some type of exercise at least four times a week. Check with your doctor before beginning any diet or exercise program.

- **Medication.** For some people, diet and exercise are just not enough. In this case, your doctor might give you medication to help lower your blood pressure.

- **Smoking.** If you smoke—QUIT!

Food Groups	1,600 Calories	2,000 Calories	2,600 Calories	3,100 Calories	Serving Sizes	Examples and notes	Significance of Each Food Group to the DASH Eating Plan
Grains[b]	6 servings	7-8 servings	10-11 servings	12-13 servings	1 slice bread, 1 oz dry cereal 1/3 cup cooked rice, pasta, or cereal[c]	Whole wheat bread, English muffin, pita bread, bagel, cereals, grits, oatmeal, crackers, unsalted pretzels, and popcorn	Major sources of energy and fiber
Vegetables	3-4 servings	4-5 servings	5-6 servings	6 servings	1 cup raw leafy vegetable 1/3 cup cooked vegetable 6 oz vegetable juice	Tomatoes, potatoes, carrots, green peas, squash, broccoli, turnip greens, collards, kale, spinach, artichokes, green beans, lima beans, sweet potatoes	Rich sources of potassium, magnesium, and fiber
Fruits	4 servings	4-5 servings	5-6 servings	6 servings	6 oz fruit juice 1 medium fruit 1/4 cup dried fruit 1/3 cup fresh, frozen, or canned fruit	Apricots, bananas, dates, grapes, oranges, orange juice, grapefruit, grapefruit juice, mangoes, melons, peaches, pineapples, prunes, raisins, strawberries, tangerines	Important sources of potassium, magnesium, and fiber
Low-fat or fat-free dairy foods	2-3 servings	2-3 servings	3 servings	3-4 servings	8 oz milk 1 cup yogurt 11/2 oz cheese	Fat-free or low-fat milk, fat-free or low-fat buttermilk, fat-free or low-fat regular or frozen yogurt, low-fat and fat-free cheese	Major sources of calcium and protein
Meat, poultry, fish	1-2 servings	2 or fewer servings	2 servings	2-3 servings	3 oz cooked meats, poultry, or fish	Select only lean; trim away visible fats; broil, roast or boil instead of frying; remove skin from poultry	Rich sources of protein and magnesium
Nuts, seeds, legumes	3-4 servings/ week	4-5 servings/ week	1 serving/ day	1 serving/ day	1/3 cup or 11/2 oz nuts 2 Tbsp or 1/2 oz seeds 1/3 cup cooked dry beans or peas	Almonds, filberts, mixed nuts, peanuts, walnuts, sunflower seeds, kidney beans, lentils	Rich sources of energy, magnesium, potassium, protein, and fiber
Fat and oils[d]	2 servings/ week	2-3 servings/ week	3 servings	4 servings	1 tsp soft margarine 1 Tbsp low-fat mayonnaise 1 Tbsp light salad dressing 1 tsp vegetable oil	Soft margarine, low-fat mayonnaise, light salad dressing, vegetable oil (such as olive, corn, canola, or safflower)	DASH has 27 percent of calories as fat (low in saturated fat), including fat in or added to foods
Sweets	0 servings	5 servings/ week	2 servings	2 servings	1 Tbsp sugar 1 Tbsp jelly or jam 1/2 oz jelly beans 8 oz lemonade	Maple syrup, sugar, jelly, jam, fruit-flavored gelatin, jelly beans, hard candy, fruit punch sorbet, ices	Sweets should be low in fat

a NIH publication No. 03-4082; Karanja NM et al. MDA 8:519-27,1999.
b Whole grains are recommended for most servings to meet fiber recommendations.
c Equals 1/2-11/4 cups, depending on cereal type. Check the product's Nutrition Label.
d Fat content changes serving counts for fats and oils: For example, 1 Tbsp of regular salad dressing equals 1 serving, 1 Tbsp of low-fat dressing equals 1/2 serving,
   1 Tbsp of a fat-free dressing equals D servings.

The DASH Eating Plan at 1,600-, 2,000-, 2,600-, and 3,000- calorie levels[a] from the Dietary Guidelines for Americans 2005 *from the National Heart, Lung, and Blood Institute, part of the National Institutes of Health and Human Services and the* Department of Health and Human Services.

How Much Sodium Is Recommended?

Many question the "one size fits all" recommendation because not everyone is salt-sensitive. However, there is no test for salt sensitivity; therefore, it makes sense for *everyone* to play it safe and follow a prudent approach.

The 2005 Dietary Guidelines recommend limiting your intake of sodium to no more than 2,300 milligrams per day. This includes both the salt you add and the sodium that is already present in foods you eat. Become familiar with the following list of high-sodium foods, and learn to balance your diet so you don't go sodium overboard. Note, if you have high blood pressure, your doctor might prescribe a more severe sodium restriction.

Common Foods That Are High in Sodium

Seasonings and Cooking Aids	Portion Size	Sodium (mg)
Baking powder	1 tsp.	426
Baking soda	1 tsp.	1,259
Table salt	1 tsp.	2,300
Garlic salt	1 tsp.	2,050
Bouillon cube, chicken	1 item	1,152
Bouillon cube, beef	1 item	864
Monosodium glutamate (MSG)	1 TB.	1,914
Salad dressing, Italian	1 TB.	116
Soy sauce	1 TB.	1,029
Low-sodium soy sauce	1 TB.	660
Butter buds	1 TB.	177

Canned Food Items	Portion Size	Sodium (mg)
Tuna, canned	3 oz.	303
Sardines, canned	3 oz.	261
Caviar, black and red	1 TB.	240
Chicken noodle soup	1 cup	1,106
Vegetable soup	1 cup	795
Veg. beef soup (low-sodium)	1 cup	57
Corn, canned	½ cup	266
Asparagus, canned	½ cup	472
Sauerkraut, canned	½ cup	780

continues

Common Foods That Are High in Sodium   (continued)

Processed/Cured and Smoked Meats	Portion Size	Sodium (mg)
Bologna	3 oz.	832
Salami	3 oz.	1,922
Hot dog	1 item	639
Smoked turkey	3 oz.	916
Smoked fish	3 oz.	619
Smoked sausage	3 oz.	853
Salted nuts	1 oz.	230
Pretzels	1 oz.	476
Corn chips	1 oz.	164
Potato chips	1 oz.	133
Popcorn	1 oz.	179
Saltines	5 crackers	180
Peanut butter	1 TB.	80

Dairy Products	Portion Size	Sodium (mg)
American cheese	1 oz.	336
Cheddar cheese	1 oz.	176
Parmesan cheese	3 Tb	329
Cottage cheese	$1/2$ cup	459
Butter	1 TB.	81
Margarine	1 TB.	132

Common Breakfast Cereals	Portion Size	Sodium (mg)
Rice Krispies	1 cup	256
Corn Flakes	1 cup	200
All-Bran	1 cup	160
Cheerios	1 cup	210
Special K	1 cup	220
Raisin Bran	1 cup	350

Source: First Databank, Nutritionist Pro 2005.

Salt-Less Solutions

Giving up salt doesn't mean giving up the pleasure of eating. However, you'll need to be a bit more selective with certain food products and much more creative in the seasoning department. The following guidelines can show you how to drastically cut the amount of salt in your food and body:

◆ Enhance the flavor of your foods with spices and herbs.

◆ Avoid putting a salt shaker on your breakfast, lunch, or dinner table.

◆ Choose fresh and frozen vegetables when possible. (The canned versions generally contain a lot of salt.) When canned is the only option, reduce the salt by draining the liquid and rinsing the vegetables in water before eating.

◆ Another plug for fresh fruit: it's naturally low in sodium and high in potassium.

◆ Go easy on condiments that contain considerable amounts of salt, including catsup, mustard, monosodium glutamate (MSG), salad dressings, sauces, bouillon cubes, olives, sauerkraut, and pickles. Stock your kitchen with low-sodium versions of soy sauce, teriyaki sauce, steak sauce, and anything else you might find in your travels.

◆ Select unsalted (or reduced salt) nuts, seeds, crackers, popcorn, and pretzels.

◆ Take it easy with cheese. Unfortunately, it not only has a lot of fat, but sodium as well. If you're feeling extra motivated, stock your fridge with low-salt/low-fat brands.

◆ Read labels carefully and choose foods lower in sodium, especially when choosing frozen dinners, canned soups, packaged mixes, and combination dishes.

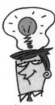

Food for Thought

Folks with recurring kidney stones (calcium-oxalate stones), should follow a low-salt diet.

Overrated-Undercooked

Be aware that some over-the-counter medicines contain a lot of sodium. For example, two tablets of dissolvable Alka-Seltzer (plop plop fizz fizz) have a whopping 1,134 milligrams of sodium. (Each single tablet provides 567 milligrams.) Instead, opt for the caplets that you swallow; they contain *only* 1.8 milligrams. Quite a drastic difference.

◆ Avoid processed luncheon cold cuts, as well as cured and smoked meats. Also be aware that most varieties of canned fish (tuna, salmon, and sardines) are extremely high in sodium.

◆ When dining in Chinese or Japanese restaurants ask for meals without MSG or added salt. Nowadays, you can also request low-sodium soy sauce for your table. If they don't have any, dilute the regular by adding a tablespoon of water.

The Least You Need to Know

◆ Salt consists of 40 percent sodium and 60 percent chloride. The mineral sodium is essential for many important functions. It maintains body fluids, controls the contraction of muscles, and transmits nerve impulses.

◆ Eating a high-sodium diet can increase blood pressure in people who are "salt-sensitive."

◆ People diagnosed with high blood pressure often need to reduce their salt intake, lose excess weight, increase exercise, and in some instances, take blood pressure–lowering medication.

◆ Because salt sensitivity is *not* something we are tested for, everyone should limit their sodium intake to less than 2,300 milligrams per day.

◆ Reduce your sodium intake by using herbs, spices, and seasonings instead of salt. Limit canned food items, salty snack foods, luncheon cold cuts, and meats that have been smoked or cured. Go easy on high-sodium condiments such as soy sauce, teriyaki sauce, mustard, catsup, olives, pickles, and sauerkraut. Also read labels carefully and opt for the lower-sodium foods.

Chapter 6

In and Out with Fiber

In This Chapter

- ◆ What is fiber?
- ◆ The different kinds of fiber
- ◆ Benefits from a fiber-rich diet
- ◆ How much do you need?
- ◆ Increasing your daily fiber intake

Say you're a little constipated? Got high cholesterol? Have I got a food for you! And you don't have to buy any special potions, formulas, or seek the advice of your local medicine man. This incredible healer is conveniently found in some of your favorite carbohydrate-rich foods.

Fiber Facts: What Is Fiber Anyway?

Fiber is a mix of many different substances found in plant cell walls and is not digestible by the human body. In it comes and out it goes. How can a substance we cannot even digest (and, by the way, has no nutritional value) be so beneficial? Might sound crazy, but once inside your body, fiber does some pretty amazing things. The term *dietary fiber*, when listed on a nutrition label, simply refers to the amount of these indigestible substances in a specific food product. This way, you can identify a food rich in fiber.

Fiber fits in two categories, insoluble and soluble, depending upon its ability to dissolve (or not dissolve) in water. Some foods contain *both* soluble and insoluble fiber, whereas others are predominant in only one. The key is to eat a variety of fiber-rich foods each day and receive the beneficial effects from both types.

Soluble Fiber

Water-soluble fiber readily dissolves in water. Technically speaking, soluble fibers include pectins, gums, and mucilages. It's obvious, however, that these terms won't be of any help to you in your grocery store. Translated into "real-food" terminology, you'll find soluble fiber in the following:

- Oats
- Brown rice
- Barley
- Oat bran
- Dried beans and peas
- Rye
- Seeds
- Vegetables (especially carrots, corn, cauliflower, and sweet potatoes)
- Fruits (especially apples, strawberries, oranges, bananas, nectarines, and pears)

Why all the hoopla? Well for starters, foods rich in soluble fiber have been shown to help decrease blood cholesterol, therefore reducing the risk of heart disease. Another benefit comes from its ability to slow the absorption of glucose (sugar in the blood), which might in turn help control blood-sugar levels in diabetics.

Insoluble Fiber

The type of fiber that does not readily dissolve in water is called water-insoluble. Insoluble fiber includes lignin, cellulose, and hemicellulose. Once again, converted into understandable food terms, we are talking about the following:

- Wheat bran

- Corn bran

- Whole-wheat breads and cereals

- Fruits

- Vegetables (especially potatoes with skin, parsnips, green beans, and broccoli)

As you can see, some foods are mentioned on both lists, indicating that they provide both soluble *and* insoluble fiber.

Insoluble fiber is primarily responsible for accelerating intestinal transit time, along with increasing and softening stools. In other words, insoluble fiber is responsible for "moving things along." In addition to promoting regularity, insoluble fiber has been shown to decrease your risk for hemorrhoids and *diverticulosis*.

Nutri-Speak

Diverticulosis is an illness or condition where tiny pouches (called diverticula) form in the wall of the colon. The condition is often without symptoms, but when the pouches become infected or inflamed, it can be painful. When this happens, the condition is known as diverticulitus, which can cause fever, abdominal pain, and diarrhea.

Overrated-Undercooked

Just because a food sounds healthy doesn't necessarily mean that it is. Some bran muffins are loaded with fat and sugar—certainly not worth the small amount of fiber they provide.

Lowering Your Cholesterol Level

If your cholesterol tends to be a bit high, or you'd just like to maintain an already low number, you might want to increase your *soluble fiber*. Soluble fibers have been shown to bind with cholesterol and pull it out of the body. Fruits, vegetables, legumes, oats, and all foods made with oat bran can therefore reduce your risk for heart and artery disease by lowering blood cholesterol. Another thought is that high-fiber foods can displace some of the high-fat, artery-clogging foods in your diet—a double impact!

Feeling Fuller with Less Food

Did you ever feel as though a plate of vegetables expanded in your stomach after you ate it? Well, it did! Eating fiber-rich foods can make you feel full because they absorb water and swell inside you. You might also feel full longer if you choose a meal with some soluble fiber. Unlike insoluble fiber, which quickly moves food through your body, soluble fiber tends to stick around a while, keeping you full and satisfied.

Does this mean you'll lose weight from eating a lot of fiber? It does if you eat these foods *instead* of the high-fat, high-calorie stuff. If you eat them in addition to all the junky food, your chance of becoming slim is slim.

How Much Fiber Do You Need?

Although there's no Recommended Daily Allowance (RDA) for fiber, most health experts agree that we should aim for 25 to 35 grams of dietary fiber each day (a mix of both soluble and insoluble). The following menu shows a few ideas to help you raise your intake of fiber.

Ready-Made Menu

This sample day provides about 31 grams of fiber:

Breakfast	Bowl of **bran cereal** with milk
	Banana
	Glass of juice
Lunch	Roast beef sandwich on wheat bread
	Cup of **vegetable barley soup**
	Apple with skin
	A lot of water
Snack	**Soy Crisps**
	Low-fat yogurt
Dinner	**Mixed green salad**
	Grilled fish with **sautéed carrots**
	Baked sweet potato
	Fresh strawberries
	Club soda with lemon

Tips to Increase the Fiber in Your Diet

As you read the following tips, keep these points in mind. It's important to increase your fiber *gradually* (sometimes over several weeks) because your body needs time to adjust. For example, if you are a newcomer to the world of fiber, start with 20 grams each day for the first week. Increase to 25 grams per day the second week, and—if your stomach can handle it—graduate to 30+ grams per day by week three. Also, drink plenty of fluids. Fiber acts as a bulking agent by absorbing some of the fluid in your body. Extra fluids will prevent you from becoming dehydrated, and most important, help that bulk to move merrily on its way.

- Read nutrition labels. Generally, a good source of fiber should have at least 2.5 grams per serving.

- Start your day with a high-fiber breakfast cereal. Supermarkets are flooded with them. Read the nutrition label and select a cereal that offers more than 4 grams per serving.

- Add a few tablespoons of wheat bran to your cereal, cottage cheese, yogurts, and salads.

- Include plenty of fresh or frozen vegetables in your day. Add them to soups, pizza, sandwiches, stir-fries, pastas, omelets, rice, and anything else you can think of.

- Eat breads and pasta made from wheat, rye, and oat products, along with brown rice, barley, and bulgur.

- Add fruit to your cereal (hot or cold), top off your pancakes and waffles with fruits, mix fruits into yogurts and salads, or simply enjoy them plain. Remember, whole fruit, with seeds and peels intact, provides more fiber than most fruit juice.

- Cook with beans and lentils. They are loaded with fiber. Enjoy them in soups, stews, salads, burritos, and a million other creative entrees.

- Get your fiber from food sources, not supplements. Food is a natural provider not only of fiber, but other essential nutrients as well.

The table on the next page lists foods rich in fiber.

How much fiber do kids need?

Although recent research suggests that kids should take in 14 grams of fiber for every 1,000 calories eaten, this may be too much for small bellies to handle. Nutritionists who work with children generally use the formula "Age plus 5" for healthy kids ages 3 to 18. For example, a 5-year-old should have 10 grams of fiber per day (5+5=10).

Foods Rich in Fiber

Fruits	Grams of Fiber
Elderberries (1 cup)	10.0
Blackberries (1 cup)	8.0
Raspberries (1 cup)	8.0
Avocado ($\frac{1}{2}$ medium)	6.0
Pear (1 medium)	5.0
Strawberries ($1\frac{1}{2}$ cups, whole)	4.5
Prunes (4)	4.0
Orange (1 large)	4.0
Dates ($\frac{1}{4}$ cup)	3.7
Blueberries (1 cup)	3.0
Figs, raw (3 medium)	3.0
Raisins ($\frac{1}{4}$ cup)	3.0
Apple (1 medium)	3.0
Banana (1 medium)	3.0
Kiwi (1 medium)	2.0
Peach (1 large)	2.0
Grapefruit ($\frac{1}{2}$ large)	2.0

Vegetables	Grams of Fiber
Artichoke, globe (1)	6.5
Edamame, shelled ($\frac{1}{2}$ cup, cooked)	5.5
Lima beans ($\frac{1}{2}$ cup, cooked)	5.0
Pumpkin, canned ($\frac{1}{2}$ cup)	5.0
Green peas ($\frac{1}{2}$ cup, cooked)	4.5
Sweet potato with skin (1 medium)	4.0
Baked potato with skin (1 medium)	4.0
Spinach (1 cup, cooked)	4.0
Corn (1 large ear)	4.0
Brussels sprouts (1 cup)	3.0
Broccoli (1 cup, chopped)	2.0
Carrot (1 medium)	2.0

Breads and Grains	Grams of Fiber
Dunkin' Donuts Reduced-Carb Bagel	14.0
Thomas' Carb Consider English Muffin	9.0
Thomas' Light English Muffin	8.0
Bulgur wheat (1 cup, cooked)	8.0
Barley (1 cup, cooked)	6.0
Whole-wheat spaghetti (1 cup, cooked)	6.0
Arnold's Bakery Light Bread (2 slices)	4.0-5.0
Brown rice (³/₄ cup, cooked)	3.0

Cereals	Grams of Fiber
Fiber One (¹/₂ cup)	14.0
Simply Fiber (1 cup)	14.0
Bran Buds (¹/₃ cup)	13.0
All Bran (¹/₃ cup)	10.0
Uncle Sam (³/₄ cup)	8.0
Kashi Heart to Heart (³/₄ cup)	5.0
Bran Flakes (³/₄ cup)	5.0
Raisin Bran (³/₄ cup)	5.0
Barbara's Puffins (1 cup)	5.0
Shredded Wheat (³/₄ cup)	4.5
Oatmeal (1 cup, cooked)	4.0
Wheat germ (2 TB.)	2.0

Beans (All Servings Equal; ¹/₂ Cup, Cooked)	Grams of Fiber
Navy	9.5
Kidney	8.2
Lentils	8.0
Pinto	8.0
Black	7.5
White	6.3
Chickpeas	6.0
Amy's Organic Burritos	6.0

Sources Include: USDA National Nutrient Database for Standard Reference, Release 17, *NutritionData.com*, USDA Dietary Guidelines for Americans 2005.

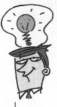

Food for Thought _____

Watch how the amount of fiber can decrease as food changes form:

Apple with peel = 3.0 grams

Apple without peel = 2.0 grams

½ cup apple juice = 0 grams

Don't Overdo It!

Can you ever eat too much fiber? You sure can, especially if your body is not used to it. I remember a client who ate half of a large box of high-fiber cereal and spent the entire day doubled over in his bathroom. Overloading on fiber can cause severe bloating, cramping, gas, diarrhea, and other abdominal discomforts. Furthermore, excessive amounts of fiber (generally 50 grams or more per day) can decrease the absorption of important vitamins and minerals—specifically calcium, zinc, magnesium, and iron. With all this in mind, once again, be sure to increase your fiber *gradually*, over a period of several weeks, and drink plenty of extra fluids to help the fiber pass through your system. The key is to pay attention to your body's response so you can figure out the amount you can handle at one time.

The Least You Need to Know

♦ Fiber is the indigestible substance found in plants and is classified in two categories: water-soluble and water-insoluble.

♦ Most foods contain combinations of both fibers. Foods particularly rich in soluble fiber include oats, oat bran, legumes, rye, fruits, and vegetables. Foods rich in insoluble fiber include wheat bran, whole wheat breads and cereals, fruits, and vegetables.

♦ Evidence suggests that soluble fiber can help lower blood cholesterol and improve the control of blood sugar in diabetics. Insoluble fiber has been reported to decrease the risk for colon cancer and diverticulosis, along with preventing hemorrhoids and constipation.

♦ The recommended fiber intake is 20 to 35 grams a day and is an important part of every well-structured food plan for the average adult.

♦ Increase your fiber gradually to give your body time to adjust. Also, be sure to drink plenty of extra fluids.

Vitamins and Minerals: The "Micro" Guys

In This Chapter

- ◆ All about vitamins and minerals
- ◆ Recommended Dietary Allowances (RDAs) and Dietary Reference Intakes (DRIs)
- ◆ Choosing foods that supply what you need
- ◆ Antioxidants and your health
- ◆ The full list of minerals—and a comprehensive look at selenium

A woman walked into my office for an initial consult. After introducing herself, she pulled open a large duffel bag filled to the rim with vitamin and mineral bottles. "I take one of each, every day," she claimed. "Why?" I asked. "Well, a neighbor told me about extra Bs, and my hairdresser recommended extra iron, and the others I can't seem to remember."

Unfortunately, this story is not uncommon. Popping pills has certainly become a popular morning ritual throughout this country. And why not? We've all heard the dramatic tales of vitamins and minerals. From health food stores to infomercials, everyone seems to be buzzing about megadosing on one thing or another. Needless to say, the vitamin industry is big business, with annual sales reaching the multi-billion-dollar level.

Do you really need all of the pills? Chances are you don't. With so much misinformation floating around, it's no wonder some people swallow exorbitant amounts of supplements they don't need. By the way, those extra supplements are literally money down the toilet because your body usually filters out the extra stuff. What's worse, some vitamins do not get flushed out and can potentially become toxic.

Don't get me wrong, vitamins and minerals are essential for normal functioning, and without them, you could not survive. However, your body requires only minute amounts of these "micro-guys," and most nutrition experts agree that the best way to get all the vitamins and minerals you need is to eat a balanced, varied diet. Although some groups of people *can* benefit from supplements (and most everyone can benefit from the backup of a multivitamin/mineral that provides 100 percent of the RDA), it is important to check with a competent health professional before running out to your nearest drugstore.

Get ready to buckle in and find out whether you are getting what your body needs. This chapter will help to clear up the facts on vitamins and minerals.

What Are Vitamins and Minerals?

In previous chapters, you became familiar with the macro-nutrients carbohydrate, protein, and fat. Now it's time to understand the micro-nutrients (in other words, vitamins and minerals) which exist *within* the macro-nutrients. Although the macro-nutrients receive top billing, these micro-guys are equally important in your diet because they perform specific jobs that enable your body to operate efficiently.

Think about carbohydrate, protein, and fat as the rock stars on stage. Now imagine the vitamins and minerals as the backup singers, the band, and all the people who help produce the concert. The big guys and little guys work together to get the job done, and the result is one dynamite show.

That's how your body works. You eat the carbohydrate, protein, and fat, which in turn supply your body with the 13 vitamins and at least 22 minerals you need. Although tiny in size and quantity, these nutrients accomplish the mighty tasks that keep your body going. Furthermore, a lack of any one will cause a unique deficiency that can only be corrected by supplying that particular nutrient.

The RDAs: Recommended Dietary Allowances

The Recommended Dietary Allowances (RDAs) are standards set by an expert committee known as the Food and Nutrition Board of the National Academy of Sciences/National Research Council. These recommendations list the average daily requirements for a variety of nutrients (in other words, vitamins and minerals) and are intended for healthy people.

Note: People with certain illnesses might require more or less of specific nutrients. The RDA guidelines are set slightly higher than the level your body actually needs, building in a precautionary safety net.

> **Food for Thought**
>
> Taking vitamin E supplements may decrease the effectiveness of certain cardiac medications—specifically the meds that work to increase HDL levels (that's the good cholesterol). Always check with your cardiologist to see if supplementation is appropriate.

The DRIs: Dietary Reference Intakes

Because scientific knowledge regarding diet and health has increased, the Food and Nutrition Board has recently expanded its framework and developed the Dietary Reference Intakes (DRIs) for several vital nutrients. These new DRI standards include the RDAs as goals for intakes, plus three new reference values: the estimated average requirement (EAR), the tolerable upper limit (UL), and the adequate intake (AI). On the two reference charts provided here, you'll notice that some nutrients are listed as DRIs, some as RDAs, and some as AIs—a bit confusing—but all you'll need to understand is the actual recommended amount.

FOOD AND NUTRITION BOARD, NATIONAL ACADEMY OF SCIENCES–NATIONAL RESEARCH COUNCIL
RECOMMENDED DIETARY ALLOWANCES,[a] Revised 1989 (Abridged)

Designed for the maintenance of good nutrition of practically all healthy people in the United States

Category	Age (years) or Condition	Weight[b] (kg)	(lb)	Height[b] (cm)	(in)	Protein (g)	Vitamin A (µg RE)[c]	Vitamin E (mg α-TE)[d]	Vitamin K (µg)	Vitamin C (mg)	Iron (mg)	Zinc (mg)	Iodine (µg)	Selenium (µg)
Infants	0.0–0.5	6	13	60	24	13	375	3	5	30	6	5	40	10
	0.5–1.0	9	20	71	28	14	375	4	10	35	10	5	50	15
Children	1–3	13	29	90	35	16	400	6	15	40	10	10	70	20
	4–6	20	44	112	44	24	500	7	20	45	10	10	90	20
	7–10	28	62	132	52	28	700	7	30	45	10	10	120	30
Males	11–14	45	99	157	62	45	1,000	10	45	50	12	15	150	40
	15–18	66	145	176	69	59	1,000	10	65	60	12	15	150	50
	19–24	72	160	177	70	58	1,000	10	70	60	10	15	150	70
	25–50	79	174	176	70	63	1,000	10	80	60	10	15	150	70
	51+	77	170	173	68	63	1,000	10	80	60	10	15	150	70
Females	11–14	46	101	157	62	46	800	8	45	50	15	12	150	45
	15–18	55	120	163	64	44	800	8	55	60	15	12	150	50
	19–24	58	128	164	65	46	800	8	60	60	15	12	150	55
	25–50	63	138	163	64	50	800	8	65	60	15	12	150	55
	51+	65	143	160	63	50	800	8	65	60	10	12	150	55
Pregnant						60	800	10	65	70	30	15	175	65
Lactating	1st 6 months					65	1,300	12	65	95	15	19	200	75
	2nd 6 months					62	1,200	11	65	90	15	16	200	75

NOTE: This table does not include nutrients for which Dietary Reference Intakes have recently been established (see *Dietary Reference Intakes for Calcium, Phosphorus, Magnesium, Vitamin D, and Fluoride* [1997] and *Dietary Reference Intakes for Thiamin, Riboflavin, Niacin, Vitamin B6, Folate, Vitamin B12, Pantothenic Acid, Biotin, and Choline* [1998]).

[a] The allowances, expressed as average daily intakes over time, are intended to provide for individual variations among most normal persons as they live in the United States under usual environmental stresses. Diets should be based on a variety of common foods in order to provide other nutrients for which human requirements have been less well defined.

[b] Weights and heights of Reference Adults are actual medians for the U.S. population of the designated age, as reported by NHANES II. The median weights and heights of those under 19 years of age were taken from Hamill et al. (1979). The use of these figures does not imply that the height-to-weight ratios are ideal.

[c] Retinol equivalents. 1 retinol equivalent = 1 µg retinol or 6 µg β-carotene.

[d] α-Tocopherol equivalents. 1 mg d-α tocopherol = 1 α-TE.

FOOD AND NUTRITION BOARD, INSTITUTE OF MEDICINE–NATIONAL ACADEMY OF SCIENCES
DIETARY REFERENCE INTAKES: RECOMMENDED INTAKES FOR INDIVIDUALS

Life-Stage Group	Calcium (mg/d)	Phosphorus (mg/d)	Magnesium (mg/d)	Vitamin D (μg/d)[a,b]	Fluoride (mg/d)	Thiamin (mg/d)	Riboflavin (mg/d)	Niacin (mg/d)[c]	Vitamin B6 (mg/d)	Folate (μg/d)[d]	Vitamin B12 (μg/d)	Pantothenic Acid (mg/d)	Biotin (μg/d)	Choline[e] (mg/d)
Infants														
0–6 mo	210*	100*	30*	5*	0.01*	0.2*	0.3*	2*	0.1*	65*	0.4*	1.7*	5*	125*
7–12 mo	270*	275*	75*	5*	0.5*	0.3*	0.4*	4*	0.3*	80*	0.5*	1.8*	6*	150*
Children														
1–3 yr	500*	460	80	5*	0.7*	0.5	0.5	6	0.5	150	0.9	2*	8*	200*
4–8 yr	800*	500	130	5*	1*	0.6	0.6	8	0.6	200	1.2	3*	12*	250*
Males														
9–13 yr	1,300*	1,250	240	5*	2*	0.9	0.9	12	1.0	300	1.8	4*	20*	375*
14–18 yr	1,300*	1,250	410	5*	3*	1.2	1.3	16	1.3	400	2.4	5*	25*	550*
19–30 yr	1,000*	700	400	5*	4*	1.2	1.3	16	1.3	400	2.4	5*	30*	550*
31–50 yr	1,000*	700	420	5*	4*	1.2	1.3	16	1.3	400	2.4	5*	30*	550*
51–70 yr	1,200*	700	420	10*	4*	1.2	1.3	16	1.7	400	2.4[f]	5*	30*	550*
> 70 yr	1,200*	700	420	15*	4*	1.2	1.3	16	1.7	400	2.4[f]	5*	30*	550*
Females														
9–13 yr	1,300*	1,250	240	5*	2*	0.9	0.9	12	1.0	300	1.8	4*	20*	375*
14–18 yr	1,300*	1,250	360	5*	3*	1.0	1.0	14	1.2	400[g]	2.4	5*	25*	400*
19–30 yr	1,000*	700	310	5*	3*	1.1	1.1	14	1.3	400[g]	2.4	5*	30*	425*
31–50 yr	1,000*	700	320	5*	3*	1.1	1.1	14	1.3	400[g]	2.4	5*	30*	425*
51–70 yr	1,200*	700	320	10*	3*	1.1	1.1	14	1.5	400	2.4[f]	5*	30*	425*
> 70 yr	1,200*	700	320	15*	3*	1.1	1.1	14	1.5	400	2.4[f]	5*	30*	425*
Pregnancy														
≤ 18 yr	1,300*	1,250	400	5*	3*	1.4	1.4	18	1.9	600[h]	2.6	6*	30*	450*
19–30 yr	1,000*	700	350	5*	3*	1.4	1.4	18	1.9	600[h]	2.6	6*	30*	450*
31–50 yr	1,000*	700	360	5*	3*	1.4	1.4	18	1.9	600[h]	2.6	6*	30*	450*
Lactation														
≤ 18 yr	1,300*	1,250	360	5*	3*	1.5	1.6	17	2.0	500	2.8	7*	35*	550*
19–30 yr	1,000*	700	310	5*	3*	1.5	1.6	17	2.0	500	2.8	7*	35*	550*
31–50 yr	1,000*	700	320	5*	3*	1.5	1.6	17	2.0	500	2.8	7*	35*	550*

NOTE: This table presents Recommended Dietary Allowances (RDAs) in **bold type** and Adequate Intakes (AIs) in ordinary type followed by an asterisk (*). RDAs and AIs may both be used as goals for individual intake. RDAs are set to meet the needs of almost all (97 to 98 percent) individuals in a group. For healthy breastfed infants, the AI is the mean intake. The AI for other life-stage and gender groups is believed to cover needs of all individuals in the group, but lack of data or uncertainty in the data prevent being able to specify with confidence the percentage of individuals covered by this intake.

a As cholecalciferol. 1 μg cholecalciferol = 40 IU vitamin D.
b In the absence of adequate exposure to sunlight.
c As niacin equivalents (NE). 1 mg of niacin = 60 mg of tryptophan; 0–6 months = preformed niacin (not NE).
d As dietary folate equivalents (DFE). 1 DFE = 1 μg food folate = 0.6 μg of folic acid (from fortified food or supplement) consumed with food = 0.5 μg of synthetic (supplemental) folic acid taken on an empty stomach.
e Although AIs have been set for choline, there are few data to assess whether a dietary supply of choline is needed at all stages of the life cycle, and it may be that the choline requirement can be met by endogenous synthesis at some of these stages.
f Because 10 to 30 percent of older people may malabsorb food-bound B₁₂, it is advisable for those older than 50 years to meet their RDA mainly by consuming foods fortified with B₁₂ or a supplement containing B₁₂.
g In view of evidence linking folate intake with neural tube defects in the fetus, it is recommended that all women capable of becoming pregnant consume 400 μg of synthetic folic acid from fortified foods and/or supplements in addition to intake of food folate from a varied diet.
h It is assumed that women will continue consuming 400 μg of folic acid until their pregnancy is confirmed and they enter prenatal care, which ordinarily occurs after the end of the periconceptional period—the critical time for formation of the neural tube.

Fat-Soluble Vitamins

Vitamins are organic compounds (compounds that contain carbon), and of the 13 that your body needs, 4 are called fat-soluble (A, D, E, and K). Fat-soluble vitamins do not dissolve in water and are stored in your body's fat and liver. As a result, these vitamins can build up in the tissues and become toxic (specifically vitamins A and D).

Vitamins fall into two classes: fat-soluble and water-soluble.

Fat-Soluble Vitamins	Water-Soluble Vitamins	
Vitamin A	B-vitamins	Folate
Vitamin D	Thiamin	Vitamin B-12
Vitamin E	Riboflavin	Pantothenic acid
Vitamin K	Niacin	Biotin
	Vitamin B-6	Vitamin C

Vitamin A (Retinol)

Like Mom always said, eat plenty of carrots and you'll see in the dark. That's because carrots contain beta-carotene, a substance that is converted into vitamin A by your body. Vitamin A promotes good vision, as well as healthy skin and the normal growth and maintenance of your bones, teeth, and mucous membranes. What Mom didn't tell you was that beta-carotene is also found in most orange-yellow fruits and vegetables, along with dark green vegetables.

Your body converts beta-carotene into vitamin A only when you need it, so eating foods rich in beta-carotene cannot cause vitamin A toxicity. However, eating huge amounts might turn your skin slightly orange. Not to worry, this condition isn't serious. Simply lay off the orange veggies for a few days and the color will disappear.

Although your body controls the creation of vitamin A from beta-carotene, it has no control when you ingest straight vitamin A, which can be found in vitamin tablets. Over-supplementation can be extremely toxic, resulting in general fatigue and weakness, severe headaches, blurred vision, insomnia, hair loss, menstrual irregularities, skin rashes, and joint pain. In extreme cases, there can be liver and brain damage. Huge doses taken in the prenatal period can cause birth defects.

What happens if you don't get enough? Vitamin A deficiency can cause night blindness, total blindness, and lowered resistance to infection because vitamin A plays a key role in the structural integrity of your cells. Here come the germs!

Foods rich in vitamin A include: liver, eggs, milk, butter, and cheese.

Foods rich in beta-carotene include: cantaloupes, carrots, sweet potatoes, winter squash, spinach, and broccoli.

Vitamin D: The Sunshine Vitamin

Vitamin D plays an indispensable role in building and maintaining strong bones and teeth. In fact, vitamin D is responsible for the body's absorption and utilization of the mineral calcium. Insufficient amounts of this key vitamin can lead to serious bone abnormalities, including rickets in children (bones that are soft and malformed) and osteoporosis or osteomalacia (softening of the bones) in adults.

Recently, vitamin D has also received a lot of attention for reasons that go far *beyond* bone health. Research indicates that vitamin D may help prevent autoimmune diseases such as multiple sclerosis, rheumatoid arthritis, psoriasis, and Type 1 diabetes. It may also be a factor in decreasing your risk for cancer of the colon, breast, and prostate.

Because of its potential to help prevent these diseases, several experts think we should be taking in a good deal more vitamin D than the current RDA. In fact, they recommend a whopping 1,000 IU per day! This is well below the tolerable upper limit (UL) of 2,000 IU per day, but some health professionals worry that 1,000 IU may still be too much. Remember—vitamin D is fat-soluble, and therefore can be stored in the body where it may build up to toxic levels. Some of the symptoms of excess vitamin D include drowsiness, diarrhea, loss of appetite, headaches, high blood pressure, high cholesterol, fragile bones, and calcium deposits throughout the body (including heart, kidneys, and blood vessels).

Food for Thought

The adequate intake (AI) for vitamin D is given in micrograms, while the vitamin D in food and supplements is usually measured in international units (IU). The conversion is one microgram = 40 IU.

Food for Thought

Your body synthesizes vitamin D when your skin is exposed to sunlight, but too much sun may also increase your risk for skin cancer, wrinkles, and age spots.

Your best bets for getting enough vitamin D:

◆ Allow yourself 5–15 minutes of unprotected sun exposure on your hands and arms every day (more if you are darker-skinned). Of course, if you have a history of skin cancer, you *must* talk to your physician before exposing yourself to UV rays.

◆ Eat foods rich in vitamin D, such as fortified milk, tuna, salmon, and canned sardines and mackerel.

◆ Take a daily multivitamin that contains 400–800 IU of vitamin D.

Vitamin E (Tocopherols)

Vitamin E aids the formation and functioning of your red blood cells, muscles, and other tissues, and protects essential fatty acids (special fats that are needed by your body). Because vitamin E is found in a variety of foods, deficiency is rare. However, an extreme case of vitamin E deficiency involves wasting of the muscles and neurological disorders. To date, there have been no shown toxic effects from taking doses well over the RDA.

Foods rich in vitamin E include vegetable oils, salad dressings, whole grain cereals, green leafy vegetables, nuts and seeds, peanut butter, and wheat germ.

Vitamin K

Thanks to vitamin K, you won't bleed to death after an injury. That's because vitamin K is essential for normal blood clotting. Current research also suggests that this vitamin might play a role in maintaining strong bones in the elderly. Where do you get this vitamin? Interestingly enough, bacteria that live in your intestines help to make 80 percent of the vitamin K that you need, and the rest can be found in a variety of foods listed here.

A vitamin K deficiency can cause hemorrhaging (uncontrollable bleeding), mainly in newborn infants because their immature intestinal tracts might not have enough bacteria to make this vitamin. In addition, people taking antibiotics might temporarily lose the ability to make vitamin K because the medication destroys all bacteria, good and bad.

Foods rich in vitamin K include turnip greens, cauliflower, spinach, beef liver, broccoli, kale, and cabbage.

Water-Soluble Vitamins

Unlike fat-soluble vitamins, water-soluble vitamins can easily dissolve in the watery fluids of your body. Because excessive amounts are generally excreted in the urine, there is less chance for toxic side effects but more chance for deficiencies. Therefore, it is important to regularly replenish these vitamins by eating healthy foods that supply ample amounts. Be extra careful during food preparation. Because some of these vitamins are easily washed away or destroyed by light, air, and heat, use small amounts of water, avoid overcooking, and only cut your fruits and vegetables right before eating them. The following provides a quick rundown on each of the nine water-soluble vitamins: eight B-vitamins and vitamin C.

Thiamin (B-1)

Thiamin is needed for the conversion of carbohydrate-rich foods into energy. B-1 also plays a role in keeping your brain, nerve, and heart cells healthy. A deficiency will lead to loss of energy, nausea, depression, muscle cramps, nerve damage, and muscular weakness. Although uncommon in the United States, a severe depletion of thiamin can result in the disease beriberi, causing potential muscle wasting and paralysis.

Foods rich in thiamin (B-1) include pork, beef, liver, peas, seeds, legumes, whole-grain products, oatmeal, and lamb.

Riboflavin (B-2)

Like its buddy thiamin, riboflavin plays a key role in the metabolism of energy. Furthermore, this vitamin is involved in the formation of red blood cells and is necessary for healthy skin and normal vision.

A riboflavin deficiency will cause dry, scaly skin, accompanied by cracks on your lips and in the corners of your mouth. If that's not enough, getting insufficient amounts can also make your eyes extremely sensitive to light.

Foods rich in riboflavin (B-2) include milk, yogurt, cheese, whole-grain breads and cereals, green leafy vegetables, meat, eggs, and beef liver.

Note: This vitamin is easily destroyed with exposure to sunlight; therefore, store these foods in the fridge, cabinet, or pantry.

Niacin (B-3)

This B-vitamin is also involved in energy-producing reactions in the cells that convert food to energy. In addition, niacin helps maintain healthy skin, nerves, and your digestive system. In some instances, you can use large doses of niacin as a cholesterol-lowering medication. However, you should only do this under the supervision of your doctor. Megadoses can cause hot flashes, itching, ulcers, high blood sugar, and liver damage.

In the rare case of a niacin deficiency, symptoms include diarrhea, mouth sores, changes in the skin, nervous disorders, and pellagra disease known to cause the "four Ds": diarrhea, dermatitis, dementia (mental confusion), and death.

Foods rich in niacin (B-3) include meat, poultry, liver, eggs, nuts, enriched breads and cereals, brown rice, baked potatoes, fish, peanut butter, milk, and whole grains.

Pyridoxine (B-6)

Vitamin B-6 is a vital component for chemical reactions involving proteins and amino acids. (Remember those protein-building blocks?) It also participates in the formation of red blood cells, antibodies, and insulin, in addition to maintaining normal brain function. Deficiency causes skin changes, convulsions in infants, dementia, nervous disorders, and anemia.

Foods rich in pyridoxine (B-6) include lean meats, fish, legumes, green leafy vegetables, raisins, corn, whole grain cereals, pork, bananas, lentils, mangos, and poultry.

Cobalamin (B-12)

Vitamin B-12 assists in the formation of red blood cells and the normal functioning of your nervous system and is required for the synthesis of DNA (your genetic resumé). Because B-12 is only found in foods of animal origin, strict vegetarians might need to take a supplement to avoid a deficiency. Furthermore, this unique vitamin needs the help of another substance called *intrinsic factor* to be absorbed. Because intrinsic factor is made by the lining of the stomach, people with gastrointestinal disorders (especially found in the elderly) might need to get B-12 shots directly into the bloodstream. Symptoms of B-12 deficiency include nervous disorders and pernicious anemia.

Because a good amount of vitamin B-12 can be stored in the liver, it might take years for a deficiency to be recognized. As a result, people should have their B-12 levels checked starting at age 60 and every decade thereafter.

Foods rich in cobalamin (B-12) include meat, fish, poultry, eggs, milk products, and clams.

Folic Acid (Folacin, Folate)

Folic acid appropriately gets its name from the word *foliage* because it's primarily found in leafy, dark green vegetables. In addition to playing a vital role in cell division and red blood cell formation, this vitamin is needed to make the genetic material DNA.

In recent years, folic acid has gained a lot of attention for its ability to reduce neural-tube birth defects in newborn babies. Needless to say, it is imperative that pregnant mothers and women of childbearing years get the appropriate amounts of folic acid by both foods and supplementation. For this reason, folic acid is a key ingredient in most prenatal vitamins. Because this nutrient is involved in cell division, a deficiency will leave you vulnerable to anemia and an abnormal digestive function because your blood cells and cells of the intestinal tract divide most rapidly. Foods rich in folic acid include spinach, liver, beans (all types), peas, asparagus, lima beans, oranges, brussels sprouts, collard greens, and avocadoes.

> **Food for Thought**
>
> Folic acid has been shown to decrease your risk for colon cancer. If you have ulcerative colitis or feel that you are at a high risk for colon cancer—speak to your physician about supplementation. Folic acid can also reduce the risk of heart disease by lowering the levels of a harmful substance called homocysteine in the blood.

> **Nutri-Speak**
>
> **Scurvy** is a disease resulting from a deficiency of vitamin C, characterized by bleeding and swollen gums, joint pain, muscle wasting, and bruises. Scurvy is now very rare, except among alcoholics, and can be cured by as little as 5 to 7 milligrams of vitamin C.

Pantothenic Acid and Biotin

Pantothenic acid and biotin are both part of the "B-vitamin gang" that participates in the metabolism of energy. In addition, pantothenic acid also plays a role in the formation of certain hormones and neurotransmitters. Although both vitamins are vital for normal functioning, as of today there isn't a set RDA for either one. This is because deficiencies are so rare, and they are both found in a wide variety of plant and animal foods.

Vitamin C (Ascorbic Acid)

Now the million-dollar question, "Can vitamin C ward off the common cold?" The scientists say no. To date, there is no documented evidence supporting this notion. Interestingly enough, this vitamin might lessen the severity of those lousy symptoms experienced during a cold because vitamin C has a mild antihistaminic effect.

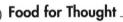

Overrated-Undercooked

For reasons that are unclear, cigarette smokers seem to require 50 percent more vitamin C than nonsmokers. Instead of popping more vitamin C, why not just quit smoking?

Food for Thought

There's no need to megadose on vitamin C because it turns out that young, healthy, nonsmokers can only absorb about 400 mg per day. Even the Linus Pauling Institute now recommends only 400 mg vitamin C per day for this group, although they caution that older people and those suffering from certain diseases may need more.

Nutri-Speak

Free radicals can be described as unstable, hyperactive atoms that literally trek around your body damaging healthy cells and tissue.

What else can vitamin C do? Let's just say if all the vitamins and minerals were on a pay scale according to the jobs they perform, vitamin C would be rolling. Vitamin C wears many hats, from helping to keep your bones, teeth, and blood vessels healthy to healing wounds, boosting your resistance to infection, and participating in the formation of collagen (a protein that helps support body structures). Another benefit from eating foods rich in vitamin C is that you increase the absorption of the mineral iron— good news for people with greater iron requirements or deficiencies.

Although vitamin C deficiency is uncommon, it can cause a lowered resistance to infection, sore gums, hemorrhages, and in severe cases, the disease *scurvy*.

Foods rich in vitamin C include melons, berries, tomatoes, potatoes, broccoli, fortified juices, guava, kiwi, mangos, papaya, yellow peppers, and citrus fruits (oranges, grapefruits, etc.)

Antioxidants and Your Health

Most of us have heard about antioxidants, but I bet a good number of people don't really know what they are and how they work. Here's the scoop: As you know, every cell in your body needs oxygen to function normally. Unfortunately, the utilization of this oxygen produces harmful by-products called *free radicals*. Free radicals are also created from environmental pollution, certain industrial chemicals, and smoking.

Outside the body, the process of oxidation is responsible for a sliced apple turning brown and the rusting of metal. Inside the body, oxidation contributes to heart disease, cancer, cataracts, aging, and a slew of other degenerative diseases. In other words, free radicals are the enemy.

So why isn't everyone falling apart? Well, in part because *antioxidants* like vitamin C, vitamin E, beta-carotene, and selenium help mop up these nasty free radicals. However, current research indicates that antioxidants may *not* be the cure-alls they were once thought to be—at least not for certain ailments.

Here's the latest on antioxidants and health:

- **Cardiovascular disease.** Several major studies have found that high doses (400 IU or more) of vitamin E do not help prevent heart disease after all. Lower doses (more like 200 IU per day) might still be helpful, but you may just want to stick to the amount in a typical multivitamin.

Food for Thought

If you are undergoing chemotherapy, you should avoid taking high-dose antioxidant supplements. A basic multivitamin is probably fine, but talk to your oncologist before taking *any* kind of dietary supplement.

- **Cancer.** Theoretically, antioxidants *should* help protect against cancer because they're great at mopping up those DNA-damaging free radicals. However, several large-scale clinical trials haven't yielded particularly promising results. Other trials are still on-going (including one on selenium, vitamin E, and prostate cancer), so stay tuned. And keep in mind that many factors influence the development of cancer, including heredity, smoking, nutritional excesses and deficiencies, and the environment.

Food for Thought

Popeye was sure on to something. With just one can of spinach (2 cups), he swallowed down about 29,000 IUs of beta-carotene, 50 milligrams of vitamin C, and 12 milligrams of vitamin E. That's one heck of a healthy sailor!

- **Macular degeneration.** Here's a winner! The Age-Related Eye Disease Study (AREDS) indicates that you can slow the progression of macular degeneration by taking 500 mg vitamin C, 400 IU vitamin E, 25,000 IU beta-carotene, as well as 80 mg zinc oxide and 2 mg copper per day. Note: 80 mg of zinc may impair your immunity, lower your "good" HDL cholesterol, and raise your risk of prostate

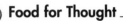

Overrated-Undercooked

Although beta-carotene is still considered a powerful antioxidant, it is no longer recommended in supplemental form. Many years ago, a study found that smokers who took beta-carotene supplements showed an increased risk of lung cancer. However, these findings certainly do not mean that you shouldn't eat plenty of *foods* rich in beta-carotene.

Food for Thought

What most people *do* know is that in large quantities, arsenic becomes a lethal poison. What most people *don't* know is that in very small amounts, arsenic is an essential mineral that your body needs to function properly.

cancer. And if you are a smoker, remember that high doses of beta-carotene may increase your risk of lung cancer.

◆ **Immunity.** Researchers theorize that antioxidants might help to strengthen the immune system by preventing the action of free radicals.

How Much Should You Take?

Your primary (and secondary) focus should be on eating *foods* rich in antioxidant vitamins. Contrary to what people might think, there are no magic bullets (or pills) to good health. Another plug for food is that scientists are constantly discovering new food substances that might help with the quest for well-being. Furthermore, future findings may even reveal that it's not just one isolated vitamin, but interactions between several food ingredients that enhance disease prevention.

The bottom line: if you decide to take antioxidant supplements, stay on top of the current research and speak with a competent health professional.

The Scoop on Minerals

Together with vitamins, at least 22 minerals are needed by your body to make things happen. Major minerals such as calcium and potassium are needed in large amounts, whereas trace minerals such as iron and zinc are only required in minute amounts. Just because a mineral is classified as "trace" doesn't mean it is any less important. The small RDA for iron is just as important to your body as the large RDA for calcium. Sort of like bread—a lot of flour with a drop of yeast—both are equally important for that perfect baked loaf.

Here's the master list of minerals. The following chapter focuses on two powerhouse players: calcium and iron.

Major Minerals	Trace Minerals	
Calcium	Iron	Chromium
Chloride	Zinc	Molybdenum
Magnesium	Iodine	Arsenic
Phosphorus	Selenium	Nickel
Potassium	Copper	Silicon
Sodium	Manganese	Boron
Sulfur	Fluoride	Cobalt

Selenium: The Newest Antioxidant and a Mineral Worth Noting!

Selenium is an important trace mineral in the human body that is essential for normal functioning of the immune system and thyroid gland. Selenium is also an imperative part of the antioxidant workforce that protects our cells against the effects of free radicals.

What Foods Provide Selenium?

Plant foods are the major dietary sources of selenium in most countries throughout the world. The amount of selenium in soil, which varies by region, determines the amount of selenium in the plant foods that are grown in that soil. Researchers know that soils in the high plains of northern Nebraska and the Dakotas have very high levels of selenium. Thus, people living in those regions generally have the highest selenium intakes in the United States. Selenium can also be found in some meats and seafood, and certain nuts, specifically Brazilian nuts, are *very* good sources of selenium.

Food Sources of Selenium

Food	Micrograms	% DV*
Brazil nuts, dried, unblanched, 1 oz.	840	1200
Tuna, canned in oil, drained, 3½ oz.	78	111
Beef/calf liver, 3 oz.	48	69
Cod, cooked, dry heat, 3 oz.	40	57
Noodles, enriched, boiled, 1 cup	35	50
Macaroni and cheese (box mix), 1 cup	32	46
Turkey, breast, oven roasted, 3½ oz.	31	44
Macaroni, elbow, enriched, boiled, 1 cup	30	43
Spaghetti w/ meat sauce, 1 cup	25	36
Chicken, meat only, ½ breast	24	34
Beef chuck roast, lean only, oven roasted, 3 oz.	23	33
Bread, enriched, whole wheat, 2 slices	20	29
Oatmeal, 1 cup, cooked	16	23
Egg, raw, whole, 1 large	15	21
Bread, enriched, white, 2 slices	14	20
Rice, enriched, long grain, cooked, 1 cup	14	20
Cottage cheese, low-fat 2%, ½ cup	11	16
Walnuts, black, dried, 1 oz.	5	7
Cheddar cheese, 1 oz.	4	6

*DV = Daily Value. DVs are reference numbers based on the Recommended Dietary Allowance (RDA). They were developed to help consumers determine if a food contains very much of a specific nutrient. The DV for selenium is 70 micrograms (mcg). The percent DV (%DV) listed on the nutrition facts panel of food labels tells adults what percentage of the DV is provided by one serving. Even foods that provide lower percentages of the DV will contribute to a healthful diet.

RDAs for Selenium

This table shows how much selenium the healthy population should be getting each day:

Life Stage	Men	Women
Ages 19 +	55 mcg	55 mcg
All ages	60 mcg	70 mcg

Should We Worry About Selenium Deficiency?

You probably don't need to worry about selenium deficiency, if you eat well and/or take a multi-vitamin/mineral. However, Keshan disease, a disease that can cause poor heart function, has been observed in low-selenium areas of China, where dietary intake is less than 19 mcg per day for men and less than 13 mcg per day for women. This intake is significantly lower than the current RDA for selenium. Also, selenium deficiency may affect thyroid function, because selenium is essential for the synthesis of active thyroid hormone.

What's more, researchers believe selenium deficiency may worsen the effects of iodine deficiency on thyroid function, and that an adequate selenium nutritional status may help protect against some of the neurological effects of iodine deficiency.

Food for Thought

Selenium and HIV/AIDS:

Selenium deficiency is commonly associated with HIV or AIDS, and has been associated with a high risk of death from this disease. Researchers believe that selenium may be important in HIV disease because of its role in the immune system and as an antioxidant. Today, scientists are actively investigating the role of selenium in HIV or AIDS, and see a need for clinical trials that evaluate the effect of selenium supplementation on HIV disease progression.

Selenium and Prostate Cancer:

Researchers have found that men with low blood levels of selenium are at a greater risk for developing prostate cancer. The large-scale SELECT trial is studying selenium (and vitamin E) to see if they protect against prostate cancer, but the trial does not end until 2013.

Who May Need Extra Selenium?

Folks with gastrointestinal disorders such as Crohn's disease, or people who have had parts of their small intestines surgically removed, may have impaired selenium absorption. Speak with your physician about possibly supplementing with extra selenium.

Furthermore, people looking to use selenium as an antioxidant in megadose form should consult with a health professional. Generally, megadoses are recommended at 200 micrograms and should *not* exceed 400 micrograms.

What Is the Health Risk of Too Much Selenium?

There is a moderate-to-high health risk of too much selenium—although selenium toxicity is rare in the United States. High blood levels of selenium can result in a condition called *selenosis*. Symptoms include gastrointestinal upsets, hair loss, white blotchy nails, and mild nerve damage. The Institute of Medicine has set a tolerable upper intake level for selenium at 400 micrograms per day for adults to prevent the risk of developing selenosis. "Tolerable upper intake levels" represent the maximum intake of a nutrient that is likely to pose no risk of adverse health effects in the general population.

The Least You Need to Know

◆ More than 13 vitamins and 22 minerals are essential for normal body function. Eating a well-balanced, varied diet will supply your body with all the right ingredients.

◆ Water-soluble vitamins (eight B-complex vitamins and vitamin C) can easily dissolve in the watery body fluids, and excessive amounts are generally excreted through the urine.

◆ Fat-soluble vitamins (A, D, E, and K) do not dissolve in water and are stored in the body's fat. As a result, these vitamins have the potential to build up in tissues and become toxic with large supplemental doses (specifically A and D).

◆ Antioxidants may enhance health by protecting against free-radical damage. Eat plenty of foods rich in vitamins C, E, beta-carotene, and selenium to reap the benefits.

Chapter 8

Mighty Minerals: Calcium and Iron

In This Chapter

- ◆ All about calcium and iron
- ◆ How much you need
- ◆ Where to find the best food sources
- ◆ Everything you need to know about calcium supplementation
- ◆ Are you a candidate for a vitamin or mineral supplement?

As you've learned from the preceding chapter, at least 22 minerals are essential for a number of vital functions and body processes. Because not a day goes by without a client or friend asking for some sort of information regarding calcium or iron, I've dedicated this entire chapter to these powerhouse minerals.

Calcium and Healthy Bones

Calcium is by far the most abundant mineral in your body, with about 99 percent of the stuff stored in your bones. The other 1 percent is located in your body fluids, where it helps to regulate functions such as blood pressure, nerve transmission, muscle contraction (including the heartbeat), clotting of blood, and the secretion of hormones and digestive enzymes. Make no bones about it: Calcium, along with vitamin D, fluoride, and phosphorus, is best known for its ability to promote strong, healthy bones. Calcium serves a vital role in bone structure, providing integrity and density to your skeleton. In turn, your bones act as a "calcium bank," releasing calcium into your blood when your diet might be deficient (which we hope is not too often).

Many people think that once you're past a certain age, you don't have to worry about getting enough calcium. Wrong! Adequate calcium is important *throughout* your life: first and foremost for optimal bone building, and later on for bone maintenance. Generally, the first 24 years are important because your body is laying down the foundation for strong skeletal bones and teeth. In the first three decades of life, your bones reach their *peak adult bone mass*. (Bones are done growing in size and density.) Children who drink plenty of milk and eat other dairy and calcium-fortified foods will enter adulthood with stronger bones than those who skimp on calcium-rich foods.

Calcium intake in the later years is equally important for maintaining healthy bones. (I hope you already did all the right things in your first 30 years.) With age, your bones gradually lose their density (that is, calcium), which is especially true in menopausal women. People who take in adequate amounts of calcium can help slow down this process and defy those brittle bones of old age.

Why bother with calcium?

Imagine your bones as your calcium bank. Over the years, you can develop quite an extensive savings account by taking in plenty of calcium-rich foods and supplementing your diet with calcium pills. Keep up the good work as an adult and your bones stay calcium-rich!

On the other hand, regularly skimp on this mineral, and you'll wind up calcium-broke! Your body fluids still need calcium to regulate normal body functions. What these fluids don't get from food must be borrowed from the calcium-bone bank. Borrowing day after day, year after year, will deplete the savings account and leave you with osteoporosis (brittle bones that break easily).

How Much Calcium Is Recommended?

The DRIs (Dietary Reference Intake) for calcium are laid out for various age categories. Here are the recommendations:

Group	DRI (mg/d)	Group	DRI (mg/d)
Infants		*Females*	
Birth–6 months	210	9–13 years	1,300
6 months–1 year	270	14–18 years	1,300
Children		19–30 years	1,000
1–3 years	500	31–50 years	1,000
4–8 years	800	51–70 years	1,200
		>70 years	1,200
Males		*Pregnancy/Lactation*	
9–13 years	1,300	18 years or less	1,300
14–18 years	1,300	19–30 years	1,000
19–30 years	1,000	31–50 years	1,000
31–50 years	1,000		
51–70 years	1,200		
>70 years	1,200		

Are You Getting Enough Calcium? The Foods to Choose

Browse through the following chart and notice that dairy foods, along with fortified juice and sardines, provide the most calcium hands down. One more thing: don't be put off by the high amounts of fat in cheese. Simply shop for the low-fat brands in your local store. They have less fat but still retain ample amounts of calcium.

The Best Sources of Calcium in Various Foods

Milk Group	Amount	Calcium (mg)
Yogurt, plain (low-fat)	1 cup	415
Yogurt, fruit-flavored (low-fat)	1 cup	345
Milk, nonfat (dry)	1/4 cup	377

The Best Sources of Calcium in Various Foods

Milk Group	Amount	Calcium (mg)
Milk, skim	1 cup	302
Milk, 1%–2%	1 cup	300
Milk, whole*	1 cup	291
Buttermilk	1 cup	285
Milk, chocolate (low-fat)	1 cup	284
Cheese, Parmesan (grated)	1/4 cup	338
Cheese, Swiss*	1 oz.	272
Cheese, Monterey Jack*	1 oz.	212
Cheese, mozzarella, low-moisture, part skim	1 oz.	207
Cheese, cheddar*	1 oz.	204
Cheese, Colby*	1 oz.	194
Cheese, American*	1 oz.	174
Ice cream*	1/2 cup	88
Cottage cheese, creamed 1%	1/2 cup	63

Fruit and Vegetable Group	Amount	Calcium (mg)
Collards, cooked	1/2 cup	168
Turnip greens, cooked	1/2 cup	134
Kale, cooked	1/2 cup	103
Spinach, cooked	1/2 cup	84
Broccoli, cooked	1/2 cup	68
Chard, cooked	1/2 cup	64
Carrot, raw	1 med.	27
Orange	1 med.	60
Dates, chopped	1/2 cup	26
Raisins	1/2 cup	22

Protein Group (Meat, Beans, Eggs)	Amount	Calcium (mg)
Sardines (canned, w/bones)	3 oz.	372
Salmon, pink (canned, w/bones)	3 oz.	165
Tofu (processed, w/calcium)	4 oz.	145

Protein Group (Meat, Beans, Eggs)	Amount	Calcium (mg)
Almonds, shelled*	1 oz.	66
Soybeans, cooked	½ cup	66
Dried beans, cooked (lima, navy, kidney)	½ cup	35–60
Egg	1 large	27
Peanut butter*	2 TB.	18
Beef patty, cooked*	3 oz.	9
Grain Group	**Amount**	**Calcium (mg)**
Calcium-fortified cereals (Total) with ½ cup milk	1 oz.	350
Calcium-fortified waffles (Eggo)	2 items	300
Farina, enriched (instant, cooked)	1 cup	189
Tortilla, corn	1 med.	60
Bread, whole wheat	1 slice	25
Calcium-Fortified Foods	**Amount**	**Calcium in mg**
Orange juice and grapefruit juice (Citrus Hill, Minute Maid, Tropicana)	8 oz.	300

Denotes foods that are also high in fat
Source: Calcium Information Center

Everything You Need to Know About Calcium Supplements

Most women can benefit from taking a calcium supplement. Before you buy your next bottle, learn all of the facts from the following information:

♦ Calcium tablets are best used by the body when taken in doses of 500 mg or less. To obtain 1,000–1,200 mg per day, take two servings—one in the morning and one in the evening for maximum absorption.

♦ Take your evening calcium supplement at bedtime—it will remain in the stomach longer.

◆ The citric acid found in orange juice and citrus fruit enhances calcium absorption, so have a piece of fruit or a small glass of juice with your supplement to maximize its benefit.

◆ Calcium and iron interfere with one another's absorption. If taking an iron or multivitamin tablet that contains iron, take your calcium at a different time.

◆ Chewable and effervescent supplements are available for those who have trouble swallowing tablets.

◆ Calcium is always paired with another compound. Calcium carbonate yields the most calcium per pill and is also cheaper and generally available in smaller tablets. Calcium citrate and calcium citrate-malate are the best absorbed, but tend to be larger tablets.

◆ Because calcium citrate takes up more space in a pill, you may need to take two citrate tablets compared to one carbonate, to get the same amount of calcium.

◆ Calcium carbonate is best absorbed when taken with meals, as it needs the stomach acid to aid in absorption, while calcium citrate can be taken between meals, without food.

◆ Calcium citrate is a good choice for older clients who have reduced stomach acid, as it dissolves and absorbs more easily in the stomach.

◆ Vitamin D is essential for calcium absorption. The latest studies suggest adults need 800 IU (International Units) per day, not 400 as previously believed. Most milk is fortified with vitamin D, and fatty fish and cod liver oil provide some, too. However, about 90 percent of the vitamin D we get is made in our skin while exposed to the sun's ultraviolet B-rays. However, reduced sun exposure and the frequent use of sun block creams have decreased this level. Therefore, for the best absorption, look for supplements that are also fortified with vitamin D.

What to Avoid in a Calcium Supplement

Calcium supplements are *not* all created equal. Read the following information so you can buy the best and leave the rest! Also, understand the contraindications with other medications and mineral supplements.

◆ Avoid natural sources of calcium such as bone meal, oyster shell, and dolomite, as they can contain harmful contaminants such as lead.

- Avoid taking calcium with meals that are high in wheat fiber—it will partly block the absorption of calcium from foods.

- Avoid taking your calcium supplement with the osteoporosis medication *Fosamax* (alendronate sodium), or the drug's effectiveness will be diminished.

- Avoid taking too much vitamin D—the upper limit is set at 2,000 milligrams, but I recommend no more than 1,000 milligrams from the sum total of all your supplements. Too much vitamin D is just as bad for your bones as too little vitamin D.

- A high calcium intake can impair zinc absorption. You may want to ensure your zinc consumption by taking a multivitamin, or eating a cereal fortified with zinc.

- The upper limit for calcium is approximately 2,500 mg per day. Be sure that you are not over-supplementing!

Iron Out Your Body

Iron deficiency is the most widespread type of vitamin or mineral deficiency in the world. Do you constantly experience sluggishness, irritability, and headaches? Perhaps you suffer from this condition. Let's take a closer look and find out.

About 70 percent of the iron in your body is located in a portion of your red blood cells known as *hemoglobin*. Hemoglobin is your oxygen delivery service, supplying every cell with the oxygen it needs to perform essential metabolic functions. Iron is also a component of *myoglobin*. Like the hemoglobin in red blood cells, myoglobin ensures adequate oxygen delivery to all your muscles. At this point, you're probably starting to understand the importance of iron in this equation: too little iron, too little oxygen. The result is fatigue, irritability, weakness, headaches, tendency to feel cold, and in the case of severe depletion, iron-deficiency anemia.

Fortunately, iron is found in a variety of animal and plant foods, making it easy to get your daily requirement. *Heme* iron, the type found in animal products (red meats, liver, poultry, and eggs), is more readily absorbed than *nonheme* iron, which can be found in vegetables and other plant foods (beans, nuts, seeds, dried fruits, and fortified breads and cereals). Interestingly enough, the body adjusts the amount it absorbs according to the body's need. In other words, a person with iron-deficient anemia will absorb about two to three times more iron after eating exactly the same meal than a person with a normal iron status.

Certain groups of people are at increased risk for developing an iron deficiency. If you think you might fall into one of the following categories, ask your doctor to check your iron status before self-prescribing supplementation. (A simple blood test can tell if you are deficient.)

Groups at risk for iron deficiency include ...

- Infants and children. Their rapid growth and finicky eating habits demand that they get iron in a variety of ways.

- Women who bleed heavily during menstruation. They lose iron-rich blood each month.

- Pregnant women with increased blood volume. They are supporting their growing babies' needs as well as their own.

- Strict vegetarians who take in only nonheme sources of iron. Remember, nonheme plant foods are *much* less absorbable than iron-rich animal foods.

- People who lose a lot of blood during surgery or other bleeding injuries.

- "Chronic dieters" who bounce from one crash diet to another. People suffering from eating disorders might not eat enough iron-rich foods to meet their requirements.

Tips to Boost Your Dietary Iron Intake

Here's information that will help you increase your iron intake and its absorption within your body.

- Make a point of eating iron-rich foods, both animal (heme) and nonanimal (nonheme) sources each day.

- When eating nonheme foods, couple them with some vitamin C. (See the list of foods that contain vitamin C in Chapter 18.) Vitamin C can increase the absorption of iron.

- Avoid drinking coffee or tea with an iron-rich meal; they inhibit the absorption of iron.

- Calcium interferes with the absorption of iron, so if you take calcium supplements, do not take them with an iron-rich meal. Try them with a snack or some juice because you usually do need some food for your calcium pills.

♦ Cook casseroles, stews, and sauces in cast iron cookware. Believe it or not, some of the iron will seep into the food.

♦ The presence of heme iron (even very small amounts) at a meal with nonheme iron will enhance the absorption of the nonheme iron.

The best sources of iron (heme) include lean red meats, turkey, chicken, pork, lamb, veal, egg yolks, and liver (although it's very high in cholesterol).

Nutri-Speak

Although not very common, **iron toxicity** is a serious problem that occurs from either a genetic abnormality causing the body to store excessive amounts or the unnecessary over-supplementation of iron. The result can be liver and other organ damage.

Good iron sources (nonheme) include beans, lentils, whole grains, dried fruit, broccoli, spinach, collard greens, nuts and seeds, chickpeas, fortified cereals, blackstrap molasses, barley, and wheat germ.

Are You a Candidate for a Supplement?

Ideally, you should be getting your daily supply of vitamins and minerals from your diet, not from pill-popping. What's more, food provides you with energy in the form of calories—something you don't get from pills. However, it's a good idea for most folks to take a daily multi-vitamin/mineral that supplies 100 percent of the RDA.

Specific groups at nutritional risk include people with these qualities:

♦ Do you constantly skip meals, grabbing only snack foods throughout the day? Do you eat fewer than five fruits and vegetables each day? You might benefit from a multivitamin/mineral supplement (supplying up to 100 percent of the RDA) to fill in the nutrition gaps. Also, consider a separate calcium supplement with vitamin D.

♦ Are you a vegan, a strict vegetarian who consumes absolutely no meat, dairy, or other animal products? You might benefit from a supplement that supplies the RDA for B-12 and the mineral calcium.

♦ Are you over 60 years old? People in this category might have a decline in the absorption of the following vitamins: B-6, B-12, C, D, E, folic acid, and the mineral calcium. A one-a-day multivitamin/mineral might provide some extra backup. Also think about some extra calcium and vitamin D if you are not eating enough calcium-rich food.

◆ Do you regularly drink alcohol or smoke? Excessive amounts of alcohol and smoking interfere with the body's ability to absorb and utilize certain vitamins and minerals. However, in this case, a supplement recommendation is not the advice—instead seek help ASAP to kick your unhealthy habit.

◆ Are you a professional dieter—on/off every wacky fad diet out there? Chances are you're cheating your body of important nutrients and would probably benefit from the backup of a one-a-day multivitamin/mineral supplement and a separate calcium supplement.

◆ Do you completely avoid specific types of foods? Some people stay away from certain foods for reasons including food allergies, intolerances, or just plain dislikes. In these cases, supplements of specific nutrients might be needed. Also, a multivitamin/mineral is a good idea for extra backup.

For women only, ask yourself these questions:

◆ Do you experience heavy bleeding during monthly menstruation? If so, you might lose iron-rich blood. Check with your doctor whether you will benefit from taking a supplement with iron. Note that iron supplements tend to cause constipation, so consider taking a stool softener as well.

◆ Are you pregnant or breastfeeding? Women in this category have greater needs for the vitamins A, C, B-1, B-6, B-12, and folic acid, as well as the minerals iron and calcium. These extra amounts are usually included in prenatal vitamins. You might need more calcium than the prenatal supplements contain, so speak with your doctor if you aren't eating enough calcium-rich food.

Are Your Supplements Absorbable?

Most people automatically assume that their supplements will absorb after they swallow them. It's a fair assumption. Unfortunately, it doesn't always work that way. Here are two ways to know whether your vitamin and mineral supplements are doing you any good.

Home Testing

You can always test your own supplements at home by immersing the individual pill in enough household vinegar to cover it, and then letting it stand for one hour. (You can stir it a bit.) The vinegar should cloud up and the pill should at least disintegrate (fall into pieces), if not completely dissolve. If it remains intact, there's a chance that it won't disintegrate in your stomach, but will pass right through you undigested.

This type of home testing might tell you something, but it's only a rough approximation of what happens in the stomach. No guarantee.

Look for the USP Stamp

The USP (U.S. Pharmacopeia) is an independent, nonprofit testing organization that tests vitamin and mineral supplements under controlled laboratory conditions, operating since 1820. This company sets legally enforceable standards for the identity, strength, quality, purity, packaging, and labeling of drug products. The USP also develops and publishes authoritative drug information for healthcare professionals, patients, and consumers. (Visit the USP website at www.usp.org/did/mgraphs.)

The USP stamp means that the product has met USP standards, including ones for disintegration, dissolution, quality, strength, and purity to name a few, and has been tested in a controlled environment. These USP tests don't guarantee the absorption of all nutrients; absorbability is very difficult to test or predict. However, if a pill does disintegrate in the digestive tract, it certainly improves the chance of the nutrients within the pill being absorbed by the body.

Unfortunately, vitamins and minerals do not have to conform to USP standards to be marketed in this country. Most brand-name vitamins are not labeled USP because the manufacturer either doesn't want to perform the tests or prefers to guarantee the vitamin through the brand name. My recommendation is to buy products with USP on the label. These tend to be generic or store brands; sometimes they're cheaper. There is no guarantee, but your chances for absorption will be *greatly* improved.

The Least You Need to Know

- Adequate calcium intake is required throughout the life cycle: the early years for bone building and the later years for bone maintenance. Make it a habit to load up on low-fat dairy products and other calcium-rich foods.
- Consider taking a calcium supplement (with extra vitamin D) if you're at risk for osteoporosis or simply don't eat enough foods rich in calcium.
- The mineral iron is responsible for delivering oxygen to every cell in your body and is found in a variety of foods.

◆ Most nutrition experts agree that a well-balanced diet should be your primary focus for optimal nutrition. However, most folks can benefit from a daily multivitamin/mineral; certain groups of people may need further supplementation.

Part 2

Making Savvy Food Choices

Decisions, decisions! With all the gazillions of foods offered in grocery stores, restaurants, delis, and even on the Internet, it's a nightmare trying to decide what to eat—let alone choosing something that's actually *nutritious*.

This section covers everything you need to know about making wise food choices *wherever* you shop or eat. You'll learn how to decode those cryptic nutrition labels, and then put your know-how into action on our "virtual tour" of a typical supermarket. You'll also learn how to master low-fat cooking techniques so you can wow your friends and family with some knockout home-cooked meals. And lest you think I want you tethered to your stove, there's a guide to eating out healthfully, whether you're dining at the finest French restaurant or the nearest fast food joint.

Bon appétit!

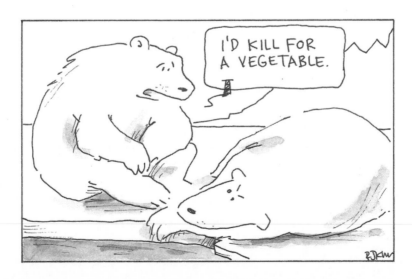

Chapter 9

Decoding a Nutrition Label

In This Chapter

- How to read a nutrition label
- Understanding the Daily Percent Values
- The scoop on organic, free range, and genetically engineered foods
- Testing your label savvy

Now that you have some solid nutrition know-how, let's put this knowledge to work and decode all that mumbo-jumbo written on prepackaged food products. Once you can interpret the information on nutrition labels, you'll become quite a detective in your local grocery store, further enhancing your skills as a healthy eater. You'll be able to make more-informed food choices, as well as compare similar food products to see which brand is nutritionally superior. Best of all, the government has set up strict food label laws and regulations to prevent companies from printing misleading or falsified claims on food items so you can actually believe what you read. This section will provide the whole truth on the foods you love to gobble down.

Serving Size

First, figure out how much food was analyzed by the folks who prepared the nutrition label. *Serving size* clearly describes this set amount of food. Of course, most packages contain more than one serving, and "Servings Per Container" refers to the number of single servings in the entire package. For example, the following label reports that a serving size is ¹/₂ cup and there are four servings per container. Therefore, there must be 2 full cups in the entire package because ¹/₂ cup × 4 = 2 cups.

Nutrition Facts
Serving Size ¹/₂ cup (114g)
Servings Per Container 4

Amount Per Serving

Calories 90   Calories from Fat 30

                                    % Daily Value*

Total Fat 3g   5%

  Saturated Fat 0g   0%

Cholesterol 0mg   0%

Sodium 300mg   13%

Total Carbohydrate 13g   4%

  Dietary Fiber 3g   12%

  Sugars 3g

Protein 3g

Vitamin A   80%   •   Vitamin C   60%
Calcium   4%   •   Iron   4%

* Percent Daily Values are based on a 2,000 calorie diet. Your daily values may be higher or lower depending on your calorie needs:

		Calories 2,000	2,500
Total Fat	Less than	65g	80g
Sat Fat	Less than	20g	25g
Cholesterol	Less than	300mg	300mg
Sodium	Less than	2,400mg	2,400mg
Total Carbohydrate		300g	375g
Fiber		25g	30g

Calories per gram:
Fat 9   •   Carbohydrate 4   •   Protein 4

Do you eat the amount of food defined as one serving? Remember, fat and calorie measurements on the label are for a single serving size only. And we know it's easy to eat more than one measly serving. Here's a perfect example of the difference between serving size and the actual servings eaten: one serving of ice cream (¹/₂ cup) has approximately 12 grams of fat. Most of the people I know can easily eat 1 cup in a sitting, and you know what that means. When you double the serving size, you double everything: the calories, protein grams, carbohydrate grams, and, of course, the fat grams. Pay close attention to the amount per serving. If you go over (or under) on servings, keep that in mind when reading the remaining information.

Calories

When calories are listed on a label, they refer to the amount of calories in a single serving. Plain and simple. The sample label shows 90 calories per serving. What about those "lo-cal" claims frequently displayed on the packaging? Luckily, the following key words are now defined by the government and must mean what they say:

- **Calorie-free** Less than 5 calories per serving.

- **Low-calorie** Forty calories or less for most food items; 120 calories or less for main dish products (lentil soup, turkey burger, chicken breast, and so on).

- **Reduced-calorie** Must have at least 25 percent fewer calories than the regular version of that food item.

Total Fat

This section lists the total number of fat grams from all types of fat—saturated, monounsaturated, and polyunsaturated. As you can see, the label reveals that there are 3 grams of fat per serving. Another listing titled "Calories from Fat" converts the total fat grams into fat calories (number of fat grams $\times$ 9 = calories coming from fat). Again, the sample label reports 30 calories from fat per serving. This is valuable information because it allows you to identify the percentage of fat in a particular food. Ideally, you should choose foods with a big difference between the total number of calories and calories coming from fat. The bigger the gap, the less the percentage of total calories coming from fat.

Here are some of the common "fat" phrases that appear on packaged food products and how they are defined by the government:

- **Fat-free** Less than 0.5 grams of fat per serving.

- **Low-fat** Three grams of fat (or less) per serving.

- **Reduced-fat** At least 25 percent less fat per serving than the original version of a food product.

> **Food for Thought** _____
>
> In 2006, trans fats will be included on food labels. Until then, the best way to determine if something contains these artery-cloggers is to check out the ingredients list. If you see the phrase "partially hydrogenated oil," put the package back on the shelf and choose something else.
>
> One exception: if the very same product with hydrogenated oil advertises "0 trans fat" or "trans fat–free," you'll know that the amount of hydrogenated oil is miniscule—and each serving has less than 0.5 gram of trans fat.

Saturated Fat

Even though saturated fat is part of the total fat in food, it gets listed by itself because it can be extremely bad for you. As you can see, the sample label shows no saturated fat—good deal! In general, avoid foods that are high in saturated fat. This type of fat is responsible for increasing your risk of heart disease and other illnesses.

Here are some of the common "saturated fat" phrases that appear on packaged food products and how they are defined by the government:

- **Saturated fat-free** Less than 0.5 gram per serving.

- **Low in saturated fat** One gram or less in a serving size or no more than 10 percent of calories coming from saturated fat.

- **Reduced saturated fat** At least 25 percent less saturated fat than the original version.

Cholesterol

Remember this waxy guy? Together with its partner in crime—fat—dietary cholesterol is a key player in raising blood cholesterol and therefore increasing your risk for heart disease. You'll notice that the cholesterol content of a food product is measured in milligrams. Budget your foods and eat less than 300 milligrams of dietary cholesterol per day.

Understand the following claims when they appear on food labels:

- **Cholesterol-free** Less than 2 milligrams of cholesterol.
- **Low-cholesterol** Twenty milligrams (or less) of cholesterol.

These cholesterol claims are only allowed when a food product contains 2 grams (or less) of saturated fat as well.

Sodium

Don't let the terminology confuse you. The label calls it sodium (300 mg reported on the sample label), but most people know it as salt. Remember, sodium is only a component of salt. However, that one component is responsible for water retention and high blood pressure in salt-sensitive people. Limit the amount of high-sodium foods in your diet, and aim for a daily intake of 2,300 milligrams or less.

Here's some sodium lingo and what it means:

- **Sodium-free** Less than 5 milligrams of sodium per serving.
- **Low-sodium** Less than 140 milligrams of sodium per serving.
- **Reduced sodium** At least 25 percent less sodium than the original food version.

Total Carbohydrate

In Chapter 2, you became well versed on the various types of carbohydrates. Now you can use the label information to identify whether a food contains a lot of simple sugar or complex carbohydrate.

First, look for the listing titled "Total Carbohydrate." This will reveal the amount of *all types* of carbs (simple and complex) in a single serving of a food. Next, look for the smaller listing located underneath "total carbohydrate" titled "Sugars." This indicates how much simple sugar is in a serving of that particular food. Obviously, the less simple sugar, the better. Now, you're ready to determine the amount of complex carbohydrate in a food by simply subtracting the total carbs from the sugars.

Overrated-Undercooked

Have you seen the terms "net carbs," "impact carbs," or "effective carbs" on packaged foods recently? This refers to carbohydrates that have less impact on your blood sugar, such as glycerine, sugar alcohols, artificial sweeteners, and fiber. The FDA has not approved any of these terms, but food manufacturers continue to use them anyway.

Let's look at the previous label for an example:

| Total Carbohydrate | 13 grams |
| Sugars | 3 grams |

These numbers indicate that the majority of carbohydrates are coming from more complex sources, 10 grams to be exact.

Located under "total carbohydrates" is "dietary fiber." Dietary fiber is predominantly found in carbohydrate-rich foods and includes both soluble and insoluble fiber sources. Because fiber promotes regularity, along with reducing the risk of heart disease and certain cancers, choose foods with at least 2.5 grams of dietary fiber per serving, and aim for a total intake of 25–35 grams each day.

Protein

As you know from Chapter 3, most Americans eat far more protein than they actually need (0.36 grams per pound of body weight). Although some of the best protein sources, unfortunately, do not carry a nutrition label (such as beef, poultry, eggs, and fish), nutrifacts posters are required in meat and produce departments, so ask your grocer and take a look. On the other hand, most dairy products and prepackaged food items do list the grams of protein in a single serving. It's interesting to see that there are even small amounts of protein in foods you might not expect.

Percent Daily Values

Now for the confusing part: what are those "%" signs floating all over the label? They're called Percent Daily Values (DV) and are based on a 2,000-calorie reference diet. In other words, these percentages indicate how much of the RDA for each nutrient is present in a single serving. Of course, your job is to ultimately eat a variety of foods that supply 100 percent of all the nutrients needed. For example, one serving of yogurt provides 35 percent of the daily calcium needed and 0 percent of the iron. It's clearly a great source of calcium, but lousy for iron.

What happens if you eat more or less than 2,000 calories? You can slightly adjust the percentages up or down if you're good with numbers (and extremely motivated). In general, the 2,000-calorie reference diet provides appropriate guidelines for almost everyone (adults and children over 4) to follow.

For total fat, saturated fat, cholesterol, and sodium, choose foods with low percent daily values. On the other hand, you want to choose foods with higher percent DVs for total carbohydrate, dietary fiber, and all vitamins and minerals.

The following are the set daily values. They are specifically used for food labels and are based on a 2,000-calorie reference diet.

Daily Values for Nutritional Items

Food Component	Daily Value
Total fat	65 grams
Saturated fat	20 grams
Cholesterol	300 mg
Sodium	2,300 mg
Potassium	3,500 mg
Total carbohydrate	300 grams
Dietary fiber	25 grams
Protein	50 grams
Vitamin A	5,000 IU
Vitamin C	60 mg
Calcium	1,000 mg
Iron	18 mg
Vitamin D	400 IU
Vitamin E	30 IU
Vitamin K	80 mcg
Thiamin	1.5 mg
Riboflavin	1.7 mg
Niacin	20 mg
Vitamin B-6	2 mg

continues

Daily Values for Nutritional Items (continued)

Food Component	Daily Value
Folate	400 mcg
Vitamin B-12	6 mcg
Biotin	0.3 mg
Pantothenic acid	10 mg
Phosphorus	1,000 mg
Iodine	150 mcg
Magnesium	400 mg
Zinc	15 mg
Copper	2 mg
Selenium	70 mcg
Manganese	2 mg
Chromium	120 mcg
Molybdenum	75 mcg
Chloride	3,400 mg

GMO (Genetically Modified Organisms)

You may notice the letters "GMO" on a food package from time to time (usually with a slash through the middle). Gaining a lot of attention, both negative and positive, these scientifically modified foods seem to be quite controversial at the moment. By altering a plant, animal, or micro-organism's genetic code, scientists are able to manipulate the speed of growth, enhance the nutritional content, and more. However, two major concerns come up with genetically altered products. The first concern is whether the new genes or proteins might produce toxins—that is, anything that can cause harm in the short or long term. The other concern is whether the introduction of a new gene might trigger an allergic reaction in a person who eats the food. On the other hand, these scientific advances may help to greatly enhance the nutritional quality of our food.

Unfortunately, you won't find labels that disclose which foods contain genetically engineered ingredients, simply because they don't have to. However, oftentimes products will go out of their way to advertise foods that do *not* contain GMOs.

Free Range *Versus* Organic

We hear the terms all the time, organic and free range. Here's exactly what they mean. *Organic* is a labeling term that means the product meets the requirements of the Organic Foods Production Act of 1990. To be certified as "organic," the poultry and/or meat must be fed certified organic feed since birth. Organic feed means grains and soybeans grown in soil that has been free of pesticides and chemical fertilizers for a period of three years. Furthermore, no drugs or antibiotics can be used in growing organic birds and animals. What's more, all organic animals must have outdoor access.

To date, the term "organic" has not yet been formally defined by the USDA, but they are working on a definition. Until a definition is available, the USDA is permitting certain animal products to be labeled as "certified organic"—the label has to be approved by the USDA and the claim must meet the criteria as outlined above.

To be labeled as *free range* poultry, the chicken must have access to the outside, and therefore not be kept in a pen 24 hours a day. However, the USDA standards don't specify how clean or large the yard must be, nor whether the chicken uses the yard or not.

The bottom line: choose organic rather than free range—it's better!

The Least You Need to Know

◆ The nutrition information provided on prepackaged food labels can help you make more informed food choices and compare similar food items for the healthier buy.

◆ All the nutrition information provided is based on one serving size. Check to see how much of a particular food is considered one serving, and if you eat more or less, adjust the nutrition information accordingly.

◆ Choose foods that have a big difference between the number of total calories and the number of fat calories. This indicates that a food is not primarily made of fat.

◆ "Daily Percent Value" refers to how much of a day's recommended amount for certain nutrients is supplied in one serving of a food product. Read carefully and generally stick with foods that have a low daily percentage for fat, cholesterol, and sodium while choosing foods that have a high daily percentage for total carbohydrate, dietary fiber, and all other vitamins and minerals.

◆ "GMO" refers to a food that has been genetically modified, "organic" refers to a food that is free of pesticides and antibiotics, and "free range" simply means that the animal has the freedom to run around.

Chapter 10

Shopping Smart

In This Chapter

- Scouting the supermarket aisle by aisle
- Selecting fresh fruits and vegetables
- Best bets for dairy, grains, and protein
- Shopping for fats, spreads, and condiments
- Stuffing your cabinet with healthy snacks

How many times have you eaten unhealthy food just because you didn't have any nutritious food in the house? Are cookies, cakes, and chips constantly on display on your shelves, or do you fill your pantry with fresh fruit and whole grains? Let's face it: When you get those midday munchies, the last thing you want to do is drive to a supermarket to buy an apple. You're going to grab whatever's closest to the couch—and who knows what that might be.

Half the battle of healthy eating is having a variety of nutritious foods on hand so when the "food mood" strikes, you've got the supplies to satisfy that growling belly with some savvy food choices. Grab a cart and read on; you're about to go grocery shopping.

The Shopping List

The nice part about food shopping today is that supermarkets are responding to nutrition-conscious consumers and shelving healthier foods than ever before. So set up a shopping list by different food categories, and get organized.

- Vegetables

- Fruits

- Dairy

- Grains (bread, cereal, pasta, and others)

- Protein foods (meats, poultry, fish, eggs, and legumes)

- Frozen meals and canned items

- Snack foods

- Condiments

- Fats, oils, dressings, and other spreads

Aisle One: Starting with the Produce Section

The produce aisle will provide you with a lot of nutritional bang for your buck. Spend a lot of time walking through and load up your wagon.

Voluptuous Veggies

Vegetables are naturally low in calories and fat, and they provide an array of vitamins, minerals, and fiber. Unfortunately, bundles of fresh produce don't carry nutrition labels, but you might see posters in the produce area revealing the benefits of specific items. Rest assured: label or no label, you can never eat too many of these guys!

Most fresh veggies can be judged for freshness and quality by their appearance. Closely examine your produce and avoid any decaying or bruising. Another piece of advice is to buy only what you need for the next few days. Fresh veggies will go bad if they sit around for a long time. If you don't shop often, or you don't have the time to wash and chop your vegetables, your best bet is to stuff your freezer. Frozen vegetables come in a variety of combinations (cut, whole, chopped, and pureed, along with medleys of premixed veggie concoctions), and all you have to do is pop them in a pot to cook. Even lazy people have no excuse. What's more, the freezer keeps the nutrients locked in, so there's no rush to eat them before they go bad. Also, frozen (and canned) vegetables have labels telling all the facts, so take advantage of this and read the impressive profile.

Here are some general shopping tips for buying produce:

♦ Buy fresh fruits and vegetables that are in season to keep the prices reasonable.

♦ Examine your fruits and vegetables for freshness; avoid bruises and other deformities.

♦ Because fresh produce is perishable, buy only what you need. If you're shopping for an extended period of time, load up on the frozen varieties.

♦ Read the labels on frozen and canned vegetables to make sure there isn't a lot of added fat or salt. Read the labels on frozen and canned fruits to make sure there isn't a lot of added sugar or heavy syrup.

♦ If you're into "super-convenience," buy the prewashed, precut bags of salad, carrots, celery, and anything else offered at your supermarket. Look for premade fruit salads in either the fresh or frozen sections of your grocery store.

♦ Check out the salad bar in your grocery store. This way you can get the exact amount of anything you need, and it's already precut and prewashed for you.

♦ Speak with the person in charge of produce at your local supermarket, ask about unfamiliar fruits and vegetables, and then try something new!

Getting to Know 'Em

Here is a quick rundown on some common vegetables and what to look for when buying fresh selections:

♦ **Artichokes** provide potassium and folic acid. Look for artichokes that are plump and heavy in relation to size. The many leaf-like parts are called "scales" and should be thick, green, and fresh-looking. Avoid artichokes with any brownish discoloration or moldy growth on the scales.

♦ **Asparagus** provides vitamins A and C, niacin, folic acid, potassium, and iron. Look for closed, dense tips with smooth, deep green spears. Avoid tips that are spread open or seem to have any mold or decay.

◆ **Broccoli** provides calcium, potassium, iron, fiber, vitamins A and C, folic acid, and niacin. Look for stalks that are not too tough with compact, firm bud clusters and that are dark green or sage green in color. Avoid broccoli with a wilted appearance, yellowish green discoloration, or bud clusters that are spread open. These are all signs of over-maturity.

◆ **Brussels sprouts** provide vitamins A and C, folic acid, potassium, iron, and fiber. Look for brussels sprouts with a bright green color and tight-fitting outer leaves. Avoid brussels sprouts that appear to be wilting or have blemishes.

◆ **Cabbage** provides vitamin C, potassium, folic acid, and fiber. Whether it's green or red, cabbage can be used in coleslaw, salads, and a variety of cooked dishes. Look for a dense, heavy head of cabbage relative to its size, with outer leaves that display a green or red color (depending on the type). Avoid cabbages with outer leaves that appear wilted or blemished.

◆ **Carrots** provide vitamin A, potassium, and fiber. Look for smooth, firm, well-formed carrots that have a rich orange color. Avoid roots that are discolored, soft, and flabby.

◆ **Cauliflower** provides vitamin C, folic acid, potassium, and fiber. Look for compact, firm curds (the edible creamy-white portion), and do not worry about green leaflets that may be scattered throughout a bunch. Although most grocers sell cauliflower without the outside jacket leaves, in the rare instance that they are left on, a nice green color reveals freshness. Avoid severe discoloration, blemishing, or spreading of the white curd.

◆ **Corn** provides vitamin A, potassium, and fiber. Although yellow-kernel is the most popular, there are varieties of white-kernel and mixed-kernel corn as well. Look for fresh green husks (the outer covering) and make sure that the silk ends are free from decay or worm injury. If the corn has already been husked (the outside covering removed), choose ears of corn that are heavily covered with bright yellow, plump kernels. Avoid kernels that appear dried or are lacking in color.

◆ **Eggplants** provide potassium. Look for firm, heavy, dark purple eggplants (although there are other colored varieties). Avoid any that are shriveled, soft, or lacking color, or that reveal decay in the form of brownish spots.

◆ **Lettuce** comes in several varieties: iceberg, butter-head, Romaine, and leaf lettuce. It provides vitamin C and folic acid. Look for bright color and crisp leaf texture when buying Romaine. For other leafy variations, select succulent, tender leaves and avoid any serious discoloration or wilting.

- **Mushrooms** provide potassium, niacin, and riboflavin. Look for closed mushroom caps around the stems, with the underneath gills (rows of paper-thin tissue located underneath the caps) colored pink or light tan. Avoid mushrooms with wide-open caps and dark, discolored gills.

- **Okra** provides vitamin A, potassium, and calcium. Look for bright green, tender pods that are under 4 $\frac{1}{2}$ inches long. Avoid stiff tips (those that resist bending) or pods with a lifeless, pale green color.

- **Onions** are not a significant source of nutrition, but they can certainly enhance the flavor of the foods you eat. With all types (red, white, and yellow), look for hard, dry onions that are free from blemishes. Avoid onions that are wet or mushy.

- **Peas** (green) provide vitamin A, folic acid, potassium, protein, and fiber. Look for a firm, fresh appearance with bright green pods. Avoid flabby, wilted pods, and any sign of decay.

- **Peppers** (sweet) provide vitamins A and C, potassium, and fiber. Although green peppers are the most common, other delicious varieties include yellow, orange, red, purple, and white. Look for firm peppers with deep characteristic color. Avoid very lightweight, flimsy peppers that have punctures or signs of decay on the outside.

- **Potatoes** provide potassium, most B-vitamins, vitamin C, protein, and fiber. Look for reasonably smooth, firm, and blemish-free potatoes. Avoid those with large bruises and soft spots and those that are sprouted or shriveled.

- **Rhubarb** provides vitamin A, calcium, and potassium. Look for firm but tender stems with a decent amount of pinkish red color. Avoid rhubarb that appears wilted or flabby.

- **Spinach** provides vitamin A, calcium, folic acid, potassium, and fiber. Look for healthy, fresh leaves that have a dark green color. Avoid spinach leaves that appear wilted or show significant discoloration.

- **Squash** (summer) provides vitamins A and C, potassium, and fiber and includes several varieties, such as yellow crookneck, large straightneck, the greenish white pattypan, and the slender green zucchini. Look for firm, well-developed, tender squash. Check for a glossy (not dull) outside, which indicates the squash is tender. Avoid dull, tough, or discolored squash.

◆ **Squash** (winter) includes acorn, butternut, buttercup, green and blue hubbard, delicious, and banana, providing vitamins A and C, potassium, and fiber. Look for squash that is heavy for its size with a tough, hard outside rind. Avoid squash with any signs of decay, including sunken spots, bruising, or mold.

◆ **Sweet potatoes** provide vitamins A and C, folic acid, potassium, and fiber. Look for firm, smooth sweet potatoes with uniformly colored skins. The moist type known as yams should have orange flesh, whereas dry sweet potatoes have a more pale appearance. Avoid discoloration, wormholes, and any other indication of decay.

> **CAUTION**
>
> **Overrated-Undercooked**
>
> Generally, canned vegetables tend to be loaded with salt. If you do buy cans occasionally, be on the lookout for labels that read "low-sodium" or "no added salt."

◆ **Tomatoes** provide vitamins A and C and potassium. Look for well-ripened, smooth tomatoes with a rich, red color. If you're not planning to eat them within the next few days, choose slightly less ripe, firm tomatoes with a pink or light red color. Only store fully ripe ones in the fridge because the cold temperature might prevent immature tomatoes from ripening. Avoid tomatoes that are over-ripened and mushy or show any signs of decay.

Fabulous Fruits

For a quick nutritious snack, a deliciously healthy dessert, or even part of a creative meal, fruit rules. Similar to its neighbor in the produce section, fruit is naturally low in calories and fat (except for avocado and coconut), while chock-full of nutrients and fiber. Get in the habit of keeping a stash of fresh fruit. Although dried fruit is another tasty option, keep in mind that it is more concentrated in calories because it has less water than its fresh counterparts. Also, beware of canned (and sometimes frozen) fruit with "heavy syrup added"; these are packed with calories and sugar. When buying canned or frozen fruit, read the labels and look for key phrases such as "no added sugar," "packed in its own juice," "packed in 100% fruit juice," or "unsweetened."

What about fruit juice? It's certainly not a substitute for whole fruit (in fact, even the brands with pulp added will be lacking in dietary fiber), but fruit juice does provide nutrients and is clearly better than colas, sweetened iced-teas, or fruit punch. Go ahead and put a couple of juice containers in your shopping cart. When available, opt for the brands with added vitamin C or the calcium-fortified varieties.

Here are some helpful hints for shopping for fresh fruits:

- **Apples** provide potassium and fiber and are available in a bunch of varieties, including Red Delicious, McIntosh, Granny Smith, Empire, Washington, and Golden Delicious. Although each kind differs in seasonal availability, taste, and appearance, some general shopping savvy is to look for crisp, firm apples with a rich color (depending upon the type). Avoid apples with bruising, soft spots, or mealy flesh.

- **Apricots** provide a lot of vitamin A, iron, and some potassium and fiber. Look for apricots that have a golden orange color and appear to be plump and juicy. Avoid apricots that are dull-looking, mushy, or overly firm or that have a yellowish green color.

- **Avocados** provide vitamin A, potassium, folic acid, and fiber. Look for avocados that are slightly tender to the touch if you plan to eat them immediately. Otherwise, buy firm avocados and let them ripen at room temperature for a few days. Avoid any with broken surfaces or dark prominent spots.

- **Bananas** provide a lot of potassium and some vitamin A and fiber. Look for firm bananas that are either yellowish green (and will ripen in a few days) or fully yellow and ready to eat. In general, bananas have their best flavor when the solid yellow color is speckled with some brown. Avoid bananas that are bruised or have a gray appearance.

- **Blueberries** provide vitamin C, potassium, and fiber. Look for plump, firm blueberries that are dark blue in color. Avoid berries that are mushy, moldy, or leaking.

- **Cantaloupes** provide vitamins A and C and potassium. Look for cantaloupes with rough skin that are slightly soft and flexible when you press on the top or bottom and that have a sweet, fresh odor. Avoid extremely hard cantaloupes (unless you want to wait for them to ripen) and any with moldy spots.

- **Cherries** provide vitamin A and potassium. Look for cherries with a dark red color, plump surfaces, and fresh stems. Avoid cherries that appear dull, shriveled, or dried.

- **Grapefruits** provide vitamins A and C and potassium. Look for firm, compact grapefruits that are heavy for their size. Do not worry about slight discoloration or skin scars; this usually does not interfere with the quality of taste. Avoid grapefruits that look extremely dull and lack color.

◆ **Grapes** provide some fiber and come in several color varieties. Look for rich-colored, plump grapes that are tightly attached to the stem. Avoid grapes that are shriveled and soft or that have brown, brittle stems.

◆ **Kiwi fruit** provides a lot of vitamin C and potassium. Look for plump kiwi fruit that yields slightly to the touch; this means it's ripe. You can ripen firm kiwi fruit at home by leaving it at room temperature for a few days. Avoid kiwi fruits that are super-soft or shriveled.

◆ **Lemons** provide vitamin C. Look for firm lemons with a rich, glossy yellow color. Avoid lemons with mold, punctures, or a dull, dark yellow coloring.

◆ **Mangos** provide vitamins A and C, potassium, and fiber. Look for orangish-yellow to red mangos that are well developed and barely soft to the touch. Avoid mangos that are rock-hard or over-ripened and mushy.

◆ **Nectarines** provide vitamin A and potassium. Look for bright-colored, plump nectarines with orange, yellow, and red color combinations. Nectarines that are hard will ripen in a few days at room temperature. Avoid nectarines that are overly soft, lacking color, or show signs of decay.

◆ **Oranges** provide a lot of vitamin C, potassium, and folic acid. Look for firm, heavy oranges (because this indicates juiciness) with relatively smooth, bright-looking skin. Avoid oranges that are very light (no juice) or that have thick, coarse, or spongy skins.

◆ **Peaches** provide vitamin A and potassium. Look for peaches that are firm but slightly soft to the touch. Avoid greenish, hard peaches that are under-ripened and mushy peaches that are over-ripened.

◆ **Pears** provide potassium and fiber. Look for pears that are firm, but not too hard. The color depends on the variety. Bartletts are pale yellow to rich yellow, Anjou or Comice are light green to yellowish green, Bosc are greenish yellow to brownish yellow, and Winter Nellis are medium to light green. Avoid wilted or wrinkled pears with any distinct spots.

◆ **Pineapples** provide vitamin C and fiber. Look for pineapples that are plump, firm, and heavy for their size and that have a fragrant aroma. Avoid pineapples that appear dull, bruised, or dried, or that have an unpleasant smell.

◆ **Raspberries** provide vitamin C, potassium, and fiber. Look for plump, tender berries with a rich, uniform scarlet color. Avoid berries that are mushy or have any mold.

- **Strawberries** provide a lot of vitamin C, along with potassium, folic acid, and fiber. Look for firm, red berries that still have the cap stem attached. Avoid berries that have large uncolored or seedy areas. Also avoid strawberries that have a shrunken appearance or any mold.

- **Tangerines** provide vitamins A and C. Look for deep yellow or orange tangerines with a bright luster (which indicates freshness and maturity). Avoid tangerines with a pale yellow or greenish color or punctures in the skin.

- **Watermelon** provides vitamin A and some vitamin C. For uncut watermelons, look for a smooth surface, well-rounded ends, and a pale green color. For cut watermelons, look for juicy flesh with a rich, red color that is free from white streaks. Avoid melons with a lot of white streaks running through pale colored flesh and light colored seeds.

Aisle Two: Down Dairy Lane

Milk products supply you with calcium (responsible for healthy bones), along with providing protein, several B-vitamins, and vitamins D and A. The problem is that whole milk also contains a lot of saturated fat, which can increase your risk for heart disease, weight gain, and other serious illnesses. What can you do? Simple: when you're at home and have control over the type of dairy that goes into your cereals, recipes, and sandwiches, use the low-fat versions that are available in most supermarkets today.

Don't throw in the towel if you don't like some of the reduced-fat items; different brands have different tastes. Just try another brand or version the next time you shop. Another thing to keep in mind is that some of the "fat-free" dairy is literally "taste-free." (Some brands even resemble plastic.) You don't have to suffer with the fat-free if you can't stand the taste; low-fat is fine, with a mere 3–5 extra grams of fat.

Food for Thought

Contrary to its name, buttermilk is actually a low-fat dairy product. In fact, buttermilk is simply skim or low-fat pasteurized milk with some added lactic acid. The consistency is thicker than regular milk and the sodium is also higher at 257 milligrams per 8 ounces (about double the amount of regular low-fat milk).

Nutri-Speak

Pasteurized milk is briefly heated to kill harmful bacteria and then rapidly chilled. Homogenized milk has been processed to reduce the size of milk fat globules so the cream does not separate and the milk stays consistently smooth and uniform.

Here's your low-fat dairy shopping list. Browse through the section and pick out the items that sound appealing:

Nonfat dry milk

Skim milk (no fat)

Evaporated skim milk

1% low-fat milk

Buttermilk

Nonfat yogurts (plain and flavored)

Low-fat yogurts (plain and flavored)

Nonfat varieties of all cheese

Low-fat varieties of all cheese

Part-skim varieties of all cheese

Reduced-fat cream cheese

Dry-curd cottage cheese

Low-fat cottage cheese

Reduced-fat sour cream

Low-fat/nonfat ice creams

Low-fat/nonfat frozen yogurts

Aisle Three: Shopping for the Whole Grains

Here are some shopping tips for buying breads and cereals:

- Stick with whole-grain varieties, including whole wheat, multigrain, rye, millet, oat bran, oat, and cracked wheat. (This goes for all types of bread: sliced bread, pita, bagels, English muffins, crackers, and so on.)

- Although "wheat" bread might sound just as healthy as "whole-wheat" bread, don't be fooled; it's merely a blend of white and whole-wheat flour. A product labeled "whole-wheat" must be made from 100 percent whole-wheat flour.

- Check the label and choose breads with at least 2 grams of fiber per slice.

- If you're looking to save calories, try the whole-wheat, reduced-calorie bread (approximately 40 calories per slice with 2 grams of fiber).

- Don't forget to check the expiration date on the label.

- Take advantage of the fiber that some cereals pack in, and choose varieties that have at least 2 grams of fiber per serving. You can usually (not always) get a sense of whether a cereal has fiber from the name on the box (Bran Flakes, All-Bran, 100% Bran, Raisin Bran, Fiber-One, Shredded Wheat, and Corn Bran).

- Some cereals pack in more sugar and salt than most people realize. Check the "Total Carbohydrates" against the "Sugars" (on the nutrition label) to make sure sugar is not a main ingredient. In fact, opt for the brands that report 6 grams of sugar or less per serving. If your kids (or spouse) insist on the sugary brand, mix it with half a bowl of a healthier look-alike (for instance, half Frosted Flakes and half Bran Flakes).

- Check the serving size. Some of the denser, heavier cereals only allot a miniscule amount for one serving. Take this into consideration if you plan to eat a normal-size bowl (and you're watching your weight). Remember, double the serving size means double the calories.

- Don't forget to throw some hot cereal into your cart. Whether you opt for the instant or the kind that requires cooking, stick with unsweetened varieties of oatmeal, grits, cream of rice, and cream of wheat. You can sweeten them with some of the fresh fruit you bought in the produce section.

- Most cereals are low in fat with the exception of granola and others that add nuts, seeds, coconut, and oils. Read the label and choose cereals with no more than 2 grams of fat per serving.

- Read the list of ingredients on your cereal box and make sure that wheat, rye, corn, or oats are listed first. Items are listed in the order of quantity.

Pasta, Rice, and More

Pasta is one of those American staple foods that everyone seems to enjoy. What's more, pasta is high in complex carbohydrates, easy to make, and inexpensive. Don't stop at the box of spaghetti; try the elbow macaroni, ziti, rigatoni, penne, fusilli, orzo, shells, bow ties, and lasagna noodles. If your supermarket has any whole-grain varieties, throw them in your basket; they're a great source of fiber.

Rice is another excellent source of complex carbohydrates and tends to be a popular standard in many homes. The most nutritious is brown rice, with a bit more fiber than the white varieties. Next in the nutrition line-up is polished white rice, and last is the instant white rice, with the fewest nutrients of all.

Try some of the not-so-common grains. Pile your cart with whole-grain couscous, barley, buckwheat, bulgur, kasha, millet, polenta, wheat berries, and cracked wheat. They are all brimming with complex carbohydrates—so jazz up your dinners and impress your family!

Aisle Four: Best Bets for Protein

When buying beef, pork, lamb, and veal, look for lean, well-trimmed cuts. Meats are graded by the USDA (United States Department of Agriculture) according to their fat content and texture. *Prime* indicates the highest in fat (unfortunately, it's usually the most tender and juicy because of the marbled fat throughout); *choice* is moderately fatty; and *select* is the leanest. Lean meats provide a lot of high-quality protein, along with iron, B-vitamins, phosphorus, and zinc.

Your leanest beef choices are the following:

Top round	Top loin steak
Tenderloin	Chuck steaks
Lean T-bone	Lean rump
Lean porterhouse	Lean flank
Sirloin	Ground beef (only extra-lean)
Eye of round	Round tip
Bottom round	

Your leanest lamb and veal choices are as follows:

Leg of lamb	Lamb roast
Foreshank	Arm chop
Lean loin chop	Veal roast
Veal loin chop	Veal cutlet

Your leanest pork choices are these:

Tenderloin	Top loin roast
Center loin chops	Canadian bacon
Lean ham	Rib chops
Sirloin roast	Shoulder blade steak

Buffalo meat and venison meat are both exceptionally lean.

Poultry

Let's not forget about poultry. Poultry can be one of your leanest animal protein sources, but lose the skin—pure fat! You can buy poultry with the skin if it's more reasonably priced. You can even cook poultry with the skin for some added moistness; just be sure to remove it before eating.

Your leanest poultry choices are these:

Skinless chicken breast

Turkey breast (white meat, no skin)

Cornish game hen (no skin)

Ground chicken or turkey breast (look for white meat only/no skin added)

Duck and pheasant (no skin)

Fish and Seafood

When choosing seafood, almost anything goes. Scout the aisle and pick up anything that looks fresh and appealing. Fresh fish and seafood should have bright skin, bulging eyes (for whole fish), firm flesh, and *no* fishy smell. You might have heard that some fish are fattier than others. It's true, but the amount of fat is so small that all fish and seafood remain great choices nutritionally. In addition, the type of fat found in fish is polyunsaturated (more specifically, omega-3 fatty acid), which has been shown to do positive things in the fight against heart disease and cancer. What's more, all types of fish supply excellent high-quality protein, along with other vitamins and minerals.

Your leanest fish choices are these:

Cod

Flounder

Sea bass

Whiting

Halibut

Red snapper

Haddock

Shellfish (crab, crayfish, lobster, and shrimp)

Monkfish

Perch

Tuna

Mullet

Mollusks (abalone, clams, mussels, oysters, scallops, and squid)

Fattier fish include the following:

Wild Salmon	Albacore tuna
Mackerel	Bluefish
Herring	Shad
Eel	Catfish
Pompano	

Eggs

Eggs are a good source of high-quality protein, iron, and vitamin A—but they also provide a lot of cholesterol, about 213 mg, to get technical. Furthermore, there are approximately 5 grams of fat in just one yolk. Not bad if you only eat whole eggs occasionally. Otherwise, think about using only the whites of the eggs, or grab a carton of the egg substitutes (no cholesterol and low in fat) that are generally sold in the frozen section. Also, some supermarkets carry straight, preseparated whites in refrigerated cartons.

Legumes (Dried Beans, Peas, and Lentils)

Definitely add some legumes to your shopping list. Legumes supply protein, calcium, iron, zinc, magnesium, and B-vitamins. Most impressive is that dried beans, peas, and lentils are the only high-protein foods that provide ample amounts of fiber. Get creative and make a meatless meal a couple of times each week.

Look for these:

Baked beans	Great northern beans
Pinto beans	Black beans
Kidney beans	Split peas
Black-eyed peas	Lentils
Tofu	Cannelloni beans
Lima beans	Vegetarian chili
Navy beans	White beans
Garbanzo beans (chickpeas)	Hummus

Aisle Five: Frozen Meals, Canned Soups, and Sauces

As mentioned earlier, frozen and canned items can be convenient and tasty. Just remember to read the labels carefully and keep the following tips in mind:

◆ For full frozen meals, always read the label and look for *less* than 400 total calories, 15 grams of fat, and 800 milligrams of sodium.

◆ When choosing soups, avoid the creamy varieties unless you have the option of mixing in your own low-fat milk. Also buy soups that say "reduced-sodium," "low-sodium," or "no added salt." Some nutritious selections include minestrone, garden vegetable, chicken noodle, split pea, tomato rice, Manhattan clam chowder, and the lentil bean combinations.

◆ To cut fat, buy sauces that are tomato- or vegetable-based. Check the labels and look for brands that have 3 grams (or less) of fat per serving.

Aisle Six: Savvy Snacks

Most of us love to nibble in between meals. If you plan to stock up your kitchen, do so with these low-fat items:

Plain popcorn kernels for air poppers

Fruit and fig bars

"Lite" or "reduced-fat" microwave popcorn

Low-fat granola bars and chewy cereal bars (preferably calcium-fortified and with 2+ grams of fiber)

Oat bran pretzels and baked chips

Lower-fat whole grain crackers

Animal crackers, ginger snaps, and graham crackers

Raisins and other dried fruit

Frozen fruit pops and sorbet

Trail mix

Flavored rice cakes

Soy crisps

Aisle Seven: Health-Conscious Condiments

The following low-fat condiments can help add pizzazz to your meals. But keep in mind that a lot of these flavor enhancers are also high in sodium. Salt-sensitive people need to pay close attention to the salt contents on the package.

Catsup	Cider vinegar
Mustard	Lemon juice
Low-sugar fruit spreads	Worcestershire sauce
Soy sauce (low-sodium)	Cocktail sauce
Teriyaki sauce (low-sodium)	Chutney
Balsamic vinegar	Salsa
Barbecue sauce	

Aisle Eight: Heart-Smart Fats, Spreads, and Dressings

When purchasing fats, remember to stick with predominantly unsaturated ones. Also, opt for the reduced-fat or fat-free versions of the original dressings and spreads. You'll substantially cut down on your fat intake (and they're usually lower in calories, too).

Here's a master list to select from:

Monounsaturated	*Others that May Come in Handy*
Olive oil	Nonstick cooking sprays
Canola oil	Fat-free and low-fat salad dressings
Low-fat dips, soft-tub margarines (regular and reduced fat)	
Plant sterol and stanol spreads	
Butter substitutes (sprays or granules)	
Low-fat mayonnaise	
Soy mayonnaise	
Natural peanut butter	
Almond butter	

The Least You Need to Know

◆ The first step to a well-stocked kitchen begins with a comprehensive, healthy shopping list. Make sure to organize your list with individual food categories.

◆ Load up your cart with fresh vegetables and fruit, but only buy what you need because fresh produce is perishable. Frozen and canned fruits and vegetables are good options for people who do not shop frequently; just check to make sure there is not a lot of added fat, sugar, and salt.

◆ Buy low-fat dairy and lean cuts of meat, poultry, and fish, and don't forget about legumes for those meatless meals. Also, look in the freezer section of your market for egg substitutes; you'll save a lot of fat and cholesterol.

◆ Scout out the grains made with whole-grain flour. When choosing cereals, read the labels and select brands that are low in sugar and provide at least 2 grams of fiber per serving.

◆ Read labels on salad dressings, fats, and other spreads. Opt for products that are reduced-fat, low-fat, or fat-free.

Now You're Cooking

In This Chapter

◆ Simple cooking modifications

◆ Great recipes for breakfast, lunch, and dinner

◆ Finding a good cookbook

Mealtime is the perfect opportunity to bond with your family, converse with friends, relax in private, or impress your date with a knockout dish. The hardest part is already done: you've stocked your kitchen with the right ingredients. So grab some pots and pans and turn on some groovin' music. This chapter offers helpful hints for recipe remodeling, plus it provides you with easy-to-make, tasty meals for breakfast, lunch, dinner, and dessert.

The Recipe Makeover: Remodeling Family Favorites

Skimming the fat in your recipe means more than just using leaner ingredients. It also means using healthful cooking techniques and tools. Here are some quick tips and tricks of the trade:

1. Use low-fat and no-fat cooking methods, such as steaming, poaching, stir-frying, broiling, grilling, microwaving, baking, and roasting as alternatives to frying.

2. Get a good-quality set of nonstick saucepans, skillets, and baking pans so you can sauté and bake without adding fat.

3. Use nonstick vegetable sprays or 1 to 2 tablespoons of defatted broth, water, juice, or wine to replace cooking oil.

4. Be aware that fat-free or reduced-fat cheeses have slightly different cooking characteristics than their fattier counterparts. For the most part, they don't melt as smoothly. To overcome this, shred these cheeses very finely. When making sauces and soups, toss the cheese with a small amount of flour, cornstarch, or arrowroot.

5. Trim all visible fat from steaks, chops, roasts, and other meat cuts before preparing them.

6. Replace one quarter to one half of ground meat or poultry in a casserole or meat sauce with cooked brown rice, bulgur, couscous, or cooked and chopped dried beans to skim the fat and add fiber.

7. Deciding to remove the skin from poultry before or after cooking depends on your cooking method. Skin helps prevent roasted or baked cuts from drying out, and studies have shown that the fat from the skin doesn't penetrate the meat during cooking. However, if you do leave the skin on, make sure any seasonings you've applied go under the skin or you'll lose the flavor when the skin is removed.

8. Skim and discard the fat from hot soups and stews, or chill the soup or stew and skim off the solid fat that forms on top.

9. Use puréed cooked vegetables, such as carrots, potatoes, and cauliflower, to thicken soups and sauces instead of cream, egg yolks, or a butter and flour roux. Also, use soft tofu to thicken sauces.

10. Select "healthier" fats when you need to add fat to a recipe. That means replacing butter, lard, or other highly saturated fats with oils such as canola, olive, safflower, sunflower, corn, and others that are low in saturates. Remember, it takes just a few drops of a very flavorful oil, such as extra-virgin olive oil, dark sesame, walnut, or garlic oil, to really perk up a dish, so go easy.

11. Skim the fat where you won't miss it, but keep the characteristic flavor of fatty ingredients such as nuts, coconut, chocolate chips, and bacon by reducing the quantity you use by 50 percent. For example, if a recipe calls for 1 cup of walnuts, use $^1/_2$ cup instead.

12. Toast nuts and spices to enhance their flavor and then chop them finely so they can be more fully distributed through the food.

13. If sugar is the primary sweetener in a fruit sauce, beverage, or other dish that is not baked, scale the amount down by 25 percent. Instead of 1 cup of sugar, use ¾ cup. If you add a pinch of cinnamon, nutmeg, or allspice, you'll increase the perception of sweetness without adding calories.

14. In baked goods, add pureed fruit instead of fat. One of the reasons fat is included in baked products is to make them moist. The high concentration of natural sweetness in pureed fruit will actually help hold on to the moisture during the baking process.

> **CAUTION**
>
> **Overrated-Undercooked**
>
> Be careful when cutting back on the amount of sugar in cakes, cookies, or other baked goods. Many times, reducing sugar will affect the texture or the volume.

Fat has flavor, but so does fruit. Fat adds liquid volume and moisture to bread or cake batter, but so does fruit. When making this substitution, if the recipe calls for ½ cup of fat, simply add ½ cup of pureed fruit. Use applesauce in apple bran muffins or cakes. Pureed, crushed pineapple works well in pineapple upside down cake. Here are some other tips:

- Dark-colored fruits, such as blueberries and prunes, are best used in dark-colored batters. You can add lighter-colored fruits, such as pears or applesauce, to almost any batter without changing its color. Adding yellow-orange fruits, such as pureed peaches or apricots, can often add an appetizing yellowish crumb.

- You can use pears and apples nearly universally in baking because their taste is mild and unnoticeable. Apricots, prunes, and pineapple add a much stronger flavor. Bananas and peaches are somewhere in the middle, adding a little flavor, but never overwhelming. Here's a secret: if you don't have a food processor to puree your own fruit, use baby food. It is already pureed, has a mild flavor, and is usually made without sugar.

15. Beat egg whites until soft peaks form before incorporating them into baked goods. This will increase the volume and tenderness.

16. Make a simple fat-free "frosting" for cakes or bar cookies by sprinkling the tops lightly with powdered sugar.

17. Increase the fiber content and nutritional value of dishes by using whole-wheat flour for at least half of the all-purpose white flour. For cakes and other baked products that require a light texture, use whole-wheat pastry flour, available in some well-stocked supermarkets.

18. Vegetables can be fat replacements in other recipes, too. Try …

   ◆ Adding baby carrot puree, roasted red pepper puree, or mashed potatoes to your pasta sauce to replace olive oil.

   ◆ Replacing some of the fat in nut breads or cakes, such as carrot cake or zucchini bread, with vegetable purees or juices, such as carrot juice or pumpkin puree.

   ◆ Substituting pureed green peas for half the amount of mashed avocado in guacamole or other dips.

   ◆ Replacing fat in soups, sauces, muffins, or cakes with mashed yams or sweet potatoes.

   ◆ Using white potatoes to thicken lower-fat milks in cream soups and bisques.

   ◆ Substituting a layer of vegetables in your favorite lasagna to replace meat or sausage.

   ◆ Topping your pizza with vegetables instead of meat.

Source: ADA. "Skim the Fat: A Practical and Up-to-Date Food Guide," 1995.

Top-10 List for Substitutions

Try some of these substitutions with your favorite recipes. They can help to reduce the fat while maintaining flavor.

1. Use nonfat plain yogurt instead of sour cream.

2. Use two egg whites instead of one whole egg.

3. Use 1% low-fat milk instead of whole milk.

4. Use $\frac{1}{2}$ the fat that a recipe calls for.

5. Use 3 TB. cocoa powder and 1 TB. oil instead of baking chocolate.

6. Use evaporated skim milk instead of cream.

7. Use fruit purees, fruit juices, or buttermilk to replace fat in a recipe.

8. Use nonfat yogurt or reduced-fat mayonnaise instead of regular mayonnaise.

9. Use diet margarine instead of regular margarine.

10. Use low-fat ricotta cheese or 1% cottage cheese instead of whole milk cream cheese or ricotta cheese.

Breakfast: Two Creative Morning Recipes

French Toast à la Mode

2 egg whites (or egg substitutes)

⅓ cup 1% low-fat milk

½ tsp. vanilla extract

1 TB. reduced-fat margarine

6 slices wheat bread

1 cup nonfat plain yogurt

1 cup fresh blueberries

Serves Three
Nutrition Information
Calories: 231
Total fat: 4 grams
Saturated fat: 0.7 gram
Fiber: 7 grams
Protein: 13 grams
Sodium: 467 mg
Cholesterol: 1 mg

From the kitchen of Carol and Victor Bauer

Beat egg whites, milk, and vanilla in a bowl. Melt margarine in a skillet over medium heat. Cut bread into diagonal slices and dip both sides evenly in the batter (made from eggs, milk, and vanilla). Next, brown each side of bread in the hot skillet by flipping individual slices. Arrange finished French toast on a plate (2 full slices or 4 halves per serving); top with scoop of yogurt and fresh blueberries.

Egg White-Veggie Omelet

8 egg whites

4 TB. low-fat milk

Pepper to taste

½ cup sliced mushrooms

½ cup sliced onions

¼ cup chopped tomato

Nonstick vegetable spray

2 oz. nonfat shredded cheddar cheese

Serves Two
Nutrition Information
Calories: 161
Total fat: 1 gram
Saturated fat: 0.2 gram
Fiber: 2 grams
Protein: 26 grams
Sodium: 445 mg
Cholesterol: 1 mg

From the kitchen of Debra, Steve, and Ben Beal

Mix egg whites together with milk and some pepper; set it aside. In a separate dish, place mushrooms, onions, and 2 tablespoons water. Cover and microwave mushrooms and onions for approximately 2–3 minutes on high (depending on how soft you like your veggies). Drain vegetables and mix in chopped tomatoes and egg mixture. Apply nonstick spray to a large skillet and cook the entire concoction over medium-high heat. When eggs begin to set, sprinkle on shredded cheese and allow it to melt. When omelet appears cooked but moist, fold over one side and gently lift onto a plate. Round off the meal with some whole-wheat toast and you're set.

Lunch—Not the Same Old Sandwich Again!

Greek Pasta Salad

Serves four
Nutrition Information
Calories: 220
Total fat: 2 gram
Saturated fat: 0 gram
Fiber: 2 grams
Protein: 10 grams
Sodium: 150 mg
Cholesterol: 0 mg

Copyright © Food for Health Newsletter, *1996. Reprinted with permission.*

3 cups uncooked bowtie (or fusilli) pasta

1 cucumber, seeded and diced ¼ inch

3 ripe plum tomatoes, seeded and diced ¼ inch

¼ cup chopped red onion

3 TB. black diced olives

2 TB. balsamic vinegar

1 grated lemon zest (the outer peel) and juice

2 TB. fresh, chopped mint leaves

Olive oil cooking spray

1 small head of Bibb or butter lettuce

Cook the pasta: Bring 2 quarts of water to a rapid boil over high heat. Add pasta slowly, stirring constantly until all pasta is in the pot. Bring back to a boil and reduce heat to medium-high. Cook according to package directions or until pasta still has a slightly firm center (about 10–13 minutes). Drain in colander and rinse with cold water.

Make the salad: Combine all vegetables (except lettuce), vinegar, lemon zest, and lemon juice in a mixing bowl. Toss in pasta and mint leaves and lightly spray with olive oil cooking spray. Toss again. Line four plates with lettuce leaves and divide pasta salad among them.

Open-Faced Tuna Melt

Serves one
Nutrition Information
Calories: 319
Total fat: 7 grams
Saturated fat: 5 grams
Fiber: 4 grams
Protein: 31 grams
Sodium: 530 mg
Cholesterol: 30 mg

From the kitchen of Glenn and Erik Music (Castlebridge Recording)

1 whole-wheat English muffin, sliced in half

3-oz. can of water-packed tuna (low sodium)

2 tsp. reduced-fat mayonnaise

Sliced tomato

2 slices low-fat American cheese

Toast both halves of muffin and set aside. Drain and mash tuna, and then mix it with low-fat mayonnaise. Spread tuna evenly over both pieces of muffin, leaving bread open-faced. Place tomato and one slice cheese on top of tuna on each piece of bread. Put open-faced sandwich in the oven until cheese is fully melted.

Dinner: Recipes to "Wow" Your Taste Buds

Shrimp and Pineapple Stir-Fry

Rice

1½ cups instant brown rice

1½ cups water

Stir-Fry

Canola vegetable oil spray

1 cup assorted sweet peppers
(red, green, yellow), diced

1 cup sliced mushrooms

½ cup snow peas

¼ cup chicken broth

½ TB. cornstarch

1 TB. light soy sauce

½ cup crushed pineapple;
drain and reserve juice

1 cup bean sprouts

½ tsp. red pepper flakes

12 ounces medium shrimp,
peeled and deveined

Serves four
Nutrition Information
Calories: 290
Total fat: 3 grams
Saturated fat: 0.5 gram
Fiber: 4 grams
Protein: 23 grams
Sodium: 290 mg
Cholesterol: 130 mg

Copyright © Food for Health
Newsletter, 1996. *Reprinted
with permission.*

Cook instant brown rice and water in microwave-proof,
covered dish for 10 minutes on medium-high power (80 percent)
in microwave.

Lightly spray a nonstick skillet with canola oil and heat over
medium-high heat. Sauté peppers until crisp-tender, about
2 minutes; add mushrooms and snow peas and allow to sauté until
crisp-tender, about 2 minutes. Combine chicken broth, cornstarch,
light soy sauce, and pineapple juice (reserved from drained,
crushed pineapple) and add to skillet along with bean sprouts.
Bring to a boil; add red pepper flakes and shrimp and cook until
shrimp is done, about 1 or 2 minutes. Serve over hot cooked rice.

Chicken Paprika

Serves six
Nutrition Information
Calories: 252
Total fat: 13 grams
Saturated fat: 3 grams
Fiber: 1 gram
Protein: 27 grams
Sodium: 65 mg
Cholesterol: 118 mg

From the kitchen of Frances Aaron

6 chicken breasts, skin removed (about 6 oz. each)

3–4 cloves of garlic, chopped

½ tsp. ground black pepper

½ tsp. paprika

1 tsp. olive oil

2 onions sliced

1–2 peppers sliced (red, yellow, and green)

1–2 carrots, cut in half and sliced lengthwise

Season chicken breasts on all sides with garlic, pepper, and paprika; set aside. Heat olive oil in deep skillet with lid. Add onions and cook for 3–5 minutes over medium heat. Add chicken and flip until all sides turn white. Add peppers and carrots; cover and simmer for 1½ to 2 hours. If you would like less sauce, remove the lid for the last 20 minutes.

Jon's Terrific Turkey Loaf
with Mashed Potatoes

Turkeyloaf

2 lbs. ground lean turkey
breast (no skin)

1 cup onions, diced

3 slices whole-wheat bread,
pulled apart

1 cup shredded fat-free
cheddar cheese

2 cups whole cranberry sauce

6 crushed cloves of garlic

1 whole egg and 2 egg
whites

5 fresh parsley sprigs

2 carrots, peeled and diced

Mashed Potatoes

5 medium-size potatoes,
peeled and quartered

2 TB. diet margarine

1 cup 1% low-fat milk

Serves eight
Nutrition Information
Calories: 498
Total fat: 4 grams
Saturated fat: 1 gram
Fiber: 6 grams
Protein: 46 grams
Sodium: 325 mg
Cholesterol: 122 mg

*From the kitchen of Jon Cohen,
Nancy Shapiro, and Camrin*

Preheat oven to 350°. Mix all turkeyloaf ingredients together in a
bowl, and then place into a loaf pan. Bake for ½ hour; drain off
oil.

In a separate pot, boil potatoes. When soft (poke with fork), mash
them and mix in margarine and milk.

Now, for the finishing touch: spread mashed potatoes across the
top of the turkeyloaf and put the combination back in the oven
for an additional 30 minutes (at 350°).

Sensational Side Dishes

Sautéed Italian Mushrooms

Serves four
Nutrition Information
Calories: 44
Total fat: 2 grams
Saturated fat: 0 gram
Fiber: 2 grams
Protein: 3 grams
Sodium: 5 mg
Cholesterol: 0 mg

From the kitchen of Grace Leder

Nonstick cooking spray

1 tsp. olive oil

2–3 garlic cloves, sliced

1 (10–12 oz.) pack of white mushrooms (or 1 lb. loose), sliced thickly

Chopped parsley

Fresh ground pepper to taste

Spray skillet with nonstick cooking spray and drizzle olive oil into the pan. Brown garlic cloves over medium-high heat and add sliced mushrooms and chopped parsley. Add plenty of fresh ground pepper (according to personal taste) and continue to sauté until mushrooms are brown and tender.

Tomato Zucchini Roast

Serves four
Nutrition Information
Calories: 35
Total fat: 0 gram
Saturated fat: 0 gram
Fiber: 2 grams
Protein: 2 grams
Sodium: 15 mg
Cholesterol: 0 mg

Copyright © Food for Health Newsletter, 1996. Reprinted with permission.

3 large, ripe plum tomatoes, diced medium

Fresh cracked black pepper

½ tsp. Italian spice mix

1½ cups sliced mustard greens

1 medium zucchini, diced medium

Olive oil cooking spray

Preheat oven to 350°. Toss all ingredients together and place into suitable-size glass or metal baking container. Bake 10–15 minutes uncovered until zucchini is tender. Stir well and serve.

Cauliflower Soup

1 head cauliflower

1 sliced onion

1 TB. olive oil

2 medium carrots, sliced

1 stalk celery, chopped

5 cups chicken stock, low-sodium

Black pepper to taste

Blanche whole cauliflower for a few minutes. Cook sliced onion in oil until it is transparent, and then add carrots, sliced cauliflower, and celery; cook slightly. Add chicken stock and black pepper. Simmer until vegetables are just tender; then puree mixture. Return to heat for a few minutes and adjust seasoning.

Serves six
Nutrition Information
Calories: 78
Total fat: 3 grams
Saturated fat: 1 gram
Fiber: 5 grams
Protein: 4 grams
Sodium: 123 mg
Cholesterol: 3 mg

From the kitchen of Frances Aaron

Decadent Desserts

Harvest Apple Cake

Serves 12
Nutrition Information
Calories: 213
Total fat: 6 grams
Saturated fat: 1 gram
Fiber: 2 gram
Protein: 3 gram
Sodium: 212 mg
Cholesterol: 35 mg

4 cups (1¼ pounds) un-peeled, chopped Golden Delicious apples, divided

1 cup firmly packed brown sugar

½ tsp. salt

¼ tsp. each ginger and cloves

¾ cup each all-purpose and whole-wheat flour

1 tsp. baking soda

1 tsp. cinnamon

¼ cup vegetable oil

2 large eggs, lightly beaten

1 tsp. vanilla extract

1 TB. confectioners' sugar

Combine 3 cups of apples and brown sugar in a bowl; let stand 45 minutes. Heat oven to 350°. Grease and flour a 6-cup fluted tube pan. Combine dry ingredients in a medium bowl. Combine oil, eggs, and vanilla in a small bowl; stir into apple-sugar mixture. Stir in dry ingredients and remaining apples until blended. Pour into the prepared pan. Bake 40–45 minutes, until a toothpick inserted in the center of cake comes out clean. Cool in the pan on a wire rack 10 minutes; unmold cake and cool completely. Sprinkle with confectioners' sugar.

Angel-Devil Smoothie

Serves four
Nutrition Information
Calories: 140
Total fat: 0 gram
Saturated fat: 0 gram
Fiber: 2 grams
Protein: 8 grams
Sodium: 135 mg
Cholesterol: 5 mg

2 cups nonfat plain yogurt

2 chocolate nonfat brownies, broken into small pieces

2 cups frozen sliced strawberries

¼ cup skim milk

Combine all ingredients in blender or food processor. Pulse until all is pureed finely. Serve immediately.

Banana-Health Split

1 banana, peeled

½ cup vanilla fat-free
   frozen yogurt

2 TB. granola cereal
   (low-fat)

Split banana lengthwise down the middle and line up the
two pieces on either side of an ice cream dish. Scoop frozen
yogurt in the middle and sprinkle granola on top. You've now
got a guilt-free banana split!

Serves one
Nutrition Information
Calories: 243
Total fat: 1 gram
Saturated fat: 0 gram
Fiber: 2 grams
Protein: 5 grams
Sodium: 65 mg
Cholesterol: 0 mg

*From the kitchen of Pam and
Dan Schloss*

Start a Cookbook Library

Check with the following resources to begin your own collection of cookbooks. You
can find healthy recipes in the following books:

Cooking With Joy: A 90/10 Cookbook, First Edition.
St. Martin's Press (January 1, 2004)

*American Heart Association Low-Fat, Low-Cholesterol Cookbook, Second Edition:
Heart-Healthy, Easy-to-Make Recipes That Taste Great (American Heart Association
Cookbook), Second Edition*
Clarkson Potter (December 29, 1997)

The Diabetes & Heart Healthy Cookbook, First Edition
American Diabetes Association (October 21, 2004)

*Healthy Cooking for Two (or Just You): Low-Fat Recipes with Half the Fuss and
Double the Taste*
Rodale Books (May 15, 1997)

The New American Plate Cookbook: Recipes for a Healthy Weight and a Healthy Life
University of California Press (March 1, 2005)

12 Best Foods Cookbook: Over 200 Recipes Featuring the 12 Healthiest Foods
Rodale Books (April 6, 2005)

365 Days of Healthy Eating from the American Dietetic Association
Wiley (December 12, 2003)

Quick Meals for Healthy Kids and Busy Parents: Wholesome Family Recipes in 30 Minutes or Less From Three Leading Child Nutrition Experts, First Edition
Wiley (August 6, 1995)

Canyon Ranch Cooks
Rodale Books (October 10, 2003)

The Moms' Guide to Meal Makeovers: Improving the Way Your Family Eats, One Meal at a Time! First Edition
Broadway (January 1, 2004)

The Least You Need to Know

◆ Simple ingredient substitutions can turn your favorite recipes into healthy, low-fat dishes.

◆ Stick with the healthier, lower-fat cooking techniques, such as steaming, poaching, stir-frying, broiling, grilling, microwaving, baking, and roasting. Jazz up the flavor with noncaloric spices and seasonings.

◆ Use puréed, cooked veggies instead of cream, butter, and egg yolks to thicken soups and sauces. For baked products, add pureed fruit instead of butter, lard, and other oils. When a recipe calls for a large amount of sugar, scale it down by 25 percent.

Restaurant Survival Guide

In This Chapter

◆ Dining out healthfully

◆ Becoming a menu detective

◆ Best bets in ethnic cuisine

Too tired to cook, or just want to get out and socialize? Join the crowd! According to the National Restaurant Association, Americans spend an average of more than $800 million a day on food away from home. Once considered a special occasion, eating out has become an everyday happening—and the food-service industry is growing by leaps and bounds. This chapter shows you that, along with convenience and atmosphere, restaurants can also provide healthy food. You just need to practice some defensive dining.

Common Restaurant Faux Pas

First, the problem of overeating. Are you the type who needs to loosen your belt buckle a couple of notches after each course? Keep in mind that this is *not* the last meal of your life, and there's no need to lick your plate clean even though your stomach is ready to explode. When you feel comfortably full, either ask the waiter to take away your plate or simply pack it up in a doggie bag and enjoy it the following day. Restaurants are notorious for their super-size portions.

What about the actual food choices? Making healthy food choices requires planning, nutrition know-how, and compromise: *planning* during the day so you can budget your fat and calories; *nutrition know-how* so you can order the healthier, lower-fat items from your favorite ethnic cuisines; and the willingness to *compromise* between the foods you should be eating and the not-so-terrific foods you looooove to chow down.

Fortunately, due to the increasing emphasis on health, most places, from fast-food joints to fancy establishments, are making an effort to prepare and offer at least a few healthy alternatives. Quite often, you will even notice a *Spa Cuisine* or *Diet* section on the regular menu listing nutrition information underneath the lower-fat, lower-cal entrees. For the restaurants that don't provide this luxury, don't be shy or embarrassed: speak up and ask for special requests such as "salad dressing or sauce on the side," "less oil and salt used during food preparation," and "substitute a baked potato or side salad instead of French fries." In fact, you may decide to order two appetizers instead of an entree, or half an order of pasta instead of the huge entree portion. Remember, good food does not have to wear the price tag of cellulite.

Become a Dining Detective

Go ahead and take on any type of restaurant. Ask yourself (and the waiter) the following five key questions before ordering something on the menu:

1. **How is the food prepared?** The same methods I advised for your own personal recipes also apply to restaurants. Whether entrees or side dishes, scout out meals that are prepared by grilling, baking, poaching, roasting, boiling, blackening, steaming, broiling, or "lightly" stir-frying. If the menu doesn't indicate the cooking technique, ask your waiter or waitress. Don't assume that a food is not fried unless the menu clearly says it isn't.

2. **Are the cuts of meat lean?** Stick with the leaner cuts of meat. For instance, loin, round, flank, shoulder, leg, and extra-lean ground beef are the preferred choices when ordering red meat. Chicken and turkey breasts are two of the leanest choices to make, and of course, all fish and seafood can be terrific when prepared in a healthful manner. When you do occasionally order steak, ask whether the chef melts butter on top before cooking. Believe it or not, some establishments do this to make the meat seem more tender.

3. **What kind of sauces come with your meal?** Ask about the ingredients used for sauces. Generally, avoid hollandaise, butter, cheese, and cream sauces that come slathered over your meal. If you're not sure about something, or it sounds delicious and hard to pass up, get it on the side and enjoy it in smaller amounts.

4. **Are the ingredients loaded with sodium?** If you're on a sodium-restricted diet for medical reasons, it's especially important to avoid entrees and side dishes that are loaded with salt. Stay away from meats and fish that are smoked, cured, pickled, or canned. Also avoid sauces, seasonings, and marinades that use soy sauce, teriyaki sauce, dried stock, MSG, or plain old table salt during preparation.

> **Q & A**
>
> Can you ever just "go whole hog" and order whatever you want without worrying about all the unhealthy ingredients?
>
> Sure you can, but save it for occasional splurges—not everyday habit. In fact, some things are so obscenely scrumptious that if you didn't periodically indulge, I'd think you were nuts!

5. **How can you balance out your meal?** If you order a pasta entree, pass up the bread. If you know that you like to splurge on dessert, order a lean grilled fish for your main dish with a lot of vegetables. If the bread basket is your thing, skip the side starch that comes with your main meal and enjoy two slices of fresh bread instead. If you like to use up calories on a few glasses of wine, skip the bread and get fresh fruit for dessert.

Ethnic Cuisine: "The Good, the Bad, and the Ugly"

Take a quick trip around the world, and check out the best bets in French, Italian, Chinese, Japanese, Mexican, Indian, and American cookery. Be adventurous and excite your palate with exotic new flavors.

I've identified the foods with the most nutrition and least amount of fat as "Include." The foods that are high in fat and calories and offer little in the way of nutrition have been labeled "Avoid." Further, I've placed an asterisk (*) next to the foods that are lower in calories, and can work for the weight-conscious diner. *Bon appétit!*

Chinese Food

Loaded with vegetables, rice, and noodles, the typical Chinese cuisine offers an assortment of healthy selections. Because most Chinese cooking is done in a wok (stir-frying), varying amounts of peanut oil are used. The good news is that peanut oil is unsaturated and won't clog up your arteries. The bad news is that excessive amounts of *any* oil can add a lot of fat calories. As you can imagine, some of the dishes have *startling* amounts.

If your thighs can't afford those extra fat calories, avoid anything fried. Try one of the steamed versions, or carefully drain off some of the fat in a stir-fried entree by taking your portion from the serving plate drenched in sauce and transferring it to your dish with rice. Another idea, if you're dining with a friend, is to order one dish in sauce and a second steamed vegetable dish. Mix the two together, and you'll have half the sauce and double the vegetables. What's more, you can better pace your eating if you use a set of chopsticks.

Another problem with Chinese food can be sodium because a lot of the sauces are high in salt. If you're on a salt-restricted diet, you should probably stick with the plain steamed dishes.

Include	Avoid
Hot and sour soup	Egg drop soup
*Wonton soup	Egg rolls
*Steamed dumplings (vegetable, chicken, and seafood)	Fried dumplings
	Fried rice
Stir-fried chicken and vegetables	Egg fu yung
*Steamed chicken and vegetables	House lo mein
Stir-fried or *steamed* beef and vegetables	Cold noodles with sesame
Stir-fried seafood and vegetables sauce	Moo-shu pork
*Steamed seafood and vegetables	Sesame chicken
Stir-fried tofu and vegetables	General Tsao chicken
*Steamed tofu and vegetables	Sweet and sour pork
*Steamed whole fish	White rice
Szechwan shrimp	Fried chicken and seafood dishes
*Moo-shu vegetables (with pancake rollups)	Seafood with lobster sauce
Steamed brown rice	Spareribs
Fortune cookies (1)	
Lychee nuts	
*Oranges and pineapple slices	
*Low-sodium soy sauce (if available)	
Duck sauce and plum sauce	

French Food

Many positive changes (nutritionally speaking) have occurred in French food during the twentieth century, from the classic *haute* cuisine that generally uses heavier cream sauces, to the newer *nouvelle* cuisine that uses a lighter and healthier approach to food preparation.

Include	Avoid
*Steamed mussels	Appetizers with olives, anchovies, or capers
*Consommé	
*Endive and watercress salads	Quiche
*French onion soup (no cheese)	French bread and baguettes
Nicoise salads	French onion soup (with cheese)
*Poached fish	Cream-based soups
*Steamed fish	Pâté
*Lightly sautéed vegetables	Fondue
*Bouillabaisse	Crèpes
Chicken in wine sauce	Brioche
*Flambéed cherries	Duck or goose with skin
*Peaches in wine	Béarnaise sauce
*Fresh and poached fruit	Hollandaise sauce
*Fruit sorbet	Béchamel sauce
Wine in moderation	Mornay sauce
Chocolate mousse (split with a friend)	Anything with the word "cream" or "au gratin"
	Chocolate mousse
	Creme caramel
	Croissants
	Pastries and éclairs

Indian Food

As with most ethnic cuisines, there are pros and cons to Indian cookery. Beginning with the pros, Indian food emphasizes complex carbohydrates such as basmati rice, breads, lentils, chickpeas, and vegetables, all accented with an array of spices. The most common veggies are spinach, cabbage, peas, onions, eggplant, potatoes, tomatoes, and green peppers. The con is that fat can easily find its way into many of the entrees, breads, and vegetable side dishes.

Scrutinize the menu and watch out for the word *ghee*, which is clarified butter used frequently in Indian cooking. Other oils that are used for sautéing and frying are sesame oil and coconut oil. Although sesame oil is unsaturated, it's quite the contrary for coconut oil—arteries beware! If salt is an issue, forego the soups, and ask the waiter to please prepare your meal without any added salt.

Include	Avoid
*Tamata salad	Anything made with ghee (clarified butter)
*Mulligatawny soup (lentils, veggies, and spices)	Coconut soups
*Chicken or beef tikka	Samosas (fried vegetable turnover)
Tandoori chicken*, beef, or fish*	Korma (meat with rich yogurt cream sauce)
Chicken*, beef, and fish* saag (with spinach)	Curries made with coconut milk or cream
Chicken*, beef, and fish*	Pakora (fried dough with veggies)
Vindaloo (with potatoes and spices)	Saag paneer (spinach with cream sauce)
Shish kabob	Creamy rice dishes
*Gobhi matar tamatar (cauliflower with peas and tomatoes)	Fried breads
Matar pulao (rice pilaf with peas)	Honeyed pastries
Papadum or papad (crispy, thin lentil wafers)	Naan (leavened, baked bread)
Coriander-, tamarind-, and yogurt-based sauces	Kulcha (leavened, baked bread)
*Chapati (thin, dry whole-wheat bread)	
*Mango, mint, and onion chutney	

Italian Food

Among my friends and family, Italian seems to be the one type of food that we can always agree upon. (It's amazing how quickly you can get into the mood.) Unfortunately, as with every other cuisine, if you take one wrong turn on the menu, you're headed for a nutritional nightmare. For instance, a salad and half order of pasta can be a terrific meal if the pasta is ordered with the right kind of sauce; stick with meatless marinara, red and white clam sauce, pomodora, white wine, and a light olive oil. On the other hand, a full-sized pasta entree swimming in one of those cream sauces is a big zero. Also watch out for super-cheesy entrees such as stuffed shells, manicotti, lasagna, and parmigiana. Of course, every once in a while, we are all entitled to indulge. Just make sure the rest of your day was pretty low-fat because some of this stuff can be lethal.

Include	Avoid
*Roasted peppers	Fried calamari and fried mozzarella
*Mussels marinara	Garlic bread
*Steamed clams	Caesar salads
*Grilled calamari	Sausage and meatball heros
*Minestrone soup	Calzones and pizza with pepperoni and sausage
*Half orders of all pastas	Antipasto salad with high-fat meats and cheese
Pasta with meatless marinara sauce	Cheese- or meat-filled ravioli and manicotti
Pasta primavera (not creamy)	Meat lasagna and cheesy vegetarian lasagna
Pasta with red and white clam sauce	Cannelloni and baked ziti
Pasta with marsala	Chicken, veal, or eggplant parmigiana
*Chicken breast with red sauce	Fettuccine alfredo and pasta carbonara
*Chicken cacciatore	Shrimp scampi
*Shrimp, chicken, or veal in wine sauce	Cannoli, spumoni, and tartufo
Chicken or veal piccatta	
Chicken or veal scaloppini	
Pizza with fresh vegetable toppings	
*Lightly marinated mushrooms	
Fresh Italian bread	
*Fresh fruit or sorbet	
Italian ices	
*Skim milk cappuccino	
Wine in moderation	

Japanese Food

The Japanese have perfected low-fat cooking with food-preparation methods that require little or no oil. Highlighting rice, vegetables, soybean-based foods, and small quantities of fish, chicken, and meat, these meals are artistic, healthy, and, best of all, delicious. What's more, once you master the art of using chopsticks, Japanese dining can be a lot of fun. The one drawback is the high-sodium marinades and traditional sauces, which include soy and teriyaki. Ask your waiter whether low-sodium soy sauce is available—and if it isn't, dilute the regular with some water.

Include	Avoid
*Miso soup (soybean-paste soup with tofu and scallions)	Vegetable tempura (battered and fried veggies)
*Steamed vegetables	Shrimp tempura
*Fish and vegetable sushi	Eel and avocado rolls
*Sashimi (raw fish served with wasabi and dipping sauce)	Tonkatsu (breaded pork cutlet)
*Hijiki (cooked seaweed)	Fried dumplings
*Oshitashi (boiled spinach with with soy sauce)	Fried bean curd
*Yaki-udon	Oyako domburi (chicken omelet over rice)
*Yakitori (skewers of chicken)	Chawan mushi (chicken and shrimp in egg custard)
*Su-udon	Yo kan (sweet bean cake)
*Sukiyaki	
Sushi and sashimi (pieces and rolls)	
*Yellowtail, *tuna, *salmon, *crab, and *shrimp	
*Edamame	
*Nabemono (a variety of casseroles)	
*Yosenabe (seafood and veggies in broth)	
*Miso-nabe	
Shabu-shabu (sliced beef, vegetables, and noodles)	
*Sumashi wan (broth with tofu and shrimp)	
*Chicken, fish, or beef teriyaki	
Steamed rice	

Mexican Food

If your taste buds cry out for hot and spicy, Mexican food is probably high on your list of favorites. Unfortunately, some typical dishes on a Mexican menu can send you straight to nutrition jail. On a positive note, Mexican food can be healthy, especially because many dishes are high in complex carbohydrate and fiber; you just need to manage the menu. For example, those fried tortilla chips can be addictive. If you typically gobble down three baskets before your food even arrives, get them off the table. Stick with cheeseless entrees that include beans, rice, and grilled chicken or fish, and use plenty of salsa in place of high-fat sour cream and guacamole. (Although guacamole made from avocado is unsaturated, it still has a lot of fat.)

Include	Avoid
*Gazpacho	Tortilla chips
Corn tortillas with salsa	Nachos with cheese
*Chicken fajitas	Chorizo (sausage)
Enchiladas	Carnitas (fried beef)
*Camarones de hacha (shrimp sautéed in tomato coriander sauce)	Refried beans
	Quesadillas with cheese
*Arroz con pollo (chicken breast with rice)	Beef tacos
Cheeseless burritos	Burritos with cheese
*Grilled fish or chicken breast	Beef and cheese enchilada
Frijoles a la charra	Chimichangas
Borracho beans and rice	Sour cream and guacamole
*Soft chicken taco	Sopapillas (fried dough with sugar)
Chicken burrito (no cheese)	Frozen margaritas and piña coladas
Chicken tostada	
*Salsa, pico de gallo, and cilantro	
*Jalapeño peppers	
*Ceviche (raw fish cooked in lime or lemon juice)	

American Food

American-style restaurants borrow an assortment of ethnic dishes from around the world. Of course, we *are* responsible for salad bars, steak and potatoes, chicken and ribs, a bunch of sandwiches, and good ol' American apple pie, but the typical American menu usually resembles the United Nations.

For example, you can usually expect to find chicken teriyaki from Japan, a stir-fried dish from China, chicken fajitas from Mexico, and a pasta dish from Italy on the spread. The nice part about such a comprehensive menu is that it offers something for everyone (even finicky kids). Placing heavy emphasis on appetizers, salads, and sandwiches, American food can certainly swing both ways.

When you're in the mood for a sandwich, stick with the unadulterated versions such as turkey, roast beef, and chicken breast—whole-wheat bread will be a bonus. Beware of white, refined breads and buns that are prebuttered before they reach your table (such as the buttery grilled cheese sandwich). Ask your waiter to substitute a side salad for those greasy French fries, and stay clear of large salad entrees that pack in more fat than you want to know about. (Read the descriptions and go easy on bacon, avocado, shredded cheese, olives, and dressings.) For standard entrees, look for the usual green-light words (grilled, broiled, and blackened); you know the routine by now.

Include	Avoid
*Shrimp/seafood cocktails	Creamy soups
*Tossed salads with light vinaigrette	Caesar salads
*Broth and vegetable-based soup	Salads with avocado, bacon, and creamy dressings
*Turkey, roast beef, and grilled chicken sandwiches on wheat bread	Buffalo/chicken wings
*Broiled, blackened, and grilled fish and chicken	Fried zucchini and mushrooms
*Plain hamburgers, turkey burgers, and veggie burgers	Cheeseburgers
*Grilled chicken on salad	Grilled cheese sandwiches
*Grilled vegetable over rice plates	Philadelphia cheese steaks
*Chicken kabobs and rice	Reuben sandwiches and tuna melts
*Sirloin steak	Tuna salad, egg salad, and chicken salad
*Buffalo burgers	Fried chicken and fish
*Baked potatoes with Dijon mustard, catsup, marinara, salsa, or small amount of butter	Hot dogs
	French fries and potato salad

Include	Avoid
*Half order pasta with tomato-based sauce	Fruit pies, cookies, cakes, and ice cream sundaes
*Steamed or lightly sautéed vegetables	
*Frozen yogurt, fruit ice, or sherbet	
*Fresh fruit	
*Angel food cake	

Fast Food

The restaurants might lack ambiance, but fast food is certainly one hopping business! It's quick, convenient, and cheap. The nice thing about fast food today is that most places offer an assortment of healthy alternatives due to the growing number of nutrition-conscious customers. Try your best to keep things simple. Generally, the items with complicated names are laden with high-fat meats and "special sauces." For example, the Bacon Double Cheeseburger Deluxe at Burger King has a whopping 39 grams of fat with 16 grams from saturated fat. Be sure to also skip the fried chicken and all sandwiches smothered with cheese. Also, don't ever assume that fish automatically gets a nutrition gold medal. Did you know that McDonald's Filet-O-Fish (breaded and fried) contains 18 grams of fat, compared to the plain hamburger, which only has 9 grams? Stick with the healthier choices to make the best of your fast-food outings.

Include	Avoid
Bagel with jelly	Biscuits and Danish
Hot cakes (no butter)	Egg sandwiches with sausage or bacon
*Grilled chicken sandwiches	Cheeseburgers
*Plain hamburgers	Jumbo burger combinations
*Turkey burgers	Fried chicken sandwiches and fried chicken nuggets
*Veggie burgers	
Vegetable pizza	Fried fish filets
*Vegetable salads with "lite" dressings	Pepperoni or sausage pizza
*Chunky grilled chicken salads	French fries
	Baked potatoes with butter, sour cream, or cheese

continues

continued

Include	Avoid
*Turkey sandwiches (no mayo)	Nachos with cheese
*Lean roast beef sandwiches (no mayo)	Onion rings and fried vegetables
*Chicken fajitas	Apple pie and milkshakes
*Baked potatoes with vegetables, salsa, catsup, or vegetarian chili	Mashed potatoes
*Grilled or steamed veggies	
*Fruit salads and fresh fruit	
*Frozen yogurt cones	
Juice or low-fat milk	
*Catsup, mustard, barbecue, and honey mustard sauce	

Your best bets in fast food:

◆ At McDonald's, try the Chicken McGrill or the Caesar salad with grilled chicken (with Newman's Own Low-Fat Balsamic Vinaigrette). For dessert, you can choose either the Fruit 'n Yogurt Parfait or a cone of vanilla reduced-fat ice cream. For breakfast, an English muffin with 2 scrambled eggs and 1% low-fat milk is your best bet.

◆ At Burger King, try the BK Veggie Burger (w/o mayo), the Chicken Whopper (w/o mayo), or the fire-grilled chicken or shrimp garden salads (with fat-free honey mustard dressing). You can wash your meal down with a bottle of Aquafina water and end with some Mott's Strawberry Flavored Apple Sauce.

◆ At Subway, try the "7 under 6" wraps or 6" subs on a whole-wheat bun (no cheese) and a bag of Baked Lay's Potato Chips.

◆ At Domino's, try a plain pizza with vegetable toppings, a side salad with "lite" dressing, and a tall glass of water.

◆ At Wendy's, try the grilled chicken sandwich on a multi-grain bun, or a baked potato with plain broccoli (or chili), and a salad tossed with "lite" dressing. Wash it down with some water or juice.

CAUTION **Overrated-Undercooked** _____

Don't let the words "salad bar" fool you. There are just as many high-fat pick-ings displayed on the buffet as there are low-fat ones. Survey the situation and load your plate with fresh vegetables, beans, whole grains, and low-fat dressings. On the flip side, watch out for the high-fat mayonnaise traps (such as tuna, egg, seafood, and chicken salads), and take it easy on the creamy dressings, bacon bits, high-fat cheeses, olives, nuts, and seeds.

Going Out for Breakfast or Brunch?

Master the following do's and don'ts.

Do order unsweetened oatmeal topped with berries or choose egg-white omelets stuffed with various veggies and whole-wheat toast. You can also enjoy unsweetened cereals with skim milk, Canadian bacon, and fresh fruit. Other healthy alternatives are English muffins with tomato and melted cheese, or a scooped-out bagel with light cream cheese, tomato, and lox. To wash it all down, opt for skim milk or a cup of green tea. Or, enjoy a skim latte.

Don't make it a habit to start your day with an unhealthy catastrophe, such as scram-bled eggs, bacon, sausage, hash browns, cheese omelets, biscuits, croissants, bagels with butter, large cake-like muffins, donuts, pancakes and waffles smothered in butter and syrup, deep-fried French toast, or steak and eggs.

The Least You Need to Know

- Once considered a luxury, dining out has become commonplace for most all Americans today.

- Remember that "eating out" does not mean "pigging out." Don't give yourself license to overeat just because you are in a restaurant. Eat slowly and selectively, and stop when you are comfortably full.

- With the proper planning, nutrition know-how, and willingness to compromise, you can fit almost any ethnic restaurant into a healthy low-fat eating plan.

- Become a dining detective and examine the menu carefully. Look for lean cuts of meat, poultry, and fish that have been prepared by low-fat cooking methods. Ask your waiter about the type of sauce that accompanies your meal. If salt is an issue, watch out for high-sodium marinades.

Chapter 13

Trimming Down the Holidays

In This Chapter

- ◆ Slicing fat and calories out of your holiday season

- ◆ Healthy menu alternatives for each major holiday

- ◆ Some great-tasting recipes

We all love holidays. There are family, friends, gifts, days off from work, and more delicious treats than we know what to do with. Doesn't it seem like we can eat whatever we want—with no consequences in the morning?

Unfortunately, overindulging leaves most of us feeling heavy, sluggish—and guilty. And suddenly you don't fit into your pants. The fact is, holidays are hard when it comes to making smart food choices, but there are ways to make it work.

Staying on Track on Holidays

No matter how much you expect to eat at Grandma's, stick with your regular meals. Skipping breakfast and barely eating lunch will only make you more ravenous and prone to overeating at a holiday party. Just because your holiday agenda involves sitting around, telling stories, and eating doesn't mean you have to stop your regular exercise routine. The more active you are around the holiday season, the better you'll feel, and hence, you'll be more likely to feed your body in a healthy manner. What's more, exercise doesn't have to mean hitting a gym: you can do little things such as parking your car a little further from your destination, taking the stairs instead of the elevator, or taking a quick walk around the block.

It's also important to be selective with your food choices. Survey the spread *before* you dive in and eat everything. Figure out what you really want, and then monitor everything else so you can balance it out. Don't deprive yourself! If you want a piece of cake, have some, but remember that quality is more important than quantity.

Follow these simple holiday menus to help cut your calories and fat intake down from one holiday to the next. Keep in mind that the nutritional info was based on real-life, *generous* holiday portions.

Easter

The spirit of Easter is all about new beginnings. It's the onset of spring; there are flowers blooming and birds returning. As the days start to get longer and the sunshine gets warmer, it's time to shed those winter doldrums, peel off those big winter sweaters, and add some spring to your step—and your meal.

Your Easter meal doesn't have to be heavy and filling; it can be light and airy, like the holiday. Just revamp your traditional menu, and lose half the calories and one third of the fat. Besides, it'll leave a little room for those sweet marshmallow chicks.

Traditional Meal
Poached salmon with cucumber dill sauce
Baked ham with pineapple, drenched in syrup
Potato and cheese gratin
Peas with black olives and hard-boiled eggs
Buttery biscuits
Vanilla ice cream
Easter candy

Nutrition Information
Calories: 1,532
Total fat: 77 grams
Saturated fat: 37 grams
Cholesterol: 366 mg
Sodium: 1,381 mg
Dietary fiber: 9 grams
Protein: 69 grams

Healthier Meal

Poached salmon with honey mustard dill sauce

Baked ham with fresh pineapple

Wild rice salad with chopped dried fruit

Asparagus with shallot vinaigrette

Whole-grain bread

Coconut sorbet

Chocolate fondue (small bowl of chocolate syrup or any other ice cream topping
with strawberries, orange slices, and banana chunks for dipping)

Nutrition Information

Calories: 867

Total fat: 27 grams

Saturated fat: 7 grams

Cholesterol: 138 mg

Sodium: 523 mg

Dietary fiber: 11 grams

Protein: 60 grams

Passover

One of the oldest and most continuously celebrated holidays, Passover commemo-
rates the Jewish exodus from Egypt after years of suffering and slavery. It is the tradition of the Jewish people to remember their ancestors with a big meal! Well, with a
few minor changes to the menu, you can still indulge in Passover with all the taste
and a lot less fat and calories. What's more, the extra fiber in the healthier version can
help to declog all of that matzo meal.

Traditional Meal

Matzo ball soup

Gefilte fish

Brisket

Roast chicken

Potato kugel

Chopped broccoli casserole

Tzimmis

Chocolate Passover Cake

Macaroons

Nutrition Information
Calories: 2,086
Total fat: 101 grams
Saturated fat: 35 grams
Cholesterol: 734 mg
Sodium: 1,768 mg
Dietary fiber: 17 grams
Protein: 116 grams

Healthier Meal
Matzo ball soup (Substitute kosher olive oil for chicken fat and use seltzer instead of liquid to get your matzo balls fluffy.)
Gefilte fish on green salad with lemon and olive oil vinaigrette (Use salmon instead of white fish; it's a great source of omega-3 fatty acids.)
Rock Cornish game hens stuffed with dried fruit and tomatoes
Sweet potato and carrot tzimmis
Artichokes stuffed with herbed matzo
Large fruit salad
Chocolate Passover Cake

Nutrition Information
Calories: 1,575
Total fat: 56 grams
Saturated fat: 11 grams
Cholesterol: 454 mg
Sodium: 1,715 mg
Dietary fiber: 27 grams
Protein: 84 grams

Fourth of July

Think fun-filled barbecues with your friends and busting out your summer attire. It's about soaking up the sun and being comfortable in your body, not feeling bloated and so heavy that you'd rather cover up and stay inside. The best way to keep yourself looking good and feeling groovy is to cut down on those heavy, high-fat foods and splurge on the fresh fruits and veggies that are in season. The traditional menu has a whopping 2,099 calories and 116 grams of fat, but the healthier menu has 985 fewer calories and 40 percent of the fat—so you can say good-bye to that beer gut and greet some great abs without feeling the least bit deprived.

Traditional Meal
Grilled hamburgers and hot dogs on buns
Cold fried chicken
Potato salad
Macaroni salad
Cole slaw
Potato chips
Brownies
Watermelon
Ice cream bars

Nutrition Information
Calories: 2,099
Total fat: 116 grams
Saturated fat: 40 grams
Cholesterol: 381 mg
Sodium: 3,741 mg
Dietary fiber: 10 grams
Protein: 72 grams

Healthier Meal
Turkey or veggie burgers on buns
Grilled tuna, salmon, or chicken filets
Pasta salad with tomato basil vinaigrette
Grilled vegetables
Health salad
Baked potato chips
Low-fat brownies
Watermelon
Frozen fruit pops

Nutrition Information
Calories: 1,411
Total fat: 55 grams
Saturated fat: 10 grams
Cholesterol: 110 mg
Sodium: 1,640 mg
Dietary fiber: 14 grams
Protein: 47 grams

Thanksgiving

It's supposed to be about giving thanks and feeling grateful for all the positive things in your life. But come on, we know it's really about the fine art of American gluttony: mounds of turkey, rich gravy, starchy stuffing, cranberry sauce, four kinds of potatoes, veggies soaked in butter and oil, pumpkin pie, apple pie, and going in for round two a few hours after your stomach finally settles. Then, there are all those leftovers: Thanksgiving eating goes on for days!

Keep your family traditions and indulge. If you make minor alterations in your meal, you'll feel a whole lot better in the morning—and maybe even have the energy to make it outside for your own game of football instead of just watching it on the tube.

Traditional Meal
Roast turkey
Stuffing with onions and sausage
Yams with marshmallows
Green bean casserole
Creamed onions
Cranberry jelly
Vanilla ice cream
Pumpkin pie

Nutrition Information
Calories: 1,713
Total fat: 59 grams
Saturated fat: 21 grams
Cholesterol: 246 mg
Sodium: 2,904 mg
Dietary fiber: 13 grams
Protein: 79 grams

Healthier Meal
Roast turkey (no skin)
Cornbread stuffing with apples, celery, and cranberries
Baked yams
Mashed potatoes made with buttermilk and roasted garlic
Roasted vegetables (drizzled with olive oil)
Cranberry chutney
Cinnamon frozen yogurt
Pumpkin chiffon pie

Nutrition Information
Calories: 1,090
Total fat: 39 grams
Saturated fat: 9 grams
Cholesterol: 143 mg
Sodium: 1,238 mg
Dietary fiber: 18 grams
Protein: 72 grams

With Thanksgiving leftovers coming out of your ears, here are some creative ways to have seconds and thirds:

Ready-Made Menu

- Turkey and cranberry risotto

- Turkey and roasted vegetables stuffed in a pita

- Turkey and rice soup

Hanukkah

For the kids, the Festival of Lights is all about the presents, but for us adults, it seems to be all about the scrumptiously fried food (and of course, commemorating the Maccabean victory over Antiochus of Syria and how the Maccabees created a miracle and lit the menorah with a drop of oil that lasted for eight long nights). Today, we're a lot more nutritionally enlightened; we realize that fried foods aren't a good base for any meal, holiday or not. With a few minor adjustments to the traditional menu, you can take the healthy route, cutting 644 calories and your fat in half, and still get your potato latkes. (A Hanukkah without them would be sacrilegious, wouldn't it?)

Traditional Meal
Chicken soup
Brisket
Potato latkes
Applesauce
Green salad with vinaigrette
Jelly donuts
Hanukkah gelt

Nutrition Information
Calories: 2,038
Total fat: 105 grams
Saturated fat: 27 grams
Cholesterol: 520 mg
Sodium: 2,896 mg
Dietary fiber: 8 grams
Protein: 114 grams

Healthier Meal
Chicken soup
Roast chicken breast, no skin
Potato latkes
Applesauce
Green salad with vinaigrette
Fresh fruit salad
Apple Streusel Pot Pie (see recipe)

Nutrition Information
Calories: 1,393
Total fat: 53 grams
Saturated fat: 11 grams
Cholesterol: 322 mg
Sodium: 1,959 mg
Dietary fiber: 13 grams
Protein: 76 grams

Low-Fat Apple Streusel Pot Pie

Honey

Canola oil

8 sheets phyllo dough

8 cups apple, sliced

½ cup golden raisins

½ tsp. nutmeg

1 tsp. cinnamon, ground

½ cup brown sugar, packed

¼ tsp. lemon juice

½ tsp. vanilla extract

1½ TB. cornstarch

Serves six
Calories/serving: 300

In a small bowl, combine equal parts honey and canola oil. Remove 4 sheets of phyllo dough, not separating leaves. Place on even surface and carve outline of serving bowl with a paring knife. Remove phyllo round to a nonstick sheet pan and brush the top with oil/honey mixture. Place in the oven and bake about 10 minutes at 350° F. (Do not let rounds get too dark.) Remove from the oven, gently flip, and brush the dry side with oil/honey mixture. Bake 2 more minutes and remove from the oven.

In a large bowl, combine apple slices, raisins, spices, brown sugar, lemon juice, vanilla, and 1 TB. canola oil. Mix well. Put in saucepan and cook over low heat, covered, for 20 minutes or until apples are soft.

Remove apples with slotted spoon and place in serving bowls. Whisk cornstarch into remaining liquid and bring to a boil. Add thickened liquid to apple mixture in bowls. Top with phyllo round and let it cool before serving.

Kwanzaa

Kwanzaa, from the African language Kiswahili, means first fruits of the harvest—contrary to how we celebrate this holiday, with foods that are high in fat and low in fruit content. As this is a relatively new holiday, now is the time to start some healthy traditions and indulge in a festive meal (with 400 fewer calories and 35 percent of the fat) that's good for you, too.

Traditional Meal
Peanut soup
Sweet potato fritters
Southern fried okra
Kale with bacon
Black-eyed peas with ham
Jerk chicken
Sweet potato pie
Benne cakes

Nutrition Information
Calories: 1,979
Total fat: 90 grams
Saturated fat: 26 grams
Cholesterol: 349 mg
Sodium: 3,933 mg
Dietary fiber: 28 grams
Protein: 101 grams

Healthier Meal
African Tomato-Avocado Soup (see recipe)
Winter squash and yams
Kale with garlic
Black-eyed peas with ham
Jerk chicken
Sweet Potato Soufflé (see recipe)
Benne cakes

Nutrition Information
Calories: 1,568
Total fat: 59 grams
Saturated fat: 18 grams
Cholesterol: 215 mg
Sodium: 2,795 mg
Dietary fiber: 28 grams
Protein: 95 grams

African Tomato-Avocado Soup

1 cup buttermilk

2 cups V8 Bloody Mary mix

2 cups chopped tomatoes

1 whole Haas avocado, peeled and pitted

½ cup cilantro leaves

½ cup low-fat plain yogurt

1 TB. lime juice

Serves six
Calories/servings: 111

In a saucepan, combine buttermilk, Bloody Mary mix, and chopped tomatoes. Heat gently; do not boil.

In a small food processor or in a bowl with a fork, mash avocado, cilantro, yogurt, and lime juice.

Serve soup in individual bowls, topped with a tablespoon of avocado mix.

Sweet Potato Soufflé

2 TB. white granulated sugar

1 cup sweet potato, canned

1 tsp. nutmeg, ground

1 tsp. cinnamon, ground

2 TB. lemon juice

5 egg whites, raw

½ tsp. cream of tartar

Serves four
Calories/serving: 125

Preheat oven to 400∞. Spray four 1-cup ramekins with spray cooking oil, sprinkle with sugar, and set aside.

Combine sweet potatoes, nutmeg, cinnamon, and lemon juice. Set aside.

Beat egg whites with cream of tartar until soft peaks form. Slowly add sugar and continue beating until stiff peaks form.

Slowly fold whites into sweet potato mixture. Spoon mixture into ramekins and place on sheet pan. Bake 10–12 minutes. Serve immediately.

Christmas

With homemade Christmas cookies, creamy veggie dishes, and what always seems like 24 hours of nibbling, you'll be praying to open up boxes of oversized sweaters from under the tree. What better way to hide all the pounds we tend to pack on during the chilly season of decked halls and tons of parties? Well, you can still splurge on warm, rich comfort foods that are good for the soul, but if you lighten up your menu just a tad, you'll be indulging in yummy eats that are good for the arteries, too. See, it can still look a lot like Christmas with almost half the calories and 20 percent of the fat!

Traditional Meal
Oyster stew
Roast beef with gravy
Yorkshire pudding
Oven-roasted potatoes
Creamed spinach
Chocolate mousse
Christmas cookies

Nutrition Information
Calories: 1,915
Total fat: 122 grams
Saturated fat: 56 grams
Cholesterol: 717 mg
Sodium: 2,516 mg
Dietary fiber: 7 grams
Protein: 107 grams

Healthier Meal
Manhattan oyster chowder
Beef tenderloin with horseradish yogurt sauce
Potato and Caramelized Onion Gratin (see recipe)
French green beans, tied with leek bow
Chocolate angel food cake
Peppermint frozen yogurt

Nutrition Information
Calories: 1,068
Total fat: 25 grams
Saturated fat: 6 grams
Cholesterol: 130 mg
Sodium: 1,620 mg
Dietary fiber: 10 grams
Protein: 66 grams

Potato and Onion Gratin

4 cups onion, sliced

1 TB. canola oil

1 TB. balsamic vinegar

4–5 large Idaho potatoes

1 tsp. table salt

1 tsp. mixed dried herbs

3 TB. sun-dried tomatoes, chopped

¾ cup fat-free chicken broth

Serves eight
Calories/serving: 134

Preheat oven to 350°. Caramelize onions: In a large nonstick sauté pan, heat oil and add onions. Cook over medium heat, stirring frequently, for about ¹/₂ hour or until onions are very soft and beginning to brown. Add 1 tablespoon balsamic vinegar and cook for another few minutes. Set aside.

Slice potatoes ¹/₄-inch thick and put in a large bowl with 1 teaspoon salt and 1 teaspoon mixed dried herbs. Do not rinse or soak potatoes in water.

In a casserole dish, sprinkle ¹/₃ of the caramelized onions and ¹/₃ of sun-dried tomatoes on the bottom of the pan. Shingle ¹/₃ of potatoes on top of that and then repeat this process two more times. Add ¾ cup chicken broth and cover with foil.

Bake for 1 hour, remove foil, and bake for 15 more minutes.

The Least You Need to Know

- The holidays are about celebration and rejoicing—not overeating and gaining weight.

- Remember to exercise, eat something before going to a party, and eat smaller portions of the higher-fat entrees and desserts.

- Try some of my menu ideas and recipes at your next holiday gathering. You and your family will enjoy the tradition with a lot less fat and fewer calories.

Part 3

The ABCs of Exercise

Exercise goes hand in hand with eating well. It can improve your balance and coordination, help prevent many diseases, and enable you to look and feel terrific. And it doesn't have to cost a thing … what a bargain!

This section provides you with the inspiration and know-how to get you moving and *keep* you moving. It's basically a crash course on becoming physically fit. In the following chapters, you'll find vital information on how to get started on an exercise program that's right for *you*. From strengthening your heart and lungs through aerobic exercise, to building muscle through weight-training—it's all in here. In addition, you'll learn how to properly fuel your body—whether for casual exercise or competitive sport.

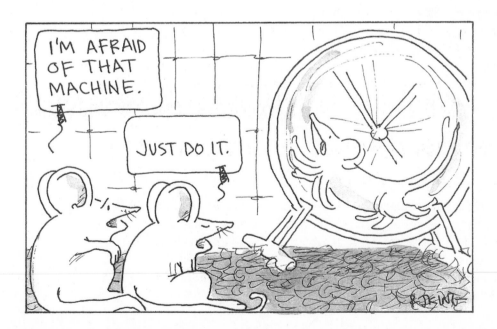

Chapter 14

Getting Physical

In This Chapter

- ◆ All the great stuff exercise can do for you
- ◆ How to properly warm up, cool down, and stretch
- ◆ All about aerobic exercise
- ◆ Getting started on a weight-training program
- ◆ Some great ideas for your personal workout plan

Throughout history, health professionals have promoted the notion that folks who regularly exercise have better overall health, improved physical functioning, and increased longevity. Even dating back to 400 B.C.E., the Greek physician Hippocrates (known as the father of medicine) addressed exercise in one of his works by writing, "Eating alone will not keep a man well; he must also take exercise." Same thought, different century!

What is exercise anyway? Exercise is formally defined as physical activity that is planned, structured, and repetitive—with the objective of improving or maintaining a level of physical fitness. Simply stated, *exercise whips your body into shape*. Put down the TV remote and say "adios" to the sofa; this chapter offers concrete guidelines and information on becoming physically active.

Of course, if you have any medical conditions, check with your physician before plunging full-force into any type of exercise program.

Why Bother Exercising?

Simply put, exercise …

♦ Makes you feel better physically.

♦ Improves self-esteem and provides a more positive mental outlook.

♦ Makes you look better and helps to control your weight.

♦ Increases your balance, coordination, and agility.

♦ Helps prevent osteoporosis, cardiovascular disease, and non–insulin-dependent diabetes.

♦ Makes you feel invigorated and more energetic.

♦ Strengthens bones and muscle, giving you the functional strength for everyday living.

Before you begin, there are some things to consider:

♦ **Have realistic expectations.** For all you beginners, don't expect to turn into Arnold Schwarzenegger or Cindy Crawford overnight. (The majority of us never will.) It's great to have a hero, but understand that people come in all shapes and sizes, and genetics plays a major role in your body makeup and proportion. Rule #1: exercise is about looking and feeling *your* best—not somebody else's best.

♦ **Set reasonable goals for yourself.** Plan reachable short-term goals each week that will not leave you overwhelmed or set you up for failure. An example of a reasonable goal is: "I will work out four days this week and eliminate all high-fat desserts."

Not a reasonable goal: "I will work out two hours every day and lose 10 pounds in three weeks."

♦ **Work exercise conveniently into your day.** You know the story: unless exercise sessions are planned during realistic time slots, your "workouts" ain't gonna "work out." Take into consideration your schedule. Are you a morning person or a night owl? Some people are lucky enough to have leisurely lunch breaks and can sneak in a quickie during their day.

♦ **Rise and shine.** Studies show that exercisers who work out in the morning are 50 percent more likely to stick with it. Basically, get it out of the way before the day wipes you out. (What's more, it can also save you an extra shower later.) If you have the capacity to endure a grueling day at the office and then *shake, rattle, and roll* in the gym—more power to you.

♦ **Keep it short and sweet.** Most people have hectic lifestyles and cannot afford to dedicate hours each day to the gym. And they shouldn't! Each workout should be short and efficient. The consistency of regular physical activity is as important as duration and intensity. Without any of these three elements, exercise is simply not effective. Furthermore, people who get carried away usually wind up with injuries or exercise burnout.

What's an Appropriate Exercise Program?

An effective exercise program has three main parts: the before, the middle, and the after. The before includes a brief warm-up; the middle, or bulk of the workout, involves aerobic activity plus weight conditioning; and the after consists of a cool-down and stretch. Let's take a closer look at each.

Warming Up

A warm-up literally *warms up* the body. By increasing your internal temperature and preparing muscles for the activity ahead, a proper warm-up can help prevent injury to muscles, joints, and connective tissue. Further, a quick 5–10 minute warm-up will increase the blood flow to the primary muscle groups so that they are ready to go.

When you think of a warm-up, do you visualize yourself sitting in a straddle position on the floor, moaning loudly while reaching for your left toe (which feels like it's somewhere south of the equator)? You're not alone. But contrary to what most people think, a warm-up doesn't necessarily involve stretching exercises. Actually, 5 to10 minutes of light aerobic activity is an effective warm-up (such as biking, rowing, walking, or even marching in place). More specifically, warm up with a lighter version of the exercise you will be engaging in.

For instance, runners can start with a 5–10 minute brisk walk, and swimmers can warm up with a couple of easy, slow laps in the pool. Even take a 5–10 minute walk on a treadmill (and include arm circles) before hitting the weight room.

> **Nutri-Speak**
>
> **Aerobics,** which is also known as *cardio,* are the exercises in which your muscles require an increased supply of oxygen.

The Cardiovascular Workout: Challenge Your Heart and Lungs

What are aerobics? If you think that aerobics are just jumping around to bad disco music, dust off your sneaks; you're way behind the times. The term *aerobic* literally means "with air." Therefore, the exercises in which your muscles require an increased supply of air (more specifically, the *oxygen* within air) are termed aerobic. Aerobic activity is also known as cardiovascular activity (or cardio) because it most definitely challenges your heart and lungs. Think about this: When you jog, the large muscles of your lower body are continuously working over an extended period of time and therefore require more than their usual supply of oxygen. Because your heart and lungs are the key players in retrieving and circulating oxygen, they go into overdrive to increase oxygen delivery. Therefore, in addition to working out the large exterior muscles, aerobic activity also provides one heck of a workout for your heart and lungs.

Normally, aerobic exercise should last 20 to 60 minutes, depending upon how much time you have and how fit you are. People who are fit can work longer and harder than those who are not, simply because they can handle the increased demand for oxygen. For all you beginners, don't let a few discouraging workouts get you down. Doing aerobics is like playing the piano; the more you practice, the better you get.

Walking briskly, biking, jogging, stair-climbing, cross-country skiing, jumping rope, and, yes, aerobic dance are all examples of aerobic activity. Generally speaking, anything involving weights and machines or a fair amount of standing in place is *not* considered aerobic activity.

What can aerobics do for you?

♦ Burn calories and help with weight management. (Most people are happy to hear that one.)

♦ Improve the functioning of your heart and lungs, therefore making you less likely to suffer from serious problems involving these key organs.

♦ Improve your circulation.

♦ Improve your sleep patterns.

♦ Improve your state of mind.

♦ Intense aerobic activity can release endorphins, in other words, the "natural" or "runner's" high—legal in all states, with no nasty side effects the day after.

How Long, How Much, How Hard?

The following guidelines have been set by the American College of Sports Medicine:

- ◆ **How long:** 20–60 minutes of aerobic activity per session

- ◆ **How much:** 3–5 times per week

- ◆ **How hard:** Low-to-moderate intensity or 60–90 percent of your maximum heart rate

Beginners should start with a modest game plan. In fact, beginners need to shoot for 40 percent of their maximum heart rate and work up from there. As you improve, you can do more activity by going longer, harder, or more frequently. But keep in mind that you should only increase the length, frequency, and intensity one at a time. Increasing all three at once is the perfect recipe for injuries and exercise burnout.

Cooling Down

The goal of a cool-down is to gradually stop the activity, allowing your heart rate, blood pressure, and body temperature to slowly return to normal. Think about how rapidly your heart is pounding and blood is pumping following an intense bout of exercise—*not* a good time to hit the shower. In fact, stopping an intense workout abruptly is a sure way to get dizzy and feel terrible after a workout. Furthermore, cooling down properly can help prevent serious health risks for older or out-of-shape participants. Take an extra 5–10 minutes and slowly reduce the intensity of the exercise you've been working on. Your body will thank you.

Stretching

Stretching is definitely important for maintaining and increasing flexibility, which in turn makes it easier for you to move around. The best time to stretch is when your body is warm, either after you have done a light aerobic warm-up or, more preferably, at the end of your workout following a cool-down period. Proper stretching allows the muscles to relax and lengthen, and it can even help alleviate some built-up body tension. What's more, it might also aid in the removal of waste products, such as lactic acid. This can prevent injury and improve muscle tone.

Some general stretching guidelines include

◆ Always get your blood pumping and body warmed up before you stretch.

◆ Stretch *all* your major muscle groups (not just the ones you think were used).

◆ Hold each stretch for at least 15 seconds; never bounce. You can still feel a good stretch with slightly bent knees.

◆ Only stretch to the point of mild tension, not agonizing pain!

◆ Ask a qualified trainer to show you the correct stretching techniques; there's a lot more to it than touching your toes.

Are You Working Hard Enough?

Let's check it out. A couple of easy ways to tell whether you are working hard enough during an aerobic workout include taking your heart rate (the number of times your heart beats per minute) and the talk test.

Follow this mathematical equation to check whether you are working in your training zone (also called the target heart-rate zone). Generally, your training heart rate falls between 60 and 90 percent of your *maximum heart rate* (the maximum times your heart can beat in one minute). Although this formula only provides an estimate, it's a great indication of whether you are working too hard or not hard enough:

> **Training heart rate formula: (220 – your age) × .60 and .90**

Let's break it up and take it step by step:

Step 1	Calculate your estimated maximum heart rate (220 – your age).
Step 2	Multiply your maximum heart rate × .60 for lower range.
Step 3	Multiply your maximum heart rate × .90 for upper range.

Here's the training zone for a 35-year-old man:

$(220 - 35) \times .60 = 111$	Lower range
$(220 - 35) \times .90 = 167$	Upper range

Therefore, his target zone would range between 111–167 beats per minute. This means if it's lower than 111, he needs to step on the accelerator, and if it's more than 167, he needs to slightly ease up.

Test Your Heart Rate and Your Math Skills

Now that you know the math, take some time during your workout and give it a whirl. Place two fingers (your pointer and middle finger) on the inside of your wrist (just to the thumb side of the large cords you feel) or on your neck (below and off to the side of your chin). If you can't find your pulse, ask for assistance. (Don't worry, you're alive.) Once you locate it, look at the second hand of your watch or a clock and count the beats in a 15-second span; then, multiply that number by four. That's your working heart rate. Just make sure it falls within the range you've calculated as your training zone—not slower, not faster.

Try the "Talk" Test

Here's a *much* easier way to tell whether you're working at an appropriate level. Can you comfortably carry on a conversation while exercising? If the answer is yes, you're doing fine. If you're so out of breath that you can't say, "Yippee! I'm rich," when someone announces you've won the lottery, you need to slow down. On the other hand, if you can belt out the chorus to "YMCA" by the Village People, you'd better step it up. In the final analysis, you should feel like you're working, but not to the point of a cardiac explosion.

Hit the Weights and "Pump Some Iron"

Let's clear something up: Weight training is *not* the same as body building. Weight training is about improving muscle strength and muscle tone. For men, who have naturally higher levels of testosterone, it usually does mean an increase in muscle size, called *hypertrophy*. On the other hand, women tend to increase the tone without significantly increasing the muscle size.

Typically, muscle conditioning uses dumb-bells and barbells (called free weights) and various types of weight machines (usually referred to by brand names such as Cybex and Nautilus).

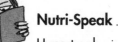

Nutri-Speak

Hypertrophy is an increase in muscle size.

What can weight training do for you?

◆ Stronger muscles can improve your posture and help keep your body in balance.

◆ Stronger muscles can prevent injuries.

◆ Weight training helps to tone, lift, firm, and shape your body.

- Stronger muscles can help with your everyday activities, such as lugging shopping bags, moving furniture, lifting kids and strollers, and so on.

- Weight training can help prevent osteoporosis.

- Weight training can help to reshape problem areas, such as your sagging arms and your butt. Unfortunately, there is no such thing as "spot reducing"— zapping off fat from specific body parts. But don't fret, because the combination of a low-fat diet and aerobic activity burns total fat from all over your body, and chances are it will eventually come off your personal pudge.

- Weight training can increase your lean body mass and therefore increase your metabolism.

Your Weekly Weight-Training Routine

Your weekly schedule is just as important as the exercises themselves. Set aside time for two to three muscle-conditioning workouts per week, targeting all of your major muscle groups. A major warning here is *not* to work the same muscles on consecutive days. Leave a day of rest in between to allow all those important biological changes to take place. In fact, resting is just as important as the workout itself. For instance, if you'd like to work all of your muscle groups on the same day, an effective schedule is Monday/Thursday/Saturday.

Another option is doing split routines. In this case, you can lift more often simply because you split up the muscles being worked over the week. In other words, train your upper body one day and your lower body the next. For those truly gung-ho types, train your chest, triceps, and shoulders on one day and your legs, back, and biceps on the next. Go ahead and plug in your abdominal exercises whichever day you like. Chest and triceps are involved in pushing-type activities, and your back and biceps are involved in pulling activities; therefore, they should be worked in pairs if you want to split up the upper-body workouts. One reason people prefer a split-routine workout is that they can devote more energy to the muscles worked on a particular day.

Food for Thought

When training with weights, your three sets should be 6–15 repetitions of 70–90 percent of the maximum weight you can lift.

Cardio and Weight Training: The Perfect Combination

Some people ask, "Which is more important, cardio or weight work?" The answer is both. You need the combination of aerobic and weight training for overall fitness. As one of my clients once said, "Weights make it hard; cardio gets rid of the lard."

Q & A
Cardio or muscle conditioning: which comes first?
If you want to do cardio and weights on the same day, that's fine. It's also fine to alternate days, whichever you fancy. There is not, as of yet, a definite rule on which you should do first—merely personal preference. Some folks like to be good and sweaty before they hit the weights, whereas others prefer to get the weight training out of the way and then loosen up with cardio afterwards. The choice is yours.

Top-Five Exercise Myths

This list will help to debunk the common misconceptions floating around the gym. Read on and learn the whole truth.

1. **No pain, no gain.** Bogus statement! It is true that both weight training and cardiovascular exercise usually involve *some* type of minor discomfort, such as feelings of slight burning or fatigue and moderate to heavy breathing. However, pain is entirely different. If you feel pain when you work out (particularly joint pain), you're doing something wrong. Stop exercising immediately, and have it checked by your physician. Pushing through agony can lead to serious trouble. If it checks out okay, seek the assistance of a qualified trainer; something is probably wrong with your exercise program or technique.

2. **Eating extra protein builds muscle.** We already went over this one in the protein chapter, but allow me to drive the point home. The increase in muscle size, known as hypertrophy, has nothing to do with eating a lot of protein. Muscles get bigger when you overload them via weight training—*not* by eating kilos of tuna. The recommended daily amounts for protein remains about .36 to .8 per pound depending on your activity level.

3. **Weight training will give you bulky muscles.** After reading that weight training causes muscles to increase in size, it's no wonder some women are hesitant to lift weights. Fear not: your lower testosterone levels cause increases in

strength and tone without all that increase in size. Incidentally, even men have to have a genetic predisposition to getting bigger. Some guys can cut and bulk quickly, whereas others work their tails off without much visible result. Stick with a moderate weight-training program, and you'll be fine.

4. **You only burn fat working cardio at a slower pace.** This myth got a lot of play back in the '80s, with exercise classes actually slowing down the pace to "burn more fat." In terms of weight loss, that's just not the case. The crucial factor for losing weight is the total amount of calories burned, and it doesn't matter whether it comes from carbs, protein, or fat. For instance, a 130-pound woman doing a high-intensity workout (such as jogging) for 30 minutes will burn approximately 350 calories; that same woman will only burn 140 calories at a low-intensity workout (such as walking).

   What if you're just starting out and can't sustain a fast pace for more than 5 to 10 minutes? In that case, you're certainly better off doing something at a slower pace for a longer length of time. Again, the reason is that you'll burn more total calories in the end.

5. **Sit-ups can burn fat off your waist.** Not a chance! Remember, there is no such thing as spot reducing or burning the fat off a particular body part. Fat comes off the body as a whole (through aerobic activity and proper nutrition) and, unfortunately, not always in the places you want it to come from first (such as "the incredible shrinking bra"). You can buy every tummy-tucker and blubber-blaster on the market. Abdominal-toning exercises *only* strengthen the tissue underneath; they don't zap off that mid-section fat (contrary to what they might say). Look on the bright side: below all the flub, you probably have some dynamite muscles—something to look forward to when you lose that outer layer.

How to Get Started: Your Personal Plan of Attack

Before embarking on an exercise program, figure out what type of plan will best fit your personality and schedule. Take a paper and pen and answer the following questions:

1. What type of activities do you enjoy doing?

2. What are your time restraints?

3. Are you a morning person or a night owl?

4. Do you like to work out alone or with people?

5. Do you prefer the indoors or outdoors?

6. What's the weather like in your neck of the woods?

7. Do you want to travel to a facility, or does the privacy of your own home sound more appealing?

8. What is within your budget?

A Million Things You Can Do to Stay in Shape

Now that you've answered the previous questions, you should have a pretty good idea of your personal preferences and limitations. Read through the possible exercise options and determine which ones are feasible. Be sure to focus on both categories: aerobic (3–5 times per week) and muscle conditioning (2–3 times per week). Remember, nothing is set in stone; mix and match often to avoid getting bored or burnt out.

Aerobic Suggestions

Activity	Where You Can Do It
Walking	Outside or treadmill (gym or at home)
Running	Outside or treadmill (gym or at home)
Biking	Outside or stationary bike (gym or at home)
Swimming	Outside or indoor pool at the gym
Skating	Outside or indoor rink
Stair climbing	Indoor staircase or stair-climbing machine (gym or at home)
Cross-country skiing	Outside or machine (home or gym)
Rowing	Outside or rowing machine (gym or home)
Aerobic classes	At the gym or at home (using videos)

Muscle Conditioning Suggestions

Activity	Where You Can Do It
Body sculpting	Classes in the gym or videos at home
Circuit/interval workouts	Classes in the gym or videos at home
Weight training	Gym or home equipment
Weight machines	Gym or home equipment
Free weights	Gym or home equipment

When Formal Exercise Is Just Not Your Thang!

Not into planned sweat? Only read this far to humor yourself? Well, you're not hopeless yet; you can still cash in on some of the benefits. In fact, everyday activities can also substantially benefit your health, even if they are done intermittently throughout the day. For example, take the stairs instead of the elevator (you live on the twenty-fifth floor—great!), walk short distances instead of driving the car, join your kids in a game of tag, do some gardening, rake the leaves, shovel the snow, and let's not forget how physical housecleaning can be. Whatever your style, formal exercise or increasing plain old daily activity, make your only life a healthy and active one.

Whether you are 18, 50, or 70 years old, invest the time to become more physically active. Regular exercise will help you to feel your best and keep you fit—while increasing bone strength, reducing your risk of disease, and helping to maintain an ideal body weight. Keep in mind, that the perfect complement to properly fueling your body is *moving* your body.

Take a look at the amount of calories you can burn doing 30 minutes of everyday chores:

Activity	130-Pound Person	183-Pound Person
Car washing	123	171
Housecleaning	111	153
Raking leaves	96	135
Shoveling snow	150	213
Wallpapering	84	120
Weeding	96	135
Window cleaning	105	147

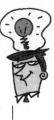

Food for Thought

Pushing your body more often than the experts recommend (unless you are in an athletic training program) can and usually does lead to injuries from over-used muscles, tendons, and joints. What's more, varying your exercise intensity and duration is also important to prevent overtraining. For example, some days you should work hard and long, but on other days make it short and sweet. Pay attention to your body's cues and make exercise an enjoyable part of your life.

The Least You Need to Know

◆ Exercise reduces your risk for certain diseases, helps you control your weight, provides you with strength and vigor for everyday activities, and makes you feel great, both mentally and physically.

◆ The important parts of an exercise program include the warm-up, aerobic activity and weight training, cool-down, and total-body stretch.

◆ Experts recommend aerobic activity 3 to 5 days each week for 20 to 60 minute sessions at a low to moderate intensity.

◆ Don't forget about your muscles! A proper weight-training program 2–3 times per week can increase your strength, reduce the risk of osteoporosis, enhance your posture, and help to reshape your body.

◆ Select activities that complement your personality and time schedule, and vary your routine often to avoid exercise burnout.

The Gym Scene

In This Chapter

- Acquainting yourself with the health-club scene
- Translating gym jargon into English
- Popular exercise equipment for cardio and weight training
- Your muscles and some exercises to work 'em out

Now that your body is rarin' to go, you might want to join a local health club. Be sure to prepare yourself for more than a physical experience: between the language barrier, high-tech equipment, scantily clad women, and members strolling around with biceps bigger than their heads, going to the gym can feel like traveling to a foreign land or outer space. But don't be intimidated. The gym scene can be terrific. Where else can you have such a tremendous variety of workout choices? There's always someone available for instruction, encouragement, and motivation. Check out the health clubs in your area and browse through the basics before hitting the locker room.

Gym Jargon 101

Here's the gym terminology you'll need to hang with the muscle-heads; it's sure to make your conversations with the locals a bit easier:

- **Reps.** Short for repetitions, meaning the number of times you do an exercise. Usually 6–15 reps make a set.

- **Sets.** A group of repetitions. Usually you do 1–3 sets per exercise. (A man working on bicep curls might do 3 sets of 10 reps. This translates to 3 full rounds of 10 bicep curls each.)

- **"He's/she's ripped."** A major compliment about a guy or gal's defined physique.

- **"You've really got great definition in your …"** A tired but effective gym come-on. Sort of gym slang for "wow" (drool, drool).

- **Being cut.** Having well-defined muscles.

- **Being pumped.** A temporary increase in the size of a muscle due to increased blood flow during exercise.

- **"Can I work in?"** Someone wants to use the weight machine you are using, and she is asking whether she can alternate sets with you. Because the gym is usually crowded, it's normal practice to share equipment. For example, you do a set of 8 reps, then someone else changes the weight to do a set, then you again, and so on. This only makes sense when you have a bunch more to go. If you only have one more set left, reply, "This is my last set"—gym slang for "Hold your horses, fella, I'm almost done."

- **"How many more sets do you have here?"** Someone is getting antsy to use the weight machine and doesn't particularly want to "work in" with you. This is a polite way of saying, "Are you planning on staying here all day? Perhaps I could order you a cappuccino."

- **"Can I get a spot?"** Basically, someone is asking you to help him do an exercise with an amount of weight he is nervous about. Politely pass on this one if you don't know how to spot the exercise. Things could get ugly if a bad spot ruins his set (or worse, the weight lands on his head).

- **Juice.** Slang for steroids. If muscle-heads are said to be "juicing," you can be sure they're not talking about fresh produce.

A Tour of the Equipment

Health clubs are loaded with amazing machinery. With all the high-tech, futuristic equipment that's available, it can almost feel like you're on *The Jetsons*. ("Hey Jane, how long you been on that Stairmaster?") Take advantage of this and try them all. Don't get stuck in that "same machine day-in, day-out" routine. Swap around from week to week and keep your workouts interesting and fun.

Get to Know the Aerobic Contraptions

All cardiovascular exercise equipment is designed to get large muscles pumping in a rhythmic fashion—to increase the heart rate and blood pressure and burn calories. What's the best piece of cardio equipment? The answer: any machine you'll use. Download some favorite tunes to your iPod, read the paper, or watch TV (*Good Morning America*, VH1, Spongebob Squarepants—whatever grabs ya), and you'll be surprised how quickly the time flies:

◆ **Treadmills.** Cardiovascular equipment that presents light-to-moderate impact on your joints, depending on whether you're walking or running. Walking on a flat grade is a good starting place for beginning exercisers. As fitness and confidence builds, you can fool around with increasing the incline and speed.

◆ **Stairclimbers.** Cardiovascular equipment that provides a challenging workout with some potential stress to your knees and lower back. (Listen carefully to your body.) This is a more advanced piece of machinery due to the importance of technique, and therefore, you need a base level of stamina and strength to use this machine, even on lower levels.

> **CAUTION**
>
> **Overrated-Undercooked**
>
> Do something too much, too hard, or too often, and sooner or later it'll get stale. Don't be afraid to vary your activities and change your program. In fact, I encourage it. Try inline skating instead of using the treadmill. Use weight machines instead of free weights. Attend an exercise class instead of riding the Life Cycle. Hey, if you want to dance around naked, I say go for it. (Just keep it at home, and close the window shades.)

◆ **Stationary bikes.** Now, they come in two flavors—the upright bike (like a regular outdoors bicycle) and the recumbent bike (legs out in front with high bucket seats lending more support for people with lower back pain). Both types provide aerobic workouts that give your joints a break because they are non–weight-bearing activities. Make sure the tension isn't too high and the seat isn't too low. If you're a beginner, ask a trainer to help you get into the proper position. When you're ready to pump up the intensity, increase your speed before increasing the tension.

♦ **Cross conditioner/cross-country ski machines.** A great aerobic exercise that uses the entire body and burns tons of calories without any jarring impact. It's also good for quick warm-ups because it gets the whole body going. There is, however, one catch: learning the movement can be tricky for some people, and let's just say the term "poetry in motion" takes on a whole new meaning.

♦ **Rowing machines.** Another good "total-body" workout (and a warm-up machine) without any impact. Be sure to get some pointers on technique; there's an easy way and the *right* way to do it. Obviously, the right way requires more energy, concentration, and muscular effort.

Become Familiar with the Weight-Training Tools

Weight-training equipment can be super high-tech (multi-muscle machinery) or super low-tech (a pair of dumbbells and a box). Don't be fooled into thinking that something more complicated means a better workout. That's not the case at all:

♦ **Weight-training machines.** In general, machines are a good starting point for beginners. They remove a lot of the guess work; you just move from machine to machine. (Adjust your seat, stick in a pin, and you're ready for action.) Several machine variations include weight stacks with pulleys and cords (such as Universal and Cybex), metal rod systems (such as Cybex and Med-X), cams and chains (such as Nautilus), or air pumps (such as Kaiser). Just name the nut and bolt, and there's a machine out there that has it. Test them all and find the one you're most comfortable with.

Q & A

Do I really need to buy all of the belts, wraps, and straps associated with weight training?

No. In fact, the only peripheral equipment you might need is a pair of gloves to help protect against calluses.

♦ **Free weights.** These, on the other hand, require a fair amount of coordination, strength, and skill because they heavily depend on your balance and body control. Although weight training with barbells and dumbbells (free weights) might seem significantly harder at first, some people claim free weights yield greater gains than machines. When embarking on a free-weight program, consult with a qualified trainer for tips on proper form and technique. *Bad* habits lead to *bad* injuries.

Learn Your Muscles and "Buff That Bod"

This section provides a quick rundown on the major muscles that conscientious gym folks tend to work out. Of course, your body is action-packed with hundreds more. Browse through the list, and become familiar with your muscles *and* the exercises that work them out. Be sure to ask a qualified trainer to personally show you the correct form and technique for each and every exercise.

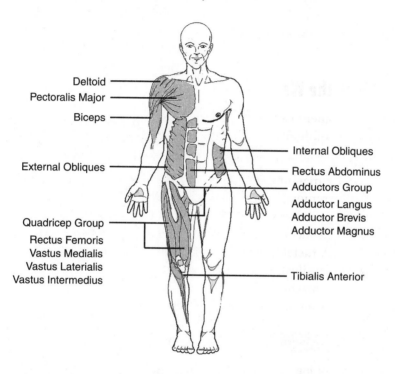

Gym Slang	Muscle Group	Exercises That Work 'Em
Traps	Trapezius	Upper traps: shoulder shrugs Mid traps: reverse flys, seated rows Lower traps: dips
Delts	Deltoids	Anterior delts: frontal raises Medial delts: lateral raises Posterior delts: reverse flys
Midback	Rhomboids Mid trapezius	Seated rows Reverse flys

continues

continued

Gym Slang	Muscle Group	Exercises That Work 'Em
Pecs	Pectoralis major	Dumbbell bench press Dumbbell flys Push-ups Dips
Lats	Latissimus dorsi	Lat pulldowns Seated row pulley rowing
Lower back	Erector spinae	Lower back lifts (on a mat) Opposite arm/leg lifts on all fours
Bis	Biceps	Bicep curls Supination curls with dumbbells
Tris	Triceps	Tricep dips Tricep pulldowns
Abs	Abdominal group: *internal obliques* *external obliques* *rectus abdominis*	Stomach crunches Oblique twist Side crunches
Butt	Gluteus maximus	Leg press/squats Hip extension (with a low pulley cable)
Outer hips	Abductor group: *gluteus medius* *gluteus minimus*	Abductor machine Side leg lifts (with a low pulley cable)
Inner thighs	Adductor group: *adductor longus* *adductor brevis* *adductor magnus*	Adductor machine Inward leg lifts (with a low pulley cable)
Quads	Quadricep group: *rectus femoris* *vastus medialis* *vastus lateralis* *vastus intermedius*	Leg press Leg extension (also includes squats, lunges, and step-ups with dumbbells)
Hams	Hamstring group: *biceps femoris* *semitendinosus* *semimembranosus*	Leg press Leg curl

Gym Slang	Muscle Group	Exercises That Work 'Em
Calves	Gastronemius soleus	Heel raises straight leg
		Toe presses straight leg
		Heel raises bent leg
		Toe presses bent leg
Shins	Tibialis anterior	Toe taps
		Toe backs

Do You Need a Personal Trainer?

Some people decide to hire a personal trainer to help them get into shape. Although some exercisers require a personal trainer only for a single show-you-the-ropes session, others enjoy continual weekly appointments that help keep them focused and motivated. If you decide to work with a trainer, be selective about whom you hire because the unfortunate truth is that *anyone* can call himself a personal trainer.

Consider hiring a personal trainer if you fall into any of the following categories:

- You are completely out of shape and haven't the slightest idea how to begin an exercise program. A trainer can acquaint you with all of the up-to-date exercise techniques and available aerobic and weight machinery.

- You are in a *huge* exercise rut and have been doing the same old routine for as long as you can remember. A trainer can show you variations on your day-to-day workout and make exercising more efficient and effective.

- You just plain lack the "umph" to exercise on your own. A trainer can help to push, motivate, and whip your butt into shape.

Seek out somebody with a B.S. (better yet, a Master's degree) in exercise physiology, physical education, or kinesiology. You can also look for a *certified* fitness trainer, which means she has studied for and passed a comprehensive training exam. Some of the most reputable organizations that provide certifications include the following:

- ACSM (American College of Sports Medicine)

- ACE (American Council on Exercise)

- NSCA (National Strength and Conditioning Association)

- ◆ AFAA (Aerobics and Fitness Association of America)
- ◆ NASM (National Academy of Sports Medicine)

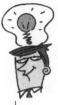

> **Food for Thought** _____
>
> Studies report that arthritis sufferers who regularly participate in strength training and stretching programs can greatly improve their balance, speed, and ability to walk, as well as reduce joint pain and fatigue. Check it out with your doctor first to be sure there's not too much joint inflammation.
>
> For more information, contact the Arthritis Foundation at 1-800-283-7800, and ask about its Aquatics and PACE program (People with Arthritis Can Exercise).

Other comprehensive fitness certifications are offered at various universities. Most of these organizations offer a variety of certifications (aerobic instructor, yoga, and so on). Make sure your trainer is specifically certified in *personal training* or *fitness instruction* and that his or her certification is up to date.

Interview a trainer before you actually set up an appointment to be sure you feel comfortable with his or her workout philosophy, personality, and fee scale. Rates vary tremendously, anywhere from $40 to $100 per workout. They can even run more than $200 if you're looking for a "trainer to the stars."

The Least You Need to Know

- ◆ Joining a local gym can be an invaluable tool in your pursuit of that "body beautiful." Take advantage of the variety of workout choices and the qualified staff of trainers who can help instruct, motivate, and encourage you.

- ◆ Some of the aerobic equipment commonly found in most gyms includes tread-mills, bikes, stairclimbers, rowing machines, and cross-country ski machines. Weight-training equipment generally involves either multi-purpose machinery (Cybex, Nautilus) or free weights (barbells and dumbbells).

- ◆ Because bad form and technique can lead to injuries, seek the assistance of a qualified trainer before embarking on any type of program.

Chapter 16

Sports Nutrition

In This Chapter

- ◆ Super-fueling your body with carbohydrates
- ◆ Where to find high carbohydrate foods
- ◆ Increased protein requirements for athletes
- ◆ What to eat before, during, and after exercise

If you've read this far, you know the basics of sports nutrition. Contrary to what some people think, there isn't any "magic" ingredient that helps optimize exercise and training (such as instant-muscle shake concoctions or endurance potions). In fact, the same healthy-eating guidelines you read about in the earlier chapters apply for competitive sport and casual exercise. You know the story: moderate-high on the carbs, low on the fat, and moderate amounts of protein. You might just need to increase your total calories to compensate for the amount you're now burning with all that activity. But don't stop reading: there's a lot more to sport-specific nutrition, and this chapter clues you in. Stay tuned for a mouthful of information that can help enhance your athletic performance and secure that competitive edge.

Carbohydrates: Fuel of Choice

Carbohydrate is the high-octane fuel for exercise and should provide at least 55 percent of an athlete's total daily calories. To get a bit more technical, you should consume approximately 3.0 to 4.5 grams of carbohydrate per pound of body weight. Where do you fit in? If your sport is pretty low-key—not a lot of nonstop running around—you should aim for 3.0 grams. On the other hand, if you participate in a super-endurance sport that involves hours of heavy training each day, you should aim for 4.5 grams.

Food for Thought

Carbohydrate-rich foods are the fuel of choice for athletes. Carbs provide the muscles with ongoing energy in the form of glucose and help maintain prolonged endurance and optimal performance.

What does that mean, anyway?

Math time—grab a calculator. Take your weight in pounds and multiply it by 3.0 grams (for moderate intensity sports) and 4.5 grams (for strenuous endurance training). Obviously, these are two extremes; most exercisers and athletes fall in the middle. In fact, give yourself a range; play around and see where your body feels most vigorous.

For example: here's the carbo requirement for a 150-pound *elite* runner training several hours each day:

150 pounds × 4.5 grams = 675 grams of carbohydrate

Because 1 *gram* of carbohydrate = 4 calories, we can now convert 675 carb grams into carb calories by using the following equation:

675 × 4 = 2,700 carbohydrate calories

Now, let's look at a typical 150-pound health club member, working out at a moderate intensity (approximately 45 minutes), 4–5 days a week:

150 pounds × 3.0 grams = 450 grams of carbohydrate

Now, convert into carb calories:

450 × 4 = 1,800 carbohydrate calories

As you can see, a more intense endurance exercise program will demand more carbohydrate. But keep in mind that the proportions of carbs, protein, and fat pretty much remain the same as in the previous chapters because in the end, you're taking in more of everything.

Develop Your Own High-Carb Diet

Need to boost your carbs? Take a look at the variety of foods you can choose from, and watch how fast you can rack up the grams.

The Starchy Carbs

Generally speaking, breads, grains, and other starchy foods contain approximately 15 grams (give or take a few) of carbohydrate per serving (1 slice bread, ¹/₂ cup pasta, 1 serving of cereal). These foods receive top billing for endurance athletes simply because it's easy to eat multiple servings in one sitting. For instance, a pasta entree can easily total five grain servings, and because one pasta serving contains about 20 grams of carb, five servings supplies a whopping 100 grams of carbohydrate. Clearly, this is the reasoning behind marathon runners "packing in the pasta" before the lengthy 26-mile run.

Fruits

Next up are fruits, also providing about the same 15 grams of carbohydrate per serving (1 medium fresh fruit, 1 cup berries/melon, ¹/₂ cup fruit juice). Why are they second? Athletes looking to load up on carbs can eat 10+ servings of grain more comfortably than 10+ servings of fruit. Remember, fruit has a lot of fiber and tends to fill you up more quickly. (You might be "bursting with fruit flavor" in more ways than one!) Incorporate a lot of fresh fruit into your regimen, but don't skimp on the grains and rely *solely* on fruit.

Milk Products

Milk products contain about 12 grams of carbohydrate per serving (1 cup milk, 1 cup yogurt) and can certainly boost your total carbs together with the starchy foods, fruits, and vegetables. What's more, milk pumps you with calcium, a key ingredient for maintaining strong, athletic bones.

Vegetables

Veggies provide approximately 5 grams of carbohydrate per serving (1 cup raw or ¹/₂ cup cooked) and are certainly packed with vitamins and minerals. Although veggies alone can't supply enough concentrated carbohydrate for increased requirements, they can sure jazz up your meals and add tremendous amounts of nutrition to your table.

Common High-Carb Foods	Carbohydrate Grams
Medium baked potato	51
Medium bagel	45
1 cup rice	44
1 cup low-fat, flavored yogurt	43
Power bars	42
1 cup beans	41
1 cup pasta (cooked)	40
Banana	27
Glass of O.J. (8 oz.)	26
1 cup cereal (ready to eat)	25
1 cup oatmeal	25
Granola bar	25
2 slices whole-wheat bread	23
2 fig cookies	23
10 crackers	21
1 oz. pretzels	21
1 cup low-fat yogurt (plain)	18
$\frac{1}{2}$ cup corn	17
1 cup low-fat milk	12
$\frac{1}{2}$ cup peas	11

Note that the carbohydrate grams are calculated for serving sizes that are commonly eaten, not the standard single serving sizes frequently listed throughout the book and within the new Dietary Guidelines.

Nutri-Speak

Muscle glycogen is the stored carbohydrate within the muscles. Athletes can use the "energy stores" during prolonged exercise.

All About Muscle Glycogen

Muscle glycogen is stored carbohydrate in your muscle. Imagine this: after you eat and digest a meal, the amount of carbohydrate that you immediately need will get used as fuel, but the rest (up to a point) will be stored in your muscles for *future* fuel. Athletes in ultra-endurance sports such as soccer, basketball, hockey, and distance running rely on high-octane muscle fuel for energy. In fact, between the grueling practice sessions and vigorous competitions, serious endurance athletes are constantly depleting and restoring their muscle glycogen stores, so they require much more carbohydrate-rich food than athletes involved in less aerobic activity (golf, archery, and martial arts).

Just because you don't compete in an ultra-endurance sport doesn't mean you can fumble in the carb department. Think about all of the laborious practice sessions that wrestlers, divers, or short-distance swimmers put in during the week. Bear in mind, it's not just the actual competition that matters, but the intensity of your training as well.

What happens if you don't replenish your muscle-glycogen stores? Simple: if you run out of glycogen, you run out of energy. The amount of muscle fuel you have determines how long you can exercise. As a car needs a full tank of gas before heading out on a long trip, an endurance athlete requires sufficient "muscle gasoline" to sustain the pace and go the distance. Always tired or run down? Obviously, a vigorous training schedule alone is enough to make you feel that way. You might also want to look into your carbohydrate consumption. Keep a food log and do the math; there could be an easy solution to your problem.

Food for Thought

You can take in more than 100 grams of carbohydrate by eating 4 bananas, or 2½ power bars, or 3 cups pasta, or 6 medium pancakes, or 2½ cups Raisin Bran cereal, or 2 medium baked potatoes, or 8 fig cookies and a glass of milk.

Overrated-Undercooked

For you nonathletes who decided to browse through this chapter, not everyone is a candidate for overdosing on carbs. Active people might continuously burn loads of carbohydrate calories, but your muscles can only store a certain amount of carbohydrate. If you're not using what is already there, you'll just end up putting on weight.

Personal Protein Requirements

It's true that athletes do need more protein than sedentary folks, but because most people already take in far more protein than the RDA, chances are you're A-okay. (You're okay unless you're one of those "carb-o-holics" who live on the "cereal-bagel-pasta" program, or you're trying so hard to carbo-load that you forget the other key ingredients for optimal performance.)

Athletes do need protein for that competitive edge. You learned the vital roles of protein in Chapter 3, but let's get sport-specific for a minute. Protein is essential for building and maintaining muscle tissue, as well as repairing the muscle damage you endure during hard workouts. Remember, dietary protein does *not* automatically build bigger muscles: *you* build bigger muscles through regular exercise and training. Dietary protein simply allows all your hard work to pay off. Following are the recommended daily intakes for protein. You'll see that athletes do have greater requirements than the RDAs for the general population (also in Chapter 3). But keep in mind that your total proportion should still be higher in carbs, moderate in protein, and low in fat. This is because you're taking in more of everything.

Find your exercise category, and then multiply your weight (in pounds) by the number of grams to the right. After you do the math and know your personal daily requirements, keep a food log for a week and tally up your daily protein totals by checking your foods in the chart located in Chapter 3.

Exercise Category	Recommended Daily Protein (Grams per Pound)
Sedentary folks	.36
Moderate exercisers	.36–.5
Endurance athletes	.5–.8
Strength athletes	.6–.8
Growing teenage athletes	.6–.9

Here are some examples:

 ◆ A 200-pound bodybuilder needs between 120 and 160 grams of protein daily.

 ◆ A 150-pound triathlete needs 75 to 120 grams of protein each day.

 ◆ A 14-year-old elite gymnast weighing 92 pounds needs 55 to 83 grams of protein each day.

 ◆ A casual 120-pound health-club member needs 43 to 60 grams of protein each day.

Notice that even though the growing gymnast might require more protein per pound than the bodybuilder, bodybuilders usually weigh a lot more and therefore tend to have greater protein requirements.

Food Before, During, and After Exercise

This section investigates favorable food choices for your pre-event meal, *plus* the recovery foods to help your body bounce back after an intense workout. It also lays out the guidelines for fueling your system throughout prolonged periods of exercise.

Pre-Event Meals

Let me begin by saying that the most outstanding meal before your sporting event won't make up for a week's worth of potato chips, French fries, and cookies! With that in mind, study the following guidelines and help make your pre-event meal a "winning beginning":

- Make your large meal (approximately 600–800 calories) at *least* 3–4 hours prior to an event. This will provide adequate time for your food to digest. (You don't want to feel heavy or nauseous, or have indigestion, while you're running around on the field.)

- Stick with carbohydrate-rich foods and moderate amounts of lean protein. The carbs are both loaded with energy and easy to digest. Avoid eating a lot of high-fat stuff; it takes much longer to leave your stomach, and you don't want food bouncing along for the ride.

- Avoid super–high-fiber foods that can cause annoying stomach gurgles, *or* send you running to the bathroom right before kickoff.

- Also limit gaseous foods such as beans, brussels sprouts, grapes, broccoli, and anything else you think might give you a gassy stomach.

- Liquid meals are also fine, especially if you have "pre-game jitters" and can't stomach solid food. Some athletes prefer liquid supplements because they don't leave you feeling as full as a large meal of equal calories does. In fact, they leave your stomach quicker than solid food.

- Also, lay off the salt. As you read in the salt chapter, some people tend to retain a lot of fluid, which can lead to puffiness and discomfort.

- Never eat something completely new before an important competition. *Always* test it during training and see how it settles in your stomach.

- Reduce the size of your food intake as you approach the time of your event. For example, 3–4 hours before, you can have a large meal (approximately

600–800 cals); 2–3 hours before, you can have a smaller meal (approximately 400–500 cals); and less than 2 hours before, you can grab some lighter snacks (cereal bars, fruit, flavored rice cakes, fruit juice, yogurts, and so on).

What time is your sporting event? Which meal will be your pre-event send-off: breakfast, lunch, or dinner? Check out the sample menus and get an idea of the foods you should choose. Keep in mind that you should *always* have a well-balanced, carbo-rich meal the night before, especially because on game day, you might get fidgety and lose your appetite.

Ready-Made Menu

> **Breakfast:** (for a late-morning or an early-afternoon competition)
> Bowl of cereal with low-fat milk
> Sliced bananas
> Toasted whole-grain English Muffin with peanut butter
> Glass of orange juice
>
> **Lunch:** (for a late-afternoon or evening competition)
> Turkey sandwich on whole-wheat bread
> Salad with light dressing (or veggie soup)
> Frozen yogurt with sliced strawberries
> Water
>
> **Dinner:** (for an early-morning or any-time-the-next-day competition)
> Grilled chicken
> Pasta with marinara sauce
> Broccoli and carrots
> Fruit salad
> 2 fig bars
> Glass of skim or 1% low-fat milk

Q & A
Is there really such a thing as "winning meals" or "winning foods" that can enhance your performance?
Yes! You see, if a particular food or meal makes you *mentally* feel at your best, then for you, that is a winning meal.

Fueling Your Body During Prolonged Endurance Activity

Some sports are so lengthy they require feedings *throughout* the event, to help supply your body with glucose when glycogen stores are running low. For example, marathon runners (and other endurance athletes, such as soccer players) need to eat about 30–60 grams of carbohydrate per hour, which translates into a mere (but important) 120–240 calories. Although it's a minuscule amount, these calories should be spread out over each hour. The simplest method is to drink one of the popular sports drinks during the event. You can hydrate and "*carbo*-hydrate" your body at the same time.

Recovery Foods

Now for the last piece of the puzzle—the aftermath nourishment. First, understand that recovery foods are not just for recovering after a competition or game. They're equally important after practice as well. In fact, athletes who regularly train long and hard should replace emptied glycogen stores, fluids, and potassium lost through sweat on a daily basis. What's more, carbohydrate and fluid repletion should begin immediately, within 30 minutes after exercise, to promote a quick recovery. Sound unrealistic? Just grab a fruit juice or sports drink while you make your congratulatory "high-fives." When you can focus on a real meal, enjoy whatever you fancy; just make sure to include the following essentials:

- Plenty of fluids: water, fruit juice, sports drinks, soups, and watery fruits and veggies (watermelon, grapes, oranges, tomatoes, lettuce, and cucumbers).

- A lot of carbohydrate-rich foods: pasta, potatoes, rice, breads, fruits, yogurts, and so on.

- Adequate lean protein.

- Potassium-rich foods such as potatoes, bananas, oranges, orange juice, and raisins.

- Do *not* attempt to replenish lost sodium by smothering your food in salt *or* by popping dangerous salt tablets. A typical meal, moderately salted, supplies enough sodium to replace the amount lost through sweat.

As you have read, food can make or break your athletic performance. While training hard is incredibly important, you'll never reach your full potential without paying close attention to balanced food choices. Remember to focus on the right mix of carbohydrate and protein, and preplan your pre-event and recovery meals. You'll feel great, and you'll have more energy and strength for a winning performance.

The Least You Need to Know

◆ Athletes need carbohydrate-rich foods such as grains, pasta, rice, fruits, and veggies. Carbohydrates supply energy for both grueling practice sessions and competitions.

◆ Athletes have greater daily protein requirements than sedentary folks—roughly .5–.8 grams per pound of body weight. However, this is easily met because their greater caloric intake usually provides proportionately more protein.

◆ Your pre-event meal is important, and you need to reduce your food intake as you get close to your event.

◆ During prolonged exercise, your body requires about 30–60 grams of carbohydrate per hour, which translates into 120–240 calories.

◆ Help your body recover after a grueling workout with plenty of fluids, carbohydrates, and potassium-rich foods.

Going That Extra Mile: Fluids and Supplements

In This Chapter

- ◆ All about fluids and proper hydration
- ◆ The nutritional content of popular sports bars
- ◆ The lowdown on a few exercise enhancers

Grab your water bottle and guzzle down. In fact, exercise places such great demands on fluid replacement that proper hydration before, during, and after intense physical activity is critical. Think about the numerous tasks that depend on fluid: your blood needs fluid to transfer oxygen to working muscles, your urine needs fluid to funnel out metabolic waste products, and your temperature regulating system needs fluid to dissipate heat through sweat.

You might feel wet, gross, and disgusting on the outside, but sweating helps keep you at a comfortable working temperature. You need to continuously replace the fluids lost through sweat so that you can prevent your body from becoming dehydrated and overheated. What's more, athletes who fail to keep up with their water requirements not only jeopardize performance, but also place themselves at risk for serious heat conditions (heat cramps, heat exhaustion, and heat stroke).

Guidelines for Proper Hydration

Unfortunately for athletes, the thirst mechanism is an unreliable indicator. First, by the time you feel thirsty, you could already be on your way to dehydration; second, the amount of fluid that quenches your thirst might not be enough to quench your body. To ensure adequate hydration, you need to follow a drinking schedule. Here's what is recommended:

♦ 16–24 ounces (or 2–3 cups) 2 hours prior to exercise

♦ 8–16 ounces (1–2 cups) 15–30 minutes *before* exercise

♦ 4–12 ounces (or ½–1½ cups) every 15–20 minutes *during* exercise

♦ 16–24 ounces (or 2–3 cups) for every pound lost *after* exercise

Here are two quick ways to tell whether you are properly hydrated:

♦ **Weigh in before and after:** Hop on the scale before and after you exercise. For each pound of fluid lost (it's just fluid, *not* fat), drink 2 cups of water (or other fluid) to properly *rehydrate* your body. You don't have to gulp it all down at once; just make sure you're fully hydrated by the next day. For example, a soccer player weighs 165 pounds before the game and 162 pounds after the game. Therefore, he must drink 6 cups of water to replace the 3 pounds of lost fluid.

♦ **Check your urine:** The color of your urine is also a good indicator of hydration. If your urine is voluminous and clear to pale yellow, you're doing just fine. On the other hand, if your urine is dark and concentrated, keep chugging that fluid; you've got a ways to go.

Sports Drinks Versus Water

Plain old H_2O is cheap, effective, and just fine for most athletes, but in some instances, you'll benefit from the added carbohydrate in a sports drink (Gatorade, PowerAde, AllSport, Boost, and so on). Spring for the loaded stuff when continuous exercise lasts longer than 60 minutes or when you're exercising in extremely hot weather. You see, water can provide straight hydration, but sports drinks can also provide some electrolytes and carbohydrate—just enough to keep you moving and grooving during those exceptionally long or hot workouts.

The Bar Exam

Sports bars (and similar products) can be convenient and advantageous for athletes trying to increase calories, carbohydrates, and protein (depending upon the brand). Here's the nutritional profile on a variety of popular bars on the market. Because most brands carry an assortment of flavors, the information might vary slightly from the list. Also, be sure to sample several brands before you form any taste opinion; they vary tremendously!

Sports Bars and Similar Products

Product	Calories	T. Fat/ Sat. gms	Protein, gms	Carbs, gms	Fiber, gms
Atkins Advantage	220	11/7	17	15	11
Atkins Diet Advantage	221	13/5.2	21	2.6	0
All-Bran Bar	130	3/0.5	2	27	5
Balance	200	6/3	15	22	<1
Balance Gold	210	7/4	15	23	<1
Boulder Bar	200	2/0	10	43	5
CarbRite	195	4/2	21	22	-
Carb solutions	240	10/3.5	24	14	1
Centrum Energy	220	5/4	9	34	<1
Clif Bar	240	5/1	12	39	5
Dr. Soy	180	3/2.5	3	27	1
E2R	210	7/2.5	15	23	1
Edge-Advant	210	4/2.5	13	31	<1
Ensure	130	3/1	6	21	2
Gatorade	260	5/1	6	48	1
Genisoy Ultimate	230	4.5/3	14	33	2
Glow by Luna	140	7/3.5	8	15	1
Harvest by Power Bar	250	5/2	7	45	3
Healthy	190	3/.5	10	32	2

continues

Sports Bars and Similar Products (continued)

Product	Calories	T. Fat/ Sat. gms	Protein, gms	Carbs, gms	Fiber, gms
Ironman	230	8/1.5	16	24	0
Jenny Craig	210	3/0	10	35	3
Kashi Go Lean	280	5/3	13	49	6
Keto-Pro by Met-Rx	300	8/3.5	32	15	0
Kudos	130	5/2.5	1	20	1
LoCarb 2	230	6/3	20	3	0
Luna	180	4.5/2.5	10	24	2
MET-Rx Protein plus	290	4/3	32	31	3
MET-Rx 100gm bar	320-340	3.5/1.5	26	52	2
Milk & Cereal	160	4/1.5	6	26	1
Mojo by Clif	200	7/.5	9	25	2
Myoplex Plus Deluxe by EAS	340	7/1.5	24	44	0
Nature Val. Granola bar	180	6/.5	4	29	2
Nat. Valley Chewey bar	140	3.5/2	2	26	1
Nutrigrain bar	140	3	2	27	1
Nutrigrain Granola chewey bars	130	3.5/1	2	22	1
Nutrigrain Muffin bar	160	4/.5	3	30	1
Nutrigrain Yogurt bar	140	3/.5	2	27	1
Odwalla	220	5/1.5	6	42	5
Power Bar	230	2/.5	10	45	3
Power Gel	110	-	-	28	-
Pria by Power Bar	110	3/2	5	16	<1
Promax	290	6/4	20	38	2
Protein Fuel	340	7/1.5	35	12	0
Protein by Prolab	190	6/2.5	19	12	0

Product	Calories	T. Fat/ Sat. gms	Protein, gms	Carbs, gms	Fiber, gms
Protein Plus by Powerbar	270	5/3	24	36	2
SF Pro. Plus by Powerbar	170	4/2.5	16	19	1
Pure Protein	270	5/3.5	30	29	<1
Quaker Chewey LF Granola Bar	110	2/.5	2	22	1
Slim Fast	220	5/3.5	8	36	2
Source One by Met-Rx	190	3/2.5	15	29	0
SnackBarz	110-130	6/2.5	1	17	0
Special K Bar	90	1.5/1	2	18	<1
Steel Bar	330	6/3	16	52	0
Stoker	210	3	9	41	?
Think	251	8/2	6	39	1.5
Tigers Milk	140	5/1	7	18	1
Tiger Sport	230	2	10	43	
Trim Advantage Pro. Bar	240	8/1	22	22	2
Ultimate Protein Bar	280	6/3.5	32	19	0
Zone Perfect	210	7/3.5	16	21	<1

What's the Story on Ergogenic Aids?

People make outrageous claims regarding substances that can help enhance performance. The word *ergogenic* literally means "work producing," and, unfortunately, there are always cockamamie advertisements selling nutritional pills and potions claiming to beef up performance. To date, there are only a few scientifically sound ergogenic aids, including a proper diet, carbo-loading, a well-trained body, a determined soul, and the right equipment.

Here's what you need to know about a few ergogenic aids in food and supplement form with scientific backup.

Thumbs Up

To date, the following substances have been shown to improve athletic performance. Of course, this doesn't mean you should start popping pills. In fact, scientists are constantly coming up with new information (good and bad), so stay on top of the current research if you decide to go with one of these supplements. Naturally, *always* check with your physician before embarking on anything new:

- ◆ **Antioxidants** (C, E, beta-carotene, and selenium)

  Claim: Protects against the tissue damage from free radical formation induced by exercise.

  Fact: Might protect against tissue damage following prolonged endurance exercise, but doesn't improve performance while you are actually exercising. Although the quantities of antioxidants found in food are somewhat small, they do help to stop the production and spread of harmful substances.

- ◆ **Caffeine**

  Claim: Improves endurance and overall athletic performance.

  Fact: Consuming as little as one hundred milligrams of caffeine an hour before a workout—the average amount of caffeine in a cup of coffee—has been shown to improve athletic performance of dedicated exercisers (casual exercisers may not experience the same boost). Researchers aren't sure why, but it may be because caffeine signals your muscles to ignore fatigue and contract differently.

- ◆ Side effects of high caffeine consumption include nausea, muscle tremors, palpitations, and headaches. Not a good idea if you have a sensitive system.

- ◆ **Creatine**

  Claim: Increases the creatine phosphate content in muscles, improves high-power performance, and increases muscle mass.

  Fact: Research has suggested that consuming 20 grams of creatine per day (5 grams, four times daily) for five days might improve performance in brief, maximal exercise lasting less than 30 seconds. After this loading dose, a maintenance dose of 5 grams per day should suffice. However, not all studies have found that creatine improves strength, sprint performance, or lean muscle mass—so it might not improve all high-power activities.

The appeal of magic pills promising bigger muscles and faster speeds is tremendous. However, it's important to know that very few supplements have credible research to back them up—in fact, most of the sport enhancers offer nothing but misleading labels. Without a doubt, the best investment for top performance is the old-fashioned mix—good eats and plenty of hard training.

The Least You Need to Know

◆ Proper hydration is essential for maintaining prolonged activity and for optimal performance.

◆ Water is the perfect fluid replacement for exercise lasting under 60 minutes. However, ultra-endurance athletes, and anyone exercising in extremely hot weather, will benefit from the added carbohydrate and electrolyte content in the popular sports drinks.

◆ Don't be misled by ads claiming to sell exercise enhancers in the shape of a pill. The way to optimize performance is to eat smart and train hard!

◆ Sports bars can be convenient and advantageous for athletes trying to increase calories, carbohydrates, and protein (depending upon the brand). Sample several brands before you form a taste opinion; they vary tremendously.

Part 4

Beyond the Basics: Nutrition for Special Needs

There are so many diseases that can be prevented or eased by proper nutrition, and new research keeps adding to our knowledge base every day.

This section provides up-to-date nutritional approaches to cancer, diabetes, heart disease, and food allergies (among other conditions). You'll also find a primer on various types of vegetarian diets, and—for those of you who want to go *au natural*—a list of herbal remedies. Whether you're interested in reducing your cancer risk, feasting purely on plants, learning about herbal "medicines," or simply understanding *why* you keep bolting for the bathroom after eating ice cream—stay tuned.

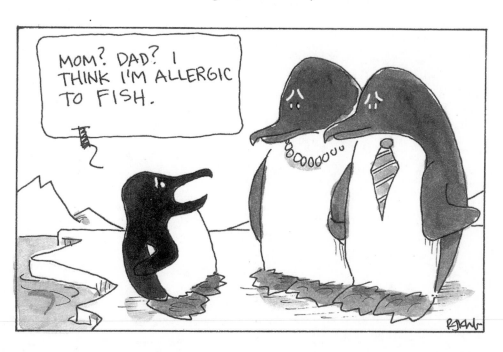

Chapter

18

Diet and Cancer

In This Chapter

- ◆ Foods that might decrease your risk of certain cancers
- ◆ Omega-3s—and how they can help
- ◆ Eating the right fish and getting the most from flaxseed
- ◆ Your best bets in vegetables and fruit
- ◆ The many benefits of soy
- ◆ Following a neutropenic diet during treatment
- ◆ Spotlight on breast cancer and prostate cancer

Over the years, there's been a lot of speculation and controversy over how eating certain foods might prevent cancer. You certainly don't need a Harvard oncologist (or a New York City nutritionist) to tell you that if you eat in a healthy manner, your body will be stronger, your immune system and organs will be in good shape, and therefore, you might be more likely to be cancer-free. But just eating tons of fruits and veggies and the right kinds of nutrients isn't a foolproof way to avoid the wrath of cancer. Unfortunately, there is no exact science linking food and cancer prevention, although we are constantly researching and studying the subject in search of some answers.

Nonetheless, while scientists and doctors learn, you can take a proactive approach to feeding your body well, giving it fuel to fight disease, and doing whatever you can to ward off this horrific illness. Even though there is no hardcore proof about which foods offer the best protection against malignancy, research has uncovered how certain foods can get in the way of a tumor's growth.

Which Fats Can Help

For years, there has been an incredible amount of hype over fat. Fat clogs your arteries, fat increases your cholesterol, fat causes weight gain—fat is the root of all evil. However, some kinds of fat are not just okay to eat—but are actually good for you. To date, the best types of fats are monounsaturated and polyunsaturated, and omega-3s. Monounsaturated fat can be found in olive oils, avocado, and most nuts. The *omega-3 fats* can be found in flaxseed, canola oil, walnuts, and fatty fish.

Nutri-Speak

The **omega-3 fats** (also known as linolenic fatty acids) are polyunsaturated—meaning their structural makeup is lacking several hydrogen atoms. Eating foods rich in omega-3 fats has been shown to have beneficial effects, such as lowering triglycerides and cholesterol, lowering blood pressure, helping alleviate arthritic pain, aiding with digestive problems, and possibly reducing the risk of certain cancers (and recurrence of them).

The Fatty Fish

Seafood lovers, rejoice! Epidemiological studies have shown a lower rate of cancer in people who eat a lot of fish. The best advice is to have a few servings of tuna, sardines, bluefish, striped bass, herring, trout, and wild salmon—the fish dishes with a rich concentration of omega-3 fats. In fact, eat them at least three times each week (even more if you can). Just make sure to avoid fish that are too high in mercury, such as swordfish, king mackerel, tilefish, and shark.

Flaxseeds and Flaxseed Oil

Flaxseed, the light brown seed from the flax plant, has received a lot of attention for its potential to protect against breast and other hormone-related cancers (in addition to lowering cholesterol and relieving constipation). Rich in omega-3s, antioxidants, lignans-phytoestrogens (which you'll read about later in this chapter), and soluble and insoluble fiber, this impressive seed has been growing in popularity.

You can buy whole flaxseeds in most health food stores and then just grind them in a coffee grinder as needed. Mix them into your cereals, salads, yogurts, cookies, muffins, pancakes, omelets, and even casseroles. Flaxseed oil is effortless, quick, and ready to pour on salad, but you'll miss out on the lignans and fiber found in the whole flaxseed. Just be sure to refrigerate ground flaxseeds and flaxseed oil because they can go rancid quickly. For more information, visit the website www.flaxcouncil.ca.

Fight Back with Antioxidants

Unfortunately, harmful agents called free radicals are produced when we breathe and process oxygen. In fact, these destructive bad guys can also be produced as a result of pollution, stress, pesticides, asbestos, x-rays, preservatives, exhaust fumes, tobacco smoke, and injury. As discussed in a previous chapter, free radicals trek all over the body and actually destroy the cells' DNA—a cancer-promoting activity. The good news is that we naturally protect ourselves by forming antioxidants, substances that help our body's defense system fight off free radicals and preserve healthy cells.

Furthermore, we know that certain foods are rich in nutrients that act as powerful antioxidants and might intensify the body's ability to degrade free radicals into harmless waste products that get eliminated before they do any damage.

Overrated-Undercooked

If you are undergoing chemotherapy, do NOT take antioxidant supplements unless advised to by your physician.

The following sections form a list of some cancer-fighting ingredients to regularly include in your diet.

Vitamins C and E, and Beta-Carotene

Vitamins C and E and beta-carotene (a form of vitamin A) are chock-full of antioxidants. You can find them in fruits and vegetables. Your best bets with each are the following:

Foods rich in Vitamin C include citrus fruits (oranges, grapefruits, and so on), melons, berries, tomatoes, potatoes, broccoli, kiwi, mangos, papayas, and yellow peppers.

Foods rich in Vitamin E include vegetable oils, salad dressings, whole-grain cereals, green leafy vegetables, nuts and seeds, peanut butter, and wheat germ.

Foods rich in Beta-Carotene include cantaloupe, carrots, sweet potatoes, winter squash, spinach, and broccoli.

Green Tea

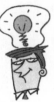

Food for Thought

Folic acid (400 milligrams per day) has been shown to reduce the risk of colon cancer.

Green tea is a traditional Asian brew, the chicken-soup, cure-all remedy that Japanese grandmas swear by—and it contains potent chemical antioxidants called polyphenols, so drink up. In fact, research has suggested that green tea might actually interfere with cancer-causing agents' ability to bind to our DNA—therefore stopping cancer activity.

Can't Get Enough of Those Fruits and Veggies

Everyone knows the nutritional value of fruits and vegetables; that's why five to nine servings a day are recommended. I've already pointed out that certain plant foods are loaded with C, E, and beta-carotene—helpful vitamins and antioxidants our bodies need to fight disease and stay strong. In addition, cruciferous veggies such as broccoli, cauliflower, cabbage, bok choy, kale, brussels sprouts, collards, mustard greens, and turnip greens may also have the potential to reduce the risk of cancer by increasing the production of certain enzymes that help carry potential carcinogens out of the body. Make sure you load your stir-fry dishes and salads with the all-mighty cruciferous ones!

Phytochemicals, Phytonutrients, and Phytoestrogens

They sound confusing but they're really quite understandable:

◆ **Phytochemicals.** Phytochemicals (meaning plant chemicals) are a group of compounds in plant foods—legumes, veggies, fruits, and whole grains—that might positively affect your body. They're naturally produced by plants to protect themselves against viruses, bacteria, and fungi. The term phytochemical includes hundreds of naturally occurring substances such as carotenoids, flavonoids, indoles, isoflavones, capsaicin, and protease inhibitors.

Their exact role in promoting health is still uncertain, but research has suggested that they might help protect against certain cancers, heart disease, and other chronic illnesses.

◆ **Phytonutrients.** Phytonutrient is a term typically used on a supplement bottle to denote that certain botanical supplements extracted from vegetables and other plant foods have been added.

There isn't enough scientific evidence to know whether supplement manufacturers have picked the "right" active substance, because there can be thousands to choose from, or if the amount contained in the pill actually offers any benefits.

◆ **Phytoestrogens.** Phytoestrogens are plant hormones similar to, but weaker than, human estrogens. They are believed to possibly reduce the risk of prostate and other cancers; they also might help protect against heart disease.

Phytoestrogens, now identified in some 300 plants, are grouped as …

Coumestans: bean sprouts, red clover, sunflower seeds.

Lignans: rye, wheat, sesame seeds, linseed, flaxseeds.

Isoflavones: many fruits and veggies but, most of all, soybeans and soy products.

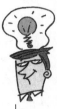

Food for Thought _____

Rosemary, turmeric, and red grapes contain Cox-2 inhibitors—compounds that may help to prevent tumor growth.

Nutri-Speak _____

Isoflavones are hormonelike substances, which are similar to estrogen and are found in plants.

The Story on Soy Products

Substituting tofu, tempeh, miso, and veggie burgers for steaks, burgers, and franks can work to your advantage. (You vegetarians are definitely on to something.) That's because soy foods contain phytoestrogens called *isoflavones*, weak estrogens that help fight against certain cancers, including prostate cancer. However, soy protein may sometimes be contraindicated for women with estrogen-positive cancers—breast, uterine, and ovarian. Always speak with your personal doctor before including them in your diet.

Although the research is preliminary regarding the amount we should consume, everyone can benefit by shifting from an animal-based to a plant-based diet. The best soy sources include soybeans, tempeh, tofu, and soy milk.

Neutropenic Diet Guidelines

The neutropenic diet was created to minimize a patient's exposure to foreign bacteria and decrease his or her risk of infection. Now, the diet is used for patients at risk for immune-related illnesses, especially cancer and AIDS patients undergoing aggressive treatment.

Here are the basic strategies to follow for the neutropenic diet.

Foods to avoid:

◆ Uncooked fruits and vegetables without peels

◆ Unpasteurized juice and milk

◆ Cheeses with molds

◆ Salads (especially from public salad bars)

◆ Dried fruits

◆ Unpackaged delicatessen food items

◆ Certain spices (especially those that are not irradiated)

◆ Foods with stem sites (they have a bacterial entry point)

Follow FDA food safety practices:

◆ Ensure that surfaces used for food preparation are clean.

◆ Discard leftovers that were at room temperature for more than two hours.

◆ Wash hands before beginning food preparation.

◆ Do not use leftovers prior to reheating to 165° F before serving. Discard any leftovers older than two days.

◆ Ensure utensils are clean.

◆ All raw foods such as meats, poultry, and entrees should be cooked until they are well-done and handled on separate surfaces to avoid cross contamination.

A separate cutting board should always be used for meats and a second one designated for cutting produce and breads. Meats should be cooked to an internal temperature of 185° F. Cold foods should be stored below 40° F and hot foods should be kept above 140° F. A home thermometer may help.

♦ Do not drink directly from cans. Cans should be rinsed and wiped down with water first and then poured into a clean glass for consumption.

♦ Wash the exteriors of products before consumption.

♦ Use sterile water to make soups, powdered drinks, and ice cubes.

♦ Baking is better at killing microorganisms than microwaving.

♦ Thaw food in the refrigerator, not on the counter or under water in the sink.

Reducing Fatigue During Chemo Treatments

Research suggests that exercise can help reduce the fatigue associated with chemotherapy. In fact, people undergoing chemotherapy felt 14 to 35 percent less fatigued on the days they exercised compared to the days they didn't. If you're undergoing chemotherapy, you may want to try the following guidelines:

♦ Participate in moderately intense activity at least 3 to 4 times each week. Some appropriate activities include brisk walking, bike riding, and swimming.

♦ Exercise sessions should be between 15 minutes and 1 hour in length. Sessions lasting longer than 1 hour have been shown to *increase* fatigue.

♦ Start your exercise regimen *before* you begin chemotherapy treatments.

♦ Begin exercising slowly and then gradually increase the intensity and duration.

♦ Do not exercise through pain and nausea. Give your body a break.

♦ You may need to rest a day or two after each treatment when the fatigue tends to be the greatest.

♦ If you feel that workouts worsen your pain or increase the fatigue, stop exercising during your full course of treatment.

Spotlight on Breast Cancer and Prostate Cancer

While the role of diet in cancer prevention is still a little murky, there *is* some promising news on the food front when it comes to these two killers.

So far, the most convincing evidence for reducing your risk of breast cancer has less to do with *what* you eat, and more to do with how *much* you eat. Studies have shown that postmenopausal women who are obese or overweight are more likely to develop breast cancer than their lean counterparts and that their survival rate may also be poorer. A few ways to cut down on your calories would be to avoid certain items that are associated with an increased risk of breast cancer, like alcohol, saturated fat, and refined carbohydrates.

Foods that may help prevent breast cancer include fruits and vegetables (because they're packed with fiber, vitamins, minerals, and phytochemicals), monounsaturated fats, omega-3 fats, and soy products. Soy is probably the most studied of all foods when it comes to breast cancer. That's because it has long been known that countries where soy is a staple have much lower rates of breast cancer than the United States. Recent studies suggest that only *whole* soy foods are cancer-busters, however, and that highly processed soy foods and supplements may actually *promote* the growth of pre-existing tumors. So—get rid of all those pills and powders and check out the *real* thing: tempeh, tofu, miso, and the incredibly yummy edamame (boiled green soy beans in the pod).

Remember—if you are at high risk for breast cancer, ONLY include soy foods in your diet if your doctor gives you the okay. If you already have breast cancer, try to avoid soy altogether (unless your doctor advises otherwise).

Weight also plays a role in prostate cancer, although in a different way than for breast cancer. A study in the March 2005 issue of the journal CANCER revealed that obese men often have lower prostate specific antigen (PSA) levels than normal-weight men, making this screening test unreliable for heavy men.

Foods and nutrients to choose when it comes to prostate cancer prevention include fish, green tea, soy foods, and foods rich in the antioxidant lycopene. The mineral selenium is also associated with a lower risk of prostate cancer (just keep your intake to no more than 200 mcg per day).

Foods and nutrients to lose include red meat and alpha-linolenic acid (ALA)—the kind of fat found in flaxseeds and flaxseed oil. You should also avoid taking in more than 1,000 mg calcium and 15 mg zinc per day.

Foods rich in selenium include Brazil nuts (eat no more than two per day), fish, sunflower seeds, and whole-wheat products.

Foods rich in lycopene include tomatoes, apricots, guava, pink grapefruit, and watermelon. Remember, cooking foods makes it easier to absorb lycopene, so your best bet is tomato sauce and other cooked tomato products.

The Least You Need to Know

- ◆ Your mom knew what she was talking about when she pushed you to eat your veggies. Plant foods are especially good for reducing the risk of cancer because they contain compounds that inhibit the growth of tumors.

- ◆ Not all fats are taboo; flaxseed, canola, olive oils, nuts, and fish oils may actually play a role in the fight against cancer.

- ◆ Drinking green tea, stewing up tomatoes, and eating foods with a high concentration of vitamins C and E, beta-carotene, and selenium will help fight harmful agents called free radicals and therefore preserve healthy cells and reduce the risk of cancer.

- ◆ Consume more high-quality soy such as tofu, miso, tempeh, and soybeans, which can help fight certain cancers.

Chapter 19

Managing Diabetes

In This Chapter

- Making the diagnosis
- Reducing your risk of diabetes
- Nutritional guidelines for people with diabetes
- Monitoring your blood sugars
- Some great sample meal plans

It's sometimes called "high sugar" or "a little bit of sugar," but diabetes is anything but sweet. The truth of the matter is that this devastating disease can strike at any age, and with serious health consequences. Babies as young as a few months can be diagnosed with diabetes, as well as slender persons in their teens and twenties. Undiagnosed, the illness can be lethal. Untreated, it leads to a whole host of health problems, such as hypertension and cardiovascular disorders.

In diabetes mellitus (the formal name), the blood-sugar level (blood glucose) is just one facet of a very complicated disorder. Diabetes is actually a group of metabolic disorders, all characterized by hyperglycemia, or high blood glucose (sugar). Hyperglycemia results from a defect in the production of the essential hormone called insulin, which is secreted by the pancreas.

In simple terms, diabetes is a disease in which insulin isn't available in sufficient amounts. This hormone is the key that allows glucose, blood sugar, to enter the cell and produce energy. With too little insulin, our primary source of fuel, glucose, can't be utilized by the body. And without glucose, cells cannot survive.

Type 1, Type 2, and More

Diabetes is most commonly known as Type 1 and Type 2 diabetes (details to come). However, there are also gestational diabetes and other specific types of diabetes associated with genetic defects, with various diseases that injure the pancreas, or with drugs or chemicals, which may induce diabetes. In addition, you may be diagnosed with impaired glucose tolerance (IGT) and impaired fasting glucose (IFG)—a metabolic stage between normal glucose balance and full-scale diabetes. People with IGT and IFG are now referred to as having "pre-diabetes." Pre-diabetes is not a clinical entity in its own right, but rather a risk factor for future diabetes, as well as cardiovascular disease.

Type 1 Diabetes

Typically diagnosed in childhood and with most cases occurring before the age of 30, type 1 diabetes can occur at any age, even in the eighth and ninth decades of life, and is the end result of an autoimmune attack. Special kinds of cells in the pancreas called beta cells are destroyed, and this means the individual can no longer produce insulin and must rely on medication (insulin) to survive. While less common (just 10 percent of all diabetics in the United States have either Type 1, gestational diabetes, or other specific types of diabetes mentioned earlier), Type 1 diabetes is also the most serious. Symptoms include weight loss, frequent urination, and thirst. If it's untreated, these same signs and symptoms can occur, along with nausea, dehydration, and vomiting.

Once diagnosed, it is imperative that blood-sugar levels be well-controlled or a number of complications, including loss of vision and kidney disease, can occur. Those with Type 1 diabetes are also at an increased risk for hypertension, stroke, heart disease, and problems with the teeth and gums. So obviously, keeping a vigilant watch on blood-sugar numbers is a constant challenge for those with Type 1 diabetes.

Type 2 Diabetes

Ninety percent of Americans with diabetes have this type, which is generally less serious than Type 1. Patients may not make enough insulin, and/or they may be resistant to the insulin that they do produce. In individuals with Type 2 diabetes, the insulin that should be produced after a meal can be decreased by as much as 50 percent. People with Type 2 usually don't have to take insulin right after diagnosis, and they may never need to. Doctors generally first prescribe a change in diet, an increase in exercise, and often times, oral medication. With Type 2, unlike Type 1, autoimmune destruction of the cells is not present.

Type 2 diabetes is often called the silent disease because out of the nearly 16 million people in this country who have it, nearly one third don't know it. In fact, Type 2 diabetes is present on average for about six and one half years before diagnosis. And even though at the time of diagnosis most Type 2 patients don't even have symptoms, they are still at significant risk for coronary heart disease, stroke, and peripheral vascular disease.

Q & A
Are you obese, overweight, or just right?
Don't rely on your bathroom scale for the answer. Experts now assess both obesity and overweight using the body mass index (BMI) because they believe that it yields a more accurate measure of total body fat than weight does. Take a look at the BMI chart at the back of the book (Appendix C) and find out where you stand.
Abdominal fat distribution—an increased percentage of body fat distributed around the belly region—is also associated with insulin resistance and therefore, an increased risk for type 2 diabetes. And you don't have to be obese to fall into this category. Abdominal obesity is defined by waist circumference over 102 cm for men (40 inches) and over 88 cm for women (over 35 inches).

The risk of developing Type 2 diabetes climbs with age, and is typically diagnosed after the age of 30. However, don't be so sure your child won't develop the disorder. Increasingly, it's being diagnosed in children and teenagers, and some authorities are predicting an epidemic among young people. What's more, Type 2 diabetes goes hand in hand with obesity. About 80 percent of Type 2 patients are obese at the time of diagnosis. Unfortunately, a growing percentage of our younger population falls into this category.

Gestational Diabetes

About 4 percent of pregnancies in the United States are complicated by gestational diabetes (GDM). This disorder, which affects 135,000 women each year, is defined as any degree of glucose intolerance during pregnancy. Most women with GDM will have a completely normal blood glucose after the baby is born, although a history of GDM means a woman is at risk for developing the disorder in subsequent pregnancies, and for possibly developing Type 2 diabetes later in life.

Diagnosing Diabetes Is Easy

In fact, it's one of the simplest disorders to diagnose. A simple finger prick yields a couple of drops of blood that are analyzed for the presence of sugar. In non-pregnant adults, the criteria for diagnosis is as follows: a blood-sugar level of greater than or equal to 200 mg/dl, a fasting blood-sugar level of greater than or equal to 126 mg/dl, or a two-hour blood-sugar level greater than or equal to 200 mg/dl during an oral glucose tolerance test.

All pregnant women should be tested for GDM between 24 and 28 weeks of gestation. The testing, called an oral glucose tolerance test (OGTT), is painless and reliable. A blood-sugar level is obtained, and then the patient drinks a glass of sugary liquid. One hour later, a second blood-sugar reading is obtained. If a mom-to-be has a fasting blood sugar of greater than or equal to 126 mg/dl, or a random blood sugar of greater than or equal to 200 mg/dl, she meets the criteria for diabetes. At this point, the physician will send the mom-to-be for further testing.

It's very important to diagnose GDM because, when treated with proper diet and possibly insulin therapy, there's a decreased risk of problems for the fetus. Complications of GDM include a higher Cesarean rate, larger babies, and chronic high blood pressure.

Q & A

Are you at risk for diabetes?

The risk of coming down with Type 1 diabetes isn't as low as you might think. In the general population, the disorder has a rate of 1 in 400 to 1 in 1,000. But there's definitely a genetic component at play, and relatives of those with diabetes have a 1 in 20 to 1 in 50 chance of developing the condition. In addition to the genetic predisposition, though, it appears that an outside trigger is necessary, and so far, experts can only speculate on what that trigger might be. One theory is that an environmental trigger is the culprit. Another is that susceptible individuals who come down with Type 1 diabetes may have an allergy to cow's milk. This is one reason why pediatricians discourage parents from giving their baby cow's milk before the first birthday. No matter what the trigger is, the presence of diabetes can be first identified by the presence of antibodies against the insulin-producing beta cells of the pancreas.

Can You Prevent Diabetes?

So far, despite a number of research studies now underway, there are no definitive answers on how to prevent Type 1 diabetes. Type 2 diabetes is another story. You can reduce many of the risk factors that increase your chances for developing the condition. Poor lifestyle habits such as a bad diet and lack of exercise can increase your chances for getting diabetes. Other non-nutrition–related risk factors for Type 2 diabetes include being over the age of 45, having a parent or sibling with the disease, being of Latino, Native American, African American, or Pacific Islander descent, and, in a woman, having polycystic ovarian syndrome.

Furthermore, there's strong evidence that even modest weight loss and exercise can significantly reduce the onset of Type 2 diabetes in people with an impaired fasting glucose (IFG) or impaired glucose tolerance (IGT). In one study, individuals who lost 5 to 7 percent of their body weight and walked for 150 minutes each week reduced their risk of developing Type 2 diabetes by 58 percent.

Becoming Proactive

You can dramatically reduce your risk of developing Type 2 diabetes by following these guidelines:

♦ Turn off the television. If you have a sedentary lifestyle and watch a lot of TV, you're at a higher risk of developing the disease. One Harvard study reports a significant connection between television-watching and the risk among men for developing Type 2 diabetes.

♦ Walk briskly or engage in some physical activity for at least 30 minutes a day.

♦ Eat whole-grain breads and cereals instead of refined breads, cereals, and sugars.

♦ Eat at least five to nine servings of fruits and vegetables (other than white potatoes, peas, or corn) each day.

♦ Reduce your total fat intake to less than 30 percent of total calories. And choose unsaturated fats over saturated.

♦ Enjoy your coffee—but without sugar! According to the Nurses Health Study and Health Professionals' Follow-up Study, long-term coffee consumption is associated with a statistically lower risk for Type 2 diabetes. However, once diagnosed with diabetes, coffee's been shown to elevate blood sugar. What's more, caffeine can temporarily raise blood pressure, so if you have hypertension or Type 2 diabetes, seek advice from your personal physician.

◆ Beginning at age 45, have your fasting glucose level tested every three years. In fact, do so more often if risk factors are present, or if your fasting blood glucose consistently exceeds 110 mg/dl.

Eating Smart When You Have Diabetes

If you're diagnosed with diabetes, you should definitely seek the nutritional advice of a registered dietitian, preferably one who is certified as a diabetes educator (credentials will read R.D., C.D.E.). The goal of nutrition therapy is to restore and maintain blood glucose levels to as near normal as possible. This means balancing your food with insulin and activity levels. What's more, you'll want to maintain appropriate cholesterol and triglyceride levels, consume the right number of calories for maintaining a reasonable weight, and improve your overall health by eating right.

Calculating Carbs

Like everyone else, people with diabetes should (and can) consume carbohydrates, which are found in starches such as breads and pastas; vegetables like corn, potatoes, peas, and winter squash; fruit; and dairy products. They should also get the same recommended amount of fiber per day: up to 25 to 35 grams.

How much carbohydrate can a diabetic eat? When figuring it out, the total amount of carbohydrate is a strong predictor of your blood sugar response. According to the American Diabetes Association (ADA), monitoring grams of carbohydrate remains a major strategy in controlling blood sugar. However, the *type* of carbohydrate also influences blood glucose level. To figure out how quickly a carbohydrate will raise your blood sugar, nutrition experts use something called the Glycemic Index (GI), a numerical rating based on how quickly a carbohydrate raises blood sugar. The higher the number, the greater the blood sugar response to a certain food, which means the quicker an increase in your blood sugar. Of course, diabetics will benefit most from foods that have a low GI. Believe it or not, certain healthy foods, like carrots and potatoes, may cause a sharper increase in blood glucose than some candy bars. Often, a healthy food has a higher GI than a less healthy food. For instance, watermelon has a GI of 72, while cheese tortellini has a GI of 50. Many factors affect the GI of a food: how you prepare it, for instance, and what other foods are consumed along with it (fat and protein). If you have watermelon for dessert right after eating a peanut butter sandwich, for example, the fat in the peanut butter will lower the GI of the watermelon. Certainly, eating food combinations that yield lower glycemic responses can be beneficial for blood sugar regulation. See Chapter 2 for more information on glycemic index and glycemic load.

Protein Power

People with diabetes who don't have good blood sugar control may need more protein than nondiabetics. But since the average protein intake in the United States is far above the Recommended Dietary Allowance (RDA), this isn't a cause for great concern. The usual protein intake (15 to 20 percent of total calories) is enough, as long as kidney function is normal. A diabetic with compromised kidney function may need to follow a protein-restricted food plan.

Fats and Oils

People with diabetes are more sensitive to cholesterol in the diet, and it's recommended that less than 10 percent of the total caloric intake should come from saturated fat. If your LDL cholesterol is greater than 100 mg/dl, then just 7 percent is recommended. It's also advisable to consume no more than 200 mg of dietary cholesterol each day (see Chapter 4). On the other hand, monounsaturated fats are terrific, as are the omega-3s. To reap the benefits of omega-3 fatty acids, it's recommended that you eat two to three servings of fatty fish each week. Or try adding ground flaxseeds to your food.

Advice on Alcohol

The same recommendations for the general public apply to people with diabetes. If you choose to drink alcohol, the daily limit should be one drink for adult women and two drinks for men.

What constitutes a drink? Either a 12-ounce beer, a 5- to 6-ounce glass of wine or $1^1/_2$ ounces of a distilled spirit like gin or rum. It's very important that alcohol be consumed with food in order to reduce the risk of hypoglycemia, or low blood sugar. And when calculating your daily food plan, don't forget to count the alcohol as part of the day's calories.

Sweeteners Beyond Sucrose

Here's a guide to the various sweeteners now on the market:

- ◆ **Fructose.** Although it doesn't raise the blood sugar as much as ordinary table sugar (sucrose), it may adversely affect the levels of fat in the blood. It's not recommended as a sweetening agent.

◆ **Sugar alcohols.** These include mannitol, sorbitol, and xylitol, all of which produce a lower glucose response than fructose or sucrose. Still, there's no evidence that they aid in weight loss or improve blood sugar control, and they may also cause diarrhea, abdominal cramping, or gas, especially in children.

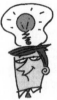

Food for Thought

Caffeine intake *before* eating carbohydrates appears to elevate blood sugars in people with Type 2 diabetes. If you've been diagnosed with Type 2, make an effort to drink decaffeinated beverages.

Food for Thought

Go for the CINNAMON! Cinnamon has been shown to improve blood sugars, triglycerides, and LDL-cholesterol in people with Type 2 diabetes. You'll need a daily dose of at least ¼ teaspoon—mix with low-fat cottage cheese, yogurt, oatmeal, sweet potato, or decaf coffee—and buy cinnamon-flavored healthy products.

◆ **Artificial sweeteners (saccharin, aspartame, acesulfame potassium, and sucralose).** The FDA has approved these for the general public, and they can be an effective tool for diabetics.

Vitamins and Minerals

While there's nothing wrong with taking a daily multi-vitamin, megadoses aren't a good idea because their long-term safety remains in question. Over the years, various supplements have been recommended for an assortment of ailments. B-vitamins, for instance, were used to treat diabetic neuropathy, but their beneficial role was never proven and they're not recommended as a therapeutic option. Although chromium piccolinate was reported to have a good effect on blood sugar control, it was never conclusively demonstrated. One antioxidant, alphalipoic acid, is a prescription drug in Germany that has been used to treat diabetic neuropathy. Although studies are underway in the United States, results will not be available for years.

Making the Nutritional Guidelines Work for You

The same nutrition recommendations that guide the general public are also appropriate for those with Type 1 or Type 2 diabetes. But diabetics on a fixed amount of daily insulin need to be vigilant about the amount of carbohydrates they eat, and how they time their meals.

You get a lot more flexibility both in meal timing and what you eat with intensive insulin therapy, in which you either take insulin injections before each meal, or with an insulin pump, which contains a continuous subcutaneous insulin infusion (CSII). Before you give yourself an injection, you determine how much carbohydrate you plan to eat and calculate the amount of insulin accordingly. There are many resources for learning the carbohydrate levels of foods, including food labels. A list of resources for carbohydrate counting and meal planning for diabetes may be found at the end of this chapter. In the following section, you'll find a carbohydrate-counting list, which shows the carbohydrate content of various foods. While a carb-counting list includes foods from the starch, fruit, and dairy groups, it does not contain foods from the fat, vegetable, and protein groups. Keep in mind that each food in the carbohydrate counting list is 15 grams of carbohydrate within the stated portion size. Vegetables—except for peas, potatoes, winter squash, and corn, which are in the starch group—have just 5 grams of carbohydrate per serving and are excluded from the list.

Help!

The American Dietetic Association (ADA) has pamphlets with step-by-step instructions on carbohydrate counting. In addition, a list of resources for meal planning is provided at the end of this chapter. When you use food labels to calculate your carb intake, be sure to look for the total grams of carbohydrates. Don't count grams of sugar on the label, since sugars are already included as part of the total carbohydrate content. And bear in mind that there is no "one size fits all" meal plan. It's best to work with a registered dietitian who is also a certified diabetes educator to learn meal planning and carbohydrate counting.

Note that the foods in the following table contain 15 grams of carbohydrate in the specified portion size.

Carbohydrate Counting

Food	Portion Size
Starch/breads/cereal/grains/starchy vegetables/miscellaneous	
Bagel	$^1/_4$
Frozen bagel	$^1/_2$
Cookies	2 medium
Potato chip	small bag
Bread, whole-wheat, white, rye, pumpernickel	1 slice

continues

Carbohydrate Counting   (continued)

Food	Portion Size
Corn chips	small bag
English muffin	$1/2$
Hamburger bun	$1/2$
Pasta, cooked	$1/2$ cup
Rice (white or brown), barley, couscous	$1/3$ cup
Bulgur, cooked	$1/2$ cup
Cold cereal (e.g., Cheerios, Bran Flakes)	$3/4$ cup
Bran cereal	$1/2$ cup
Legumes, cooked (dried beans, peas, or lentils)	$1/3$ cup
Corn, sweet potato	$1/2$ cup
White potato, baked or broiled	1 small (3 oz.)
Pretzels	$3/4$ oz.
Popcorn, air-popped or lite microwave	3 cups
Fruit	
Apple	1 small
Banana	1 small or $1/2$ reg.
Blueberries	$3/4$ cup
Cherries	12
Grapes	15
Grapefruit	$1/2$
Honeydew	1 cup of cubes
Kiwi	1 medium
Mango	$1/2$
Orange	1 small
Peach	1 medium
Pineapple	$3/4$ cup
Strawberries	$1 1/4$ cup
Tangerines	2 small

Food	Portion Size
Dairy (12 grams of carbohydrate, but 15 grams are assigned to the following portions, for ease of counting)	
Milk	8-oz. cup
Yogurt	8-oz. cup
Ice cream	$^1/_2$ cup

The next table is a sample menu that is based on the Carbohydrate (CHO) Counting System. It's based on a meal plan of 1,800 calories with 50 percent of the calories coming from carbohydrates.

Food	Amount	Grams CHO
Breakfast (Total of approximately 45 grams of CHO)		
Skim milk	1 cup	15
Cheerios	1 cup	15
Banana	$^1/_2$	15
Lunch (Total of approximately 45 grams of CHO)		
Whole-wheat bread	2 slices	30
Strawberries	1 cup	15
Turkey	4 oz.	0
Low-fat mayonnaise	1 TB.	0
Salad with dressing	1 cup	0
Snack (Total of approximately 30 grams of CHO)		
Fat-free fruit yogurt (artificially sweetened)	1 cup	15
Apple	1 small	15
Dinner (Total of approximately 75 grams of CHO)		
Brown rice	1 cup	45
Fresh fruit salad	1 cup	30
Shrimp or chicken	4 oz.	>0
Salad with low-fat dressing	1 cup	>0
Asparagus	$^1/_2$ cup	>0

continues

continued

Food	Amount	Grams CHO
Snack (Total of approximately 15 grams of CHO)		
Graham cracker	1$^1/_2$	15
Tea, plain	1 cup	0

The Exchange System

A major drawback of counting only carbs is that it de-emphasizes the fat and overall nutrient content of foods. For those with Type 2 diabetes, weight loss is a central goal. Many people are on oral medication rather than insulin, and they've been told by their health-care provider to reduce fat and calories. For them, the exchange system is a more logical approach.

With this system, foods are categorized into groups based on the same or similar nutritional value. For example, all foods in the starch group contain 15 grams of carbohydrate, 3 grams of protein and 0–1 gram of fat. The following table provides exchange lists. Carbohydrate counting is an extension of the exchange system. It simply focuses solely on carbs. An exchange plan offers balance—meals are consistent in calories, fat, and protein along with carbohydrates, and it offers a variety of food choices.

Exchange System: Foods and Their Portion Sizes

Food	Portion Size
Starch (breads/cereal/grains/starchy vegetables): 80 calories, 15 grams CHO, 3 grams protein, and 0–1 gram of fat per serving.	
Bagel, large	$^1/_4$
Bagel, small frozen	$^1/_2$
Bread	1 slice
*French fries	16–25 (3 oz.)
Pancake, 4 inches across	2
English muffin	$^1/_2$
*Cookies (small oatmeal, chocolate chip)	2

Food	Portion Size
Hamburger bun	$^1/_2$
Pasta, cooked	$^1/_2$ cup
Cake, unfrosted	2-inch square
Rice (white or brown), barley, couscous	$^1/_3$ cup
Bulgur, cooked	$^1/_2$ cup
Cold cereal (e.g., Cheerios, Puffins)	$^3/_4$ cup
Grapenuts	$^1/_4$ cup
Bran cereal	$^1/_2$ cup
Legumes, cooked (dried beans, peas, or lentils)	$^1/_3$ cup
Corn, sweet potato	$^1/_2$ cup
White potato, baked or broiled	1 small (3 oz.)
Pretzels	$^3/_4$ oz.
Popcorn, air-popped or microwave (80 percent light)	3 cups
Fruit: 60 calories, 15 grams CHO per serving	
Apple	1 small
Banana	1 small or $^1/_2$ reg.
Blueberries	$^3/_4$ cup
Cantaloupe	1 cup cubes
Cherries	12
Grapefruit	$^1/_2$
Grapes	15
Honeydew	1 cup of cubes
Kiwi	1 medium
Mango	$^1/_2$
Orange	1 small
Peach	1 medium
Pineapple	$^3/_4$ cup
Strawberries	$1^1/_4$ cup
Tangerines	2 small
Watermelon	$1^1/_4$ cup cubes

continues

Exchange System: Foods and Their Portion Sizes   (continued)

Food	Portion Size
Vegetables: 25 calories, 5 grams CHO, 2 grams protein per serving	
Asparagus	¹/₂ cup cooked
Beans (green, wax)	¹/₂ cup cooked
Beets	¹/₂ cup cooked or 1 cup raw
Broccoli	¹/₂ cup cooked or 1 cup raw
Cabbage	¹/₂ cup cooked
Carrots	¹/₂ cup cooked or 1 cup raw
Cauliflower	¹/₂ cup cooked or 1 cup raw
Celery	¹/₂ cup cooked or 1 cup raw
Cucumber	1 cup
Eggplant	¹/₂ cup cooked
Onions	¹/₂ cup cooked or 1 cup raw
Peppers	¹/₂ cup cooked or 1 cup raw
Salad (Romaine, spinach, endive, escarole)	1 cup
Summer squash	¹/₂ cup
Tomato	¹/₂ cup cooked/ juice or 1 cup raw
Tomato sauce	¹/₂ cup cooked
Zucchini	¹/₂ cup cooked
Fat-free and very low-fat milk: 90 calories, 12 grams CHO, 8 grams protein, 12 grams of carbohydrate per serving	
Milk, fat-free or 1%	8-oz. cup
Yogurt, plain nonfat	³/₄ cup
Yogurt, artificially sweetened	1 cup
Very lean protein or lean protein: 35–55 calories, 1–3 grams of fat, 7 grams of protein per serving	
Turkey breast or chicken breast, skin removed	1 oz.
Chicken, dark meat, skin removed	1 oz.
Fish fillet (flounder, cod, scrod, sole, haddock, halibut)	1 oz.
Turkey, dark meat, skin removed	1 oz.
Tuna, canned in water	1 oz.

Food	Portion Size
Salmon, swordfish, catfish, trout	1 oz.
Shellfish (clams, lobster, scallop, shrimp)	1 oz.
Lean beef (roast beef, flank steak, London broil)**	1 oz.
Cottage cheese, nonfat or low-fat	$1/4$ cup
Egg whites	2
Egg substitute	$1/4$ cup
Pork, tenderloin, fresh ham	1 oz.
Fat-free cheese	1 oz.
Beans, cooked (black beans, kidney, chickpeas, lentils)	$1/2$ cup
Low-fat cheese (3 grams fat or less per oz.)	1 oz.
Medium-fat meats: 75 calories, 5 grams of fat per serving	
Beef (any prime cut), ground beef***	1 oz.
Pork chop	1 oz.
Whole egg**	1 medium
Mozzarella cheese	1 oz.
Ricotta cheese	$1/4$ cup
Tofu	4 oz. (note that this is heart-healthy choice)
Fats: 45 calories, 5 grams of fat per serving	
Oil (olive, canola, corn, etc.)	1 tsp.
Cream cheese, light	2 TB.
Butter	1 tsp.
Avocado	$1/8$
Margarine	1 tsp.
Black olives	8 large
Mayonnaise	1 tsp.
Bacon	1 slice
Reduced-fat margarine or mayonnaise	1 TB.
Peanuts	10
Salad dressing	1 TB.
Cream cheese	1 TB.

These starches are prepared with fat (count as 1 starch exchange plus 1 fat).
**Limit to 1 to 2 times per week (count as 1 starch and 1 very lean protein).*
***Choose these very infrequently.*

The next set of tables presents five different meal patterns that explain how many servings of food to have from each food group. These meal patterns provide 1,200, 1,400, 1,600, 1,800, and 2,200 (for gestational diabetes) calories, with 50 to 55 percent of calories from CHO, 20 percent from protein, and 25 to 27 percent from fat.

Suggested Daily Food Exchanges

Exchange List	1,200	1,400	1,600	1,800	2,200
Skim Milk	2	2	2	2	3
Vegetable	4	4	3	4	4
Protein	4	5	6	7	8
Starch	4	6	7	8	10
Fruit	3	3	4	4	4
Fat	2	2	3	4	5

Plan 1

1,200 Calorie Menu	Exchange for:
Breakfast	
* ³/₄ cup whole-grain cereal	1 starch
* 1 cup blueberries	1 fruit
* 1 cup skim milk	1 milk
Lunch	
* 2 oz. tuna	2 very lean protein
* 2 cups salad with a mix of peppers and tomatoes and balsamic vinegar	2 vegetable
* 1 cup melon chunks	1 fruit
* 1 cup yogurt (artificially sweetened), add cinnamon	1 milk
Snack	
* 2 small chocolate cookies	1 starch, 1 fat

1,200 Calorie Menu	Exchange for:
Dinner	
* 2 oz. shrimp	2 very lean protein
* 1 cup wheat pasta (mix with the shrimp)	2 starch
* ½ cup marinara sauce	1 vegetable
* ½ cup broccoli rabe sautéed in	1 vegetable
* 1 tsp. olive oil and garlic	1 fat
* 15 frozen grapes	1 fruit

Plan 2

1,400 Calorie Menu	Exchange for:
Breakfast	
* 1 cup non-fat, plain yogurt (add some cinnamon)	1 milk
* ¼ cup Grapenuts	1 starch
* 1 cup cut fruit	1 fruit
Lunch	
* 2 oz. turkey wrapped in	2 very lean protein
* 1 (2 oz.) soft tortilla	2 starch
* 1 cup mixed greens	1 vegetable
* 1 TB. vinaigrette dressing	1 fat
* 1 peach	1 fruit
Snack	
* 2-inch square of cake	1 starch, 1 fat
Dinner	
* 3 oz. broiled salmon	3 lean protein

1,400 Calorie Menu	Exchange for:
* 2 small potatoes roasted with oil spray and rosemary	2 starch
* 1 cup steamed asparagus	2 vegetable
* 1 cup mixed berries	1 fruit
Snack	
* 1 cup non-fat, vanilla yogurt (artificially sweetened), add cinnamon	1 milk

Plan 3

1,600 Calorie Menu	Exchange for:
Breakfast	
* Whole-grain English muffin	2 starch
* 2 scrambled egg whites (use Pam Spray with $\frac{1}{2}$ cup onions and peppers)	1 very lean protein
* 1 orange	1 fruit
Lunch	
* 2 oz. chicken salad	2 very lean meat
* 1 tsp. mayonnaise, celery in whole-wheat pita bread	1 fat, 2 starch
* 1 cup lettuce and tomato	1 vegetable
* 1 kiwi	1 fruit
Snack	
* $\frac{3}{4}$ cup plain, nonfat yogurt (add cinnamon)	1 milk
* 1 cup fruit salad	1 fruit
Dinner	
* 4 oz. filet mignon	4 lean meat
* 1 medium baked potato	2 starch
* 1 tsp. soft tub, trans-free margarine	1 fat
* 1 cup steamed carrots	2 vegetable

1,600 Calorie Menu	Exchange for:
* 1 cup salad	1 vegetable
* 1 tsp. olive oil	1 fat
* 1 plum	1 fruit
Snack	
* ½ cup nonfat sugar-free ice cream	1 milk

Plan 4

1,800 Calorie Menu	Exchange for:
Breakfast	
* 1 cup cooked oatmeal (add cinnamon)	2 starch
* 1 cup skim milk (cooked with the oatmeal or on the side)	1 milk
* 1 small banana	1 fruit
Lunch	
* 1 small slice thin-crust pizza	2 starch, 2 protein
* 2 cups salad	2 vegetable
* 1 TB. Italian dressing	1 fat
* 1 small apple	1 fruit
Snack	
* 2 small cookies	1 starch, 1 fat
* 1 cup skim milk	1 milk
Dinner	
* 6 oz. grilled salmon	6 lean meat
* ⅔ cup brown rice	2 starch
* 1 tsp. soft tub, trans-free margarine	1 fat
* 1 cup sautéed spinach	2 vegetable
* 1 tsp. olive oil	1 fat
Snack	
* ¾ oz. bag of pretzels	1 starch

Note, the following is a two-day menu for a woman diagnosed with gestational diabetes. Each day provides 2,200 calories.

Plan 5

2,200 Calorie Menu	Exchange for:

Day One

Breakfast (note that fruit is to be avoided in the morning in gestational diabetes)

* 1½ cups whole-grain cereal	2 starch
* 1 cup 1% milk	1 milk
* 3 scrambled egg whites in	1 very lean protein
* 1 tsp. olive or canola oil with a small handful of vegetables	1 fat, 1 vegetable

Mid-morning Snack

* 1 slice whole-wheat toast	1 starch
* 1 oz. low-fat cheese	1 lean meat

Lunch

* Pasta salad (1 cup cooked)	2 starch
* 2 oz. diced chicken breast	2 very lean meat
* 1 cup cooked vegetables mixed in	2 vegetable
* 2 TB. Italian dressing	2 fat
* ½ mango	2 fruit

Mid-day Snack

* 1 cup 1% milk	1 milk
* 3 graham cracker halves	1 starch
* 12 cherries	1 fruit

Dinner

* 3 oz. pork tenderloin	3 lean meat
* 1 cup couscous	3 starch
* 2 tsp. soft tub, trans-free margarine	2 fat
* 1 cup steamed carrots	2 vegetable
* 1 cup cantaloupe cubes	1 fruit

Evening Snack

* $1/2$ sandwich (1 oz. cheese on 1 slice whole-wheat bread)	1 medium-fat meat, 1 part-skim mozzarella starch
* 1 cup skim milk	1 milk

Day Two

Breakfast

* Toasted whole-grain English muffin	2 starch
* 3 egg whites	1 protein
* 2 tsp. soft tub, trans-free margarine	2 fat
* 1 cup 1% milk	1 milk

Mid-morning Snack

* 1 slice whole-wheat toast	1 starch
* 1 TB. peanut butter**	1 protein, 1 fat

Lunch

* Chef salad with 2 cups salad greens	2 vegetable
* 3 oz. mix of low-fat cheese, roast beef, and turkey	3 lean meat
* 2 TB. vinaigrette dressing	2 fat
* $1/2$ banana or medium apple	1 fruit

Mid-day Snack

* $3/4$ cup plain low-fat yogurt	1 milk
* 1 cup strawberries	1 fruit
* $1/4$ cup Grapenuts	1 starch

Dinner

* Stir-fry with 4 oz. sliced chicken	4 very lean meat
* 1 cup mixed vegetables (snow peas, bok choy, mushrooms)	2 vegetable
* 2 tsp. sesame oil and lite soy sauce (mix with vegetables)	2 fat
* 1 cup brown rice	3 starch
* 1 cup blueberries	1 fruit

2,200 Calorie Menu	Exchange for:
Evening Snack	
* ³/₄ cup whole-grain cereal	1 starch
* 1 cup 1% milk	1 milk

Food for Thought

Resources for Meal Planning

- *The Corrine T. Netzer Carbohydrate Counter*, Dell Publishing, www.amazon.com
- *The Complete Book of Food Counts* by Corrine T. Netzer, Dell Publishing, www.amazon.com
- *Month of Meals*, American Diabetes Association: 1-800-232-3472 or www.diabetes.org
- *Carbohydrate Counting: Level 1, level 2, level 3*, American Dietetic Association: 1-800-877-1600 or www.eatright.org
- *Exchange Lists for Meal Planning*, American Dietetic Association and American Diabetes Association: 1-800-DIABETES (342-2383) or www.diabetes.org

Children and Adolescents

Nutrient requirements for children and teenagers with diabetes are the same as they are for kids who don't have diabetes. It's crucial that their families work with a health professional to organize an eating strategy, as schedules, appetites, and activity levels can vary greatly.

Food for Thought

Children and teenagers are now developing Type 2 diabetes more often than they used to. In fact, the prevalence of Type 2 diabetes in children is now as high as that of Type 1 diabetes. The culprit, as with grown-ups, is obesity. American children now watch an average of four hours of television per day, leaving little time for valuable exercise. They are also eating more high-fat, refined-carbohydrate, and calorie-laden restaurant meals than previous generations of children. This paves the way for overweight and obesity, which can contribute to the development of Type 2 diabetes.

Glucose Monitoring

Monitoring your blood sugar is critical. Without constant monitoring, optimal control cannot be achieved. Your health-care provider will tell you how often to test your blood. For those with Type 1 diabetes, it's usually recommended that blood sugar be tested at least 3 times per day. If the blood glucose is 250 mg/dl or higher, urine testing for ketones should be done. For Type 2 diabetes, the choice for glucose testing will be up to you and your doctor. However, blood glucose monitoring is an empowering tool. Using it, a diabetic can learn the effects of foods and exercise on his or her blood sugar levels. This can help to adjust the diet accordingly and ultimately achieve optimal blood sugar numbers.

Measurement Tools

Blood sugar control on a day-to-day basis is evaluated by using a glucose monitor. However, it is also recommended that a Hemoglobin A1C (A1C) test be performed at least twice a year in patients who are meeting their blood sugar goals and every three months in individuals whose blood sugar levels are *not* well controlled. The A1C is a simple blood test which shows the average blood glucose level over a three-month period. The following table provides guidelines for blood sugar and A1C goals.

	Normal	Goal	Additional Action Suggested*
Blood glucose before meals (mg/dl)	<100	80–120	<80/>140
Average bedtime glucose (mg/dl)	<110	100–140	<100/>L160
A1C (%)	<6	<7	>8

* Values above or below these levels are not acceptable in most patients. They indicate the need for a significant change in the treatment plan. The individual may require a referral to an endocrinologist, a change in medication, or more frequent contact with an R.D. or nurse educator.

The Least You Need to Know

◆ You can have Type 2 diabetes for several years and not have any symptoms at all. Since the risk for coming down with the disorder increases with age, anyone over the age of 45 should undergo glucose testing regularly.

◆ Anyone who is overweight or obese is at an increased risk for developing diabetes. To help reduce your risk, exercise regularly and eat right.

◆ As the obesity rate in children rises, more youngsters than ever before are coming down with Type 2 diabetes. Don't let your kids be couch potatoes. Whether they play soccer, swim, or jog, be sure to get them moving!

◆ If you're pregnant, make sure your doctor has you undergo glucose testing to see if you have gestational diabetes, a form of the disease that afflicts 135,000 women annually.

◆ It's a myth that candy and cookies should never be eaten by a person with diabetes. However, it's incredibly important that diabetics monitor their sum total of carbohydrates each day.

Chapter 20

Don't Eat Your Heart Out

In This Chapter

- ◆ Understanding heart disease
- ◆ Optimal cardiac numbers (total cholesterol, LDL and HDL cholesterol, cholesterol ratio, triglycerides, homocysteine, C-reactive protein, and blood pressure)
- ◆ How certain foods can protect your heart
- ◆ A heart-smart, seven-day meal plan
- ◆ Exercise for your heart

Heart disease is our nation's leading killer—claiming one life every *34 seconds*. About 1.5 million Americans suffer a heart attack and 500,000 a stroke (brain attack) annually. And listen up, ladies, heart disease is not just for men—it's also the number one killer of *women* in America. The good news is that many strokes and heart attacks could be prevented if people took better care of themselves.

If you smoke, you are five times more likely to have a heart attack than if you don't smoke. If you are one of the estimated 107 million adults with a total cholesterol of 200 mg/dL or higher, a mere 10 percent reduction could reduce your risk of heart disease by *30* percent. If you are overweight, inactive, or eat poorly, you are also at greater risk for heart disease.

In this chapter, you'll find information that will help you understand your personal cardiac numbers, and you'll also learn how to eat smart and exercise right for long-term heart health.

Understanding Your Blood Test: OptimalCardiac Numbers

We hear lots of numbers being tossed around when it comes to cardiovascular health, and without a clear understanding of what they *mean*, this information can be down-right overwhelming. Key players include total cholesterol, LDL and HDL cholesterol, cholesterol ratio, triglycerides, homocysteine, C-reactive protein, and blood pressure.

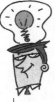

Food for Thought

The American Heart Association (AHA) recommends that healthy people limit their dietary cholesterol to less than 300 mg per day, and that people with heart disease shoot for less than 200 mg per day. The AHA also recommends that no more than 30 percent of your day's calories come from fat, and that your saturated plus trans fat intake not exceed 10 percent of total calories. (If you have heart disease, keep that number to less than 7 percent.)

Total Cholesterol

Total cholesterol is the most common measurement of blood cholesterol, and is usually expressed in milligrams per deciliter of blood (mg/dL). Knowing your total blood cholesterol level is an important *first* step in determining your risk for heart disease. You should make a point of having your cholesterol measured every five years, and more often if you are a man over 45 or a woman over 55.

If your total cholesterol is less than 200 mg/dL, good news!—your heart attack risk is relatively low (unless you have other risk factors). But even if you're not at high risk, it's still smart to eat quality foods and to get plenty of physical activity.

If your total cholesterol is 200-239 mg/dL it is considered borderline-high, and if it gets to 240 mg/dL or more, then it is flat-out high. In both cases, you should take steps to lower it.

LDL Cholesterol

LDL cholesterol is another vital part of the picture, and the lower it is, the better. If you are a healthy individual, your LDL should be around 130 mg/dL or lower. If you are at high risk for heart disease, your goal is an LDL below 100 mg/dL, and if you are at *very* high-risk, experts now say you should aim for a level below 70 mg/dL.

You are considered to be at high risk if you have …

> Coronary heart disease (CHD) or the risk equivalent—which includes diseases of the blood vessels to the brain or extremities and diabetes.
>
> or
>
> Two or more other risk factors.

You are at very high risk if you have …

> CHD or the risk equivalent
>
> and
>
> Multiple risk factors or severe and poorly controlled risk factors.

Risk factors include …

- Age (45 years or older for men; 55 years or older for women, or premature menopause)
- High blood pressure
- Low HDL cholesterol
- Smoking
- A family history of cardiovascular disease

Food for Thought

If your LDL cholesterol is too high, your doctor may advise you to reduce your intake of saturated fat, trans fat, and dietary cholesterol, while increasing foods rich in soluble fiber. It's also important that you exercise regularly and lose weight if you're overweight. If you still can't lower your LDL, medications are available.

HDL Cholesterol

HDL cholesterol is the "good" type—in fact, it's the *only* good kind of cholesterol. Some folks are genetically blessed with high HDL readings, a lucky inherited gene which significantly reduces their risk for heart disease. Other folks have to work at increasing their numbers. Desirable HDL cholesterol levels are 40 mg/dL or higher.

If you learn that you have low HDL cholesterol, you can help raise it by not smoking, losing weight or maintaining a healthy weight, choosing monounsaturated fats (olive oil, almonds, avocadoes), and by being physically active for at least 30–60 minutes a day.

Cholesterol Ratio

The American Heart Association recommends using the absolute numbers for total blood cholesterol and HDL cholesterol levels. To the physician, they're more useful than the cholesterol ratio when choosing an appropriate treatment protocol.

However, it's still a good idea to understand the ratio because some physicians and health professionals use the ratio of total cholesterol to HDL cholesterol in place of total blood cholesterol. The ratio is obtained by dividing HDL cholesterol into the total cholesterol. For example, if a person has a total cholesterol of 200 mg/dL and an HDL cholesterol of 50 mg/dL, the ratio would be stated as 4:1. The goal is to keep the ratio *below* 5:1.

Triglycerides

The triglyceride level is yet another reading. You want your triglycerides to be under 150 mg/dL because higher levels can contribute to heart disease. If your triglycerides are 150–199 mg/dL, that's borderline-high; if they are 200–499 mg/dL, they're high; and a reading of 500 mg/dL or more is considered *extremely* high.

People with high blood triglycerides usually have lower HDL cholesterol and a higher risk of heart attack and, indirectly, of stroke. Furthermore, many people with high triglycerides have underlying diseases or genetic disorders. If this applies to you, the main therapy is to change your lifestyle by controlling your weight; eating foods low in cholesterol, saturated fats, and trans fats (choose monounsaturated fats instead); exercising regularly; not smoking; and drinking little to no alcohol. Because carbs raise triglycerides and lower HDL cholesterol, your doctor may also tell you to limit your intake of refined sugar and total carbohydrates to no more than 40–50 percent of total calories.

> **Food for Thought**
>
> Omega-3 fats—the kind found in salmon, sardines, and fish oil supplements—are a great, non-prescription way to help lower your triglycerides. If you want to try supplements, best talk to your doctor or a registered dietitian first.

Homocysteine

There's a lot of interest today in this sulfur-containing amino acid. That's because clinical studies have shown that having an elevated level of homocysteine can damage blood vessel walls and increase your risk of cardiovascular disease.

Factors that contribute to elevated homocysteine levels include smoking, excessive alcohol consumption, excessive coffee drinking, a sedentary life lifestyle, and a deficiency of folate and/or vitamins B-6 and B-12. What's more, medications that interfere with the absorption of folate and vitamins B-6 and B-12 can lead to increased homocysteine levels.

Generally speaking, men tend to have higher homocysteine levels than women the same age. And in women, homocysteine levels often increase after menopause, which can lead to a heightened risk of cardiovascular disease. Furthermore, homocysteine increases with impaired metabolism of homocysteine by the kidney. For this reason, total homocysteine levels are much higher in patients with chronic kidney disease.

Normal homocysteine levels range from 5–16 mg/dL. But optimally you should strive for an upper limit of 10 mg/dL, which you can achieve by eating foods loaded with folic acid, and vitamins B-6 and B-12.

If you've been diagnosed with an elevated homocysteine level, the most simple and effective treatment is to take a supplemental dose of folic acid with an additional B-complex. But deciding on the recommended supplemental dose can be tricky, so speak with your personal physician.

C-Reactive Protein

C-reactive protein (CRP) is a protein produced primarily in the liver that is released into the bloodstream when there is inflammation anywhere in your body. Normally, there is little to no CRP in the blood, but if you have a cut, infection, or certain inflammatory diseases (like rheumatoid arthritis), levels can become elevated.

So—where does CRP fit in when it comes to *heart disease*, you might ask? Well, it has been known for some time now that inflammation plays a key role in just about every stage of atherosclerosis (hardening of the arteries)— from plaque formation, to the rupture of those plaques, which can lead to a heart attack or stroke. CRP may also be an independent risk

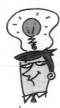

Food for Thought

Women, take note: CRP levels may be elevated in late pregnancy or if you take oral contraceptives.

factor for the development of hypertension, which further increases your chances of suffering a heart attack or stroke. And to make matters worse, if you have high CRP levels you may have more trouble lowering your blood cholesterol through diet than someone with low CRP levels.

Okay—so now that you know how bad CRP is, you probably want to know what you can do to keep your levels nice and low (that's below 1.0 mg/dL). I hate to sound like a broken record, but here goes: lose weight if you are overweight, quit smoking if you smoke, and exercise, exercise, exercise!

In terms of diet, it's probably best to follow an overall heart-smart diet. In other words—avoid trans and saturated fats, increase omega-3 fat intake (salmon, sardines, flaxseeds, fish oil supplements), and eat lots of fruits and vegetables.

When it comes to fruits and veggies, the richer the color the better. Colorful plants tend to have the most antioxidants, which are great at clearing out the nasty free radicals that are produced when inflammation is present in the body. One more thing you can do to keep your CRP levels low is to practice good oral hygiene. Flossing and brushing regularly reduces the risk of gum disease, which is a source of chronic inflammation.

Blood Pressure

One out of every four American adults (nearly 60 million people) has high blood pressure, which is known as the "silent killer" because it kind of creeps up without any warning. High blood pressure can greatly increase your risk of cardiovascular disease. As your heart beats, blood is pumped into your arteries, creating a pressure within them. When too much pressure is placed on the artery walls, high blood pressure, or hypertension, is the result. Over time, your arteries can be so damaged by such constant pressure that the end result could be a heart attack, brain attack (stroke), or kidney disease. The following table provides blood pressure guidelines, as recommended by the National Heart, Lung, and Blood Institute (NHLBI).

Blood Pressure Guidelines for Adults from the National Heart, Lung, and Blood Institute

Classification	Systolic	Diastolic
Normal	<120 mmHg	<80
Prehypertension	120–139	80–89

Classification	Systolic	Diastolic
Hypertension		
Stage 1	140–159	90–99
Stage 2	160 or higher	100 or higher

Follow these tips for lowering your numbers:

◆ Exercise at least 30 minutes a day most days of the week.

◆ Lose weight if you are overweight.

◆ Follow the DASH diet (see Chapter 5).

◆ Don't salt your food, and avoid processed and fast foods—they're usually loaded with sodium.

◆ Get 1,200–1,500 mg/d of calcium from supplements or food (taken with at least 400 IU vitamin D to aid absorption).

◆ Avoid excessive alcohol intake.

◆ Cut back on caffeine.

◆ Reduce stress—try yoga, Pilates, therapy, massage, or long walks.

◆ Eat foods rich in potassium and magnesium.

Potassium

Food	Potassium (mg)	Calories
Sweet potato, baked, 1 potato (146 g)	694	131
Tomato paste, ¼ cup	664	54
Beet greens, cooked, ½ cup	655	19
Potato, baked, flesh, 1 potato (156 g)	610	145
White beans, canned, ½ cup	595	153
Yogurt, plain, non-fat, 8-oz container	579	127
Tomato puree, ½ cup	549	48
Clams, canned, 3 oz	534	126
Yogurt, plain, low-fat, 8-oz container	531	143

continues

Potassium (continued)

Food	Potassium (mg)	Calories
Prune juice, $3/4$ cup	530	136
Carrot juice, $3/4$ cup	517	71
Blackstrap molasses, 1 TB	498	47
Halibut, cooked, 3 oz	490	119
Soybeans, green, cooked, $1/2$ cup	485	127
Tuna, yellowfin, cooked, 3 oz	484	118
Lima beans, cooked, $1/2$ cup	484	104
Winter squash, cooked, $1/2$ cup	448	40
Soybeans, mature, cooked, $1/2$ cup	443	149
Rockfish, Pacific, cooked, 3 oz	442	103
Cod, Pacific, cooked, 3 oz	439	89
Banana, 1 medium	422	105
Spinach, cooked, $1/2$ cup	419	21
Tomato juice, $3/4$ cup	417	31
Tomato sauce, $1/2$ cup	405	39
Peaches, dried, uncooked, $1/4$ cup	398	96
Prunes, stewed, $1/2$ cup	398	133
Milk, non-fat, 1 cup	382	83
Pork chop, center loin, cooked, 3 oz	382	197
Apricots, dried, uncooked, $1/4$ cup	378	78
Rainbow trout, farmed, cooked, 3 oz	375	144
Pork loin, center rib, lean, roasted, 3 oz	371	190
Buttermilk, cultured, low-fat, 1 cup	370	98
Cantaloupe, $1/4$ medium	368	47
1%–2% milk, 1 cup	366	102—122
Honeydew melon, $1/8$ medium	365	58
Lentils, cooked, $1/2$ cup	365	115
Plantains, cooked, $1/2$ cup slices	358	90
Kidney beans, cooked, $1/2$ cup	358	112
Orange juice, $3/4$ cup	355	85
Split peas, cooked, $1/2$ cup	355	116
Yogurt, plain, whole milk, 8 oz container	352	138

Magnesium

Food	Magnesium (mg)	Calories
Pumpkin and squash seed kernels, roasted, 1 oz	151	148
Brazil nuts, 1 oz	107	186
Bran ready-to-eat cereal (100%), 1 oz	103	74
Halibut, cooked, 3 oz	91	119
Quinoa, dry, 1/4 cup	89	159
Spinach, canned, 1/2 cup	81	25
Almonds, 1 oz	78	164
Spinach, cooked from fresh, 1/2 cup	78	20
Buckwheat flour, 1/4 cup	75	101
Cashews, dry roasted, 1 oz	74	163
Soybeans, mature, cooked, 1/2 cup	74	149
Pine nuts, dried, 1 oz	71	191
Mixed nuts, oil roasted, with peanuts, 1 oz	67	175
White beans, canned, 1/2 cup	67	154
Pollock, walleye, cooked, 3 oz	62	96
Black beans, cooked, 1/2 cup	60	114
Bulgur, dry, 1/4 cup	57	120
Oat bran, raw, 1/4 cup	55	58
Soybeans, green, cooked, 1/2 cup	54	127
Tuna, yellowfin, cooked, 3 oz	54	118
Artichokes (hearts), cooked, 1/2 cup	50	42
Peanuts, dry roasted, 1 oz	50	166
Lima beans, baby, cooked from frozen, 1/2 cup	50	95
Beet greens, cooked, 1/2 cup	49	19
Navy beans, cooked, 1/2 cup	48	127
Tofu, firm, 1/2 cup	47	88
Okra, cooked from frozen, 1/2 cup	47	26
Soy beverage, 1 cup	47	127
Cowpeas, cooked, 1/2 cup	46	100
Hazelnuts, 1 oz	46	178
Oat bran muffin, 1 oz	45	77

continues

Magnesium (continued)

Food	Magnesium (mg)	Calories
Great northern beans, cooked, ½ cup	44	104
Oat bran, cooked, ½ cup	44	44
Buckwheat groats, roasted, cooked, ½ cup	43	78
Brown rice, cooked, ½ cup	42	108
Haddock, cooked, 3 oz	42	95

Source: Agricultural Research Service (ARS) Nutrient Database for Standard Reference, Release 17.

Heart-Smart Eating

You can take a proactive role in preventing cardiovascular disease by paying attention to what you eat. Indeed, one of the best ways to protect your heart is to make sure you're getting a healthy diet. Instead of reaching for high-fat potato chips, for instance, choose baby carrots and salsa. Think of meat as a garnish rather than a main course. And when you eat out, avoid fried foods and instead ask for roasted, grilled, or stir-fried.

Fruits and Veggies

Both fruit and vegetables are loaded with vitamins and minerals, as well as plenty of soluble fiber. That fiber not only makes you feel full longer, but it also helps to lower your blood cholesterol. Eat fruits and veggies often as an alternative to high-fat snacks.

Whole Grains Over Refined

Whole-grain foods provide more overall nutrition and fiber than their refined counterparts. What's more, the fiber can help with weight management, lowering cholesterol levels, and managing problematic triglycerides. Choose whole-grain breads, pitas, English muffins, and crackers. Buy cereals that have at least 4–5 grams of fiber per serving. Choose oatmeal and sweeten it with fresh fruit. Buy brown rice instead of white rice, and try some different kinds of grains like couscous, barley, bulgur, kasha, millet, and polenta.

Soluble Fiber

Studies have confirmed that you can lower your cholesterol level by eating foods rich in soluble fiber. One possible explanation may be that soluble fiber binds to cholesterol and bile acids, carrying them out of the body into the feces. The National Cholesterol Education Program (NCEP) recommends getting 10–25 grams of soluble fiber each day.

The following table takes a look at the foods rich in soluble fiber.

Food	Soluble Fiber (g)	Total Fiber (g)
Breads and Cereals		
Bread, cracked wheat, reduced calorie (1 slice)	1.4	3.36
Oat Bran cereal (1 cup)	2.65	5.67
Oatmeal, regular or quick-cooking (1 cup)	1.85	3.98
98% fat-free granola (1 cup)	3.01	6.00
Roll, pumpernickel or rye (1 roll)	1.08	2.09
Fruits		
Avocado, black skin (1 medium)	3.11	8.65
Blackberries (1 cup)	1.44	7.63
Dried apricots, uncooked (1 cup)	5.72	11.7
Dried figs, uncooked (1 cup)	5.50	15.00
Grapefruit, pink or white (1 medium)	2.30	2.82
Orange, fresh (1 medium)	1.83	3.14
Pear, fresh (1 medium)	2.16	3.98
Prune juice (1 cup)	1.28	2.56
Apple (1 medium)	1.0	3.0
Vegetables		
Artichoke, regular globe, cooked (1 cup)	6.60	9.07
Beans, lima, cooked from dried (1 cup)	4.50	9.00
Beans, soybeans, boiled (1 cup)	3.50	8.00
Brussels sprouts, cooked (1 cup)	3.88	6.35
Collard greens, cooked (1 cup)	3.23	5.32

continues

continued

Food	Soluble Fiber (g)	Total Fiber (g)
Green peas, cooked (1 cup)	2.56	8.80
Mixed veggies (corn, lima beans, peas, carrots), 1 cup	3.82	8.01
Squash, acorn, cooked (1 cup)	3.50	6.00
Nuts and Seeds		
Coconut, fresh (1/2 medium)	2.0	18.0
Flax seeds (1/2 cup)	7.0	13.0
Peanuts (1/2 cup)	1.4	6.5
Pistachio nuts (1/2 cup)	1.75	6.5
Sunflower seeds (1/2 cup)	1.25	6.5

Low-Fat Dairy and Lean Proteins

When you consume dairy products and protein foods with less fat, you'll automatically be eating less saturated fat and fewer overall calories.

Choose skim and 1% milk, low-fat cream cheese, low-fat and nonfat yogurt, low-fat hard cheese, 1% low-fat cottage cheese, and part-skim mozzarella. Choose low-fat and nonfat frozen yogurt and low-fat and nonfat ice cream.

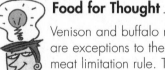

Food for Thought

Venison and buffalo meat are exceptions to the red meat limitation rule. They may be eaten more often.

Your best bets in lean protein include tofu, egg whites, egg substitutes, chicken breast, turkey breast, fish, and seafood. If you have more than one cardiac risk factor, limit red meat consumption to one meal a week.

Your leanest beef choices are top round, top loin steak, tenderloin, and chuck steaks, along with lean flank, lean porterhouse, and lean sirloin. Your leanest pork choices include the tenderloin, loin chops, lean ham, top loin roast, Canadian bacon, rib chops, and shoulder blade steak.

Try to always remove the skin from poultry before you eat it. Your best poultry bets are skinless chicken breast, no-skin turkey breast, lean ground chicken or turkey breast, and skinless duck and pheasant.

The Better Fats

You've heard all the bad news about fat. Now for the good news: some fats can actually have a beneficial effect on your heart. Monounsaturated fat, for instance, may help to lower your bad cholesterol and increase your good cholesterol. Olive oil, peanut oil, sesame seed oil, canola oil, and avocados all are high in monounsaturated fat. You still need to use these in moderation, especially if you are watching your weight, as even these "good" fats have the same number of calories as other fats (including butter!).

Another type of unsaturated fat is polyunsaturated, which has also been shown to help reduce the risk of heart disease. The best sources for polyfats are omega-3 fatty acids, polyunsaturated fats found in many fish, flaxseeds, and walnuts.

Dietary Cholesterol

Cholesterol is a waxy substance that contributes to the formation of many essential compounds, *and* some *less* essential ones—namely the arterial plaque that contributes to heart disease. All animal-origin foods and beverages contain cholesterol. Eggs, meat, fish, cheese, milk, and poultry all are sources of cholesterol. Plant foods, however, do not contain cholesterol. The liver is responsible for making most of the cholesterol that ends up in your blood, but it's still wise to limit the amount of cholesterol you get from food—especially if you have high blood cholesterol levels. The American Heart Association recommends that healthy people take in no more than 300 mg dietary cholesterol per day, and that people with cardiovascular disease aim for less than 200 mg per day. So—read labels and try not to overdo it.

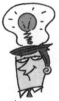

Food for Thought

Consider starting drugs if your LDL-cholesterol is greater than 130—and you've already tried eating right and exercising.

You may wonder about whether or not to eat liver. Although high in cholesterol, liver is extremely low in fat and loaded with protein, vitamin A, B-vitamins, iron, and zinc. But unfortunately, a 3-ounce serving provides nearly two times the recommended dose for dietary cholesterol—so don't eat it more than once every two to three weeks.

Decreasing Salt

Salt tends to increase blood pressure in people who are salt-sensitive. And because it's tough to tell who is and who isn't, it's always a good idea to watch the amount you take in. The American Heart Association recommends that folks with high blood pressure decrease their salt consumption to no more than 2,300 mg each day (that's about 1 teaspoon).

However, don't think that giving up salt means giving up taste and flavor. You just need to be more creative in the seasoning department—and a little more selective with certain food products. See Chapter 5 for more information on reducing the salt in your diet.

- Enhance food with spices and herbs. Try allspice, basil, chives, cinnamon, dill, fresh garlic, onion, rosemary, nutmeg, turmeric, mace, and sage.

- Eliminate the salt shaker at mealtime.

- Choose fresh or frozen vegetables whenever possible, because canned vegetables typically contain a lot of salt. If canned is the only option, reduce the salt by draining off the liquid and rinsing the vegetables in water before eating.

- Go easy on condiments that have a lot of salt, such as catsup, mustard, salad dressings, soy sauce, olives, sauerkraut, and pickles. Monosodium glutamate (MSG) is also rich in salt. Instead, stock your cabinets with low-sodium soy sauce, steak sauce, and teriyaki sauce, and buy unsalted (or reduced-salt) nuts, seeds, crackers, popcorn, and pretzels.

- Eat processed luncheon cold cuts sparingly. Ditto for cured and smoked meats, because they're saturated with sodium.

Folic Acid—Plus B-6 and B-12

Together with B-6 and B-12, folic acid can help to protect the heart by breaking down and lowering homocysteine levels.

Folate and folic acid are forms of a water-soluble B-vitamin. Folate occurs naturally in food, while folic acid is the synthetic form of this vitamin, found in supplements and fortified foods. The richest sources of folate are leafy greens like spinach and turnip greens, dry beans and peas, fortified cereals and grain products, and citrus fruits (oranges and grapefruits).

Foods rich in B-6 include fortified cereals, whole grains, oats, pork, poultry, fish, bananas, peanuts, and soybeans.

Foods rich in B-12 include fortified cereals, meats, poultry, fish, eggs, dairy, and soy products.

Plant Sterols or Stanols

You may know them as "Take Control," "Benecol," or "Cholest-Off." Whatever name they go by, these new margarinelike spreads and supplements may turn out to be promising weapons in the war against elevated total and LDL cholesterol levels. Plant sterol esters or stanol esters are natural substances found in wood pulp, leaves, nuts, vegetable oils, corn, rice, and some other plants. Now there is some evidence that the spreads (and salad dressings) made with plant sterols or stanols can actually reduce cholesterol absorption and decrease the LDL cholesterol levels. For people trying to lose weight, "light" versions of these spreads are also available.

Nutri-Speak
Numerous studies have suggested that drinking red wine may help protect your heart.

Putting the Guidelines to the Test

To help you follow a heart-smart diet, here's a seven-day food plan that incorporates lean proteins and low-fat dairy products, unsaturated fats, loads of fresh fruit and vegetables, and plenty of fiber. Plus, it's easy to follow. This meal plan is based on approximately 1,800 calories, so if your doctor recommends you lose weight, you may need to scale down portions and trim off a few foods. On the other hand, if your weight is stable (or you could stand to gain a few pounds), increase the lean protein portions and add some more olive oil, fruits, and veggies.

Seven-Day Food Plan

> **Breakfast options:**

> **Day 1   Oatmeal and fruit:** 1 serving of oatmeal (¹/₂ cup dry oatmeal) prepared with water, 3 tablespoons of raisins, or 1 banana, or 1¹/₂ cups of berries or melon—mixed with 1 tablespoon of ground flaxseeds—plus 1 slice of whole-wheat bread, toasted and topped with a spread of plant sterol or stanol margarine (e.g., Benecol or Take Control).

Day 2   **Cereal/milk/fruit:** 1 cup high-fiber cereal (any brand that provides 5+ grams fiber and 120 calories or less per serving)—1 cup skim, 1% low-fat milk or soymilk—plus 1 serving of any type of fruit (½ banana, 1 cup berries, or 2 tablespoons of raisins)—plus 1 slice of whole-wheat toast, topped with a spread of plant sterol or stanol margarine (e.g., Benecol or Take Control).

Day 3   **Tomato/cheese toast with fruit:** 2 slices of whole-wheat bread, toasted and topped with tomato slices and 2 slices of melted low-fat or nonfat cheese—plus 1 serving of any type of fruit.

Day 4   **Egg white omelet:** 5 egg whites, or a small container of egg substitute, with any kind of vegetable thrown in (for example: onion, tomato, and pepper)—use nonstick cooking spray to fry eggs—plus 2 slices of whole-wheat toast with a spread of plant sterol or stanol margarine. Also, you have the option of 1 fruit serving.

Day 5   **Yogurt and fruit:** One container (8-oz.) of nonfat, flavored yogurt (or 1 cup 1% cottage cheese)—mixed with 1 serving of any type of fruit—plus 2 tablespoons ground flaxseeds and 2 tablespoons wheat germ—plus 1 slice of whole-wheat toast, with a spread of plant sterol/stanol margarine.

Day 6   **Toast/tomato/salmon with fruit:** 2 slices of whole-wheat toast topped with a thin spread of light cream cheese, sliced tomato, and salmon. Also, 1 serving of fruit.

Day 7   **Soy/Fruit smoothie:** 1 cup soymilk mixed with 1 cup frozen strawberries, ½ banana, and ice cubes; place in a blender and mix. With 1 slice of whole-wheat toast topped with 2 teaspoons of natural peanut butter.

Breakfast beverages: Coffee or tea with skim milk—and of course, water. Try to avoid all fruit juice.

Morning snack options (choose only one):

- 1 piece of fruit, with 1 slice of low-fat cheese, or tofu cheese
- 1 sliced apple with 1 tsp. of natural peanut butter
- Small bag of oat bran pretzels
- 1 oz. of walnuts or almonds
- Nonfat flavored yogurt (8-oz. container)
- 1 cup baby carrots with 2 TB. hummus
- Large pear

Lunch Options:

Day 1   Soup and pita bread: A bowl of noncreamy, vegetable-based soup (approximately 2 cups)—try tomato, minestrone, lentil, chicken noodle, vegetarian chili, tomato rice, etc.—you'll need to avoid the versions that use cream, whole milk, or cheese in the ingredients. With that, 1 regular-size whole-wheat pita bread and a vegetable salad with 1 tablespoon of vinaigrette dressing (or 1 teaspoon olive oil and unlimited vinegar).

Day 2   Sandwich and salad: 3–5 ounces of lean turkey breast, grilled chicken, lean ham, or low-fat tuna salad—on 2 slices of whole-wheat or rye bread, with 1 slice low-fat cheese, lettuce, tomato, and mustard, catsup, barbecue sauce, or low-fat mayonnaise. With that, one side salad with 1 tablespoon of vinaigrette dressing (or 1 teaspoon of olive oil and unlimited vinegar).

Day 3   Grilled fish and vegetables: 3–4 ounces of grilled or barbecued chicken breast (no skin)—or any type of grilled fish with a side of steamed or lightly grilled vegetables (2 cups)—plus a medium sweet potato.

Day 4   Japanese food: A salad with ginger dressing (go easy), an order of edamame (soybeans), plus 4 pieces of sushi and 5 pieces of sashimi. Use low-sodium soy sauce and unlimited fresh ginger.

Food for Thought

Consider taking a low-dose aspirin every day if you're at risk for heart disease. Aspirin can help fight harmful blood clots. BUT, as always, speak with your physician before you do anything new.

Day 5   Chinese food: An order of *steamed* chicken or tofu with mixed vegetables. Ask for the garlic sauce on the side and use 1–2 tablespoons on your dish, then sprinkle additional low-sodium soy sauce—plus ½ cup of brown rice.

Day 6   Large salad entree: Unlimited raw vegetables—topped with 3–5 ounces plain tuna, grilled salmon, grilled shrimp, chicken breast, turkey breast, or tofu—plus ½ cup of chickpeas, beans, or corn—plus 1 tablespoon of chopped walnuts—and 2–3 teaspoons of olive oil and unlimited vinegar. Also, 1 whole-wheat pita.

Day 7   Potato and chili: Plain baked potato with 2 cups of vegetarian chili and low-fat sour cream.

Afternoon snack options (choose only one):

◆ Fresh fruit

◆ 1 oz. nuts

◆ 1 cup edamame (soybeans in the pod)

◆ Baby carrots and salsa

◆ Any of the morning snacks

Drink water or noncaloric, flavored seltzers throughout the day.

Dinner guidelines: Choose one from each category:

Appetizers: Salads (use olive oil and vinegar, or vinaigrette), or shrimp cocktail with red sauce, or mussels marinara, or steamed artichokes, or sliced tomatoes, or vegetables (mushrooms, asparagus, etc.).

Entree: 5 ounces of grilled/broiled/baked chicken breast, fish, seafood, tofu, turkey breast, lean pork, (red meat 1 time per week; however, you *can* have buffalo and venison more frequently), veggie burgers, turkey burgers, or soy burgers.

Unlimited vegetables: Anything goes! Steamed or lightly grilled with olive oil or vegetable oil, or with plant sterol margarine spread.

Starch: $^{1}/_{2}$–1 cup of whole-grain starch; brown rice, couscous, or whole-wheat pasta with olive oil or marinara sauce, or small sweet potato.

Optional alcohol: 1 glass of red or white wine.

Dessert options: Fresh fruit, or a scoop of fruit sorbet, or 6–8 ounces of a low-fat frozen yogurt or light ice cream. Also, you may choose to have any frozen low-fat pop that is 100 calories or less.

Lots of seltzer water or any other type of water with your dinner.

Exercise!

Not only does regular exercise make you look and feel better, it helps prevent cardio-vascular disease. Furthermore, regular physical activity puts you in the right mindset for making better food choices during your day. Double bonus. For a truly effective workout, you need to challenge your heart and lungs with aerobic activity. You can read more about the specifics in Chapter 14. But the bottom line is to find something that's enjoyable and realistic so that it becomes an everyday part of your life.

Now that you know what a tremendous effect your lifestyle has on your heart health, it's time to make some changes in your life. Some are nearly painless, while others will be more of a challenge. Just keep your ultimate goal (a healthy heart) in sight, and remember: you're worth it!

The Least You Need to Know

- Heart disease remains one of the leading causes of death in America. One and a half million people will suffer a heart attack each year.

- Cardiac risk factors include diabetes, high blood pressure, elevated levels of LDL cholesterol, triglycerides, homocysteine, and CRP, low HDL cholesterol, smoking, and family history.

- HDL cholesterol is the good cholesterol and should be 40 mg/dL or higher. You can increase your HDL level with regular aerobic exercise, adding mono-unsaturated fat to your diet, and/or by taking medication.

- Since sensitivity to salt isn't something we are tested for, folks with high blood pressure should limit sodium intake to less than 2,300 mg per day.

- Heart-smart eating revolves around a diet rich in lean protein, fresh fruit and vegetables, soluble fiber, whole grains, low-fat dairy, unsaturated fats, plant sterols, and foods rich in B-vitamins.

- Fats are not created equal. Monounsaturated fats may help to lower blood cholesterol, while saturated and trans fats can raise your blood cholesterol, which, in turn, can lead to heart disease.

Chapter 21

Food Allergies and Other Ailments

In This Chapter

- The lowdown on food allergies
- Diagnosing a true food allergy
- Different food sensitivities
- Living with lactose intolerance
- Learning about celiac disease
- Managing migraines
- Strategies for alleviating PMS

Do you break out in hives at the mere mention of a peanut? Do you bolt for the bathroom after ingesting anything made with milk? Does the smell of seafood make your stomach churn? Hey, even my Grandma Mary sneezes repeatedly after devouring her favorite ice cream.

For millions of Americans, symptoms such as these turn the pleasurable act of eating into an uncomfortable and sometimes dangerous situation. In fact, an estimated two out of five American adults have some type of food sensitivity, ranging from severe food allergies to less serious (but often still bothersome) food intolerances. This chapter provides an inside look at the variety of food hypersensitivities and sorts through the confusion, controversy, and skepticism in the world of tasty offenders.

Understanding Food Allergies

A true *food allergy* is a hypersensitive reaction that occurs when your immune system responds abnormally to harmless proteins in food. That is, your body misinterprets something good as an intruder and produces antibodies to "halt" the invasion. Remember the episode of *Three's Company* when Jack sneaked in late one night, and Chrissy and Janet mistook him for a robber and clobbered him over the head? It's the same thing with food allergies, only you're the one who gets clobbered.

The most common food culprits linked to allergic reactions are wheat, shellfish, nuts, soybeans, corn, the protein in cow's milk, and eggs. Furthermore, the organs most commonly affected are the skin (symptoms include skin rashes, hives, itching, and swelling), the respiratory tract (symptoms include difficulty breathing and "hay fever"), and the gastrointestinal tract (symptoms include nausea, bloating, diarrhea, and vomiting). Some allergic reactions are so severe they can even provoke anaphylactic shock, a life-threatening, whole-body response that requires immediate medical attention.

Here's a list of terms to know:

+ **Food sensitivity** is a general term used to describe any abnormal response to a food or food additive.

Food for Thought

Statistics report that up to 7 percent of all infants and small children are allergic to certain foods, a much higher incidence than among American adults (less than 2 percent).

+ **Food allergy** is an overreaction by the body's immune system, usually triggered by protein-containing foods (such as cow's milk, nuts, soybeans, shellfish, eggs, and wheat).

+ **Anaphylactic shock** is a life-threatening, whole-body allergic reaction to an offending substance. Symptoms include swelling of the mouth and throat, difficulty breathing, a drop in blood pressure, and loss of consciousness. In other words, get help fast!

- **Food intolerance** is an adverse reaction that generally does not involve the immune system (such as lactose intolerance).

- **Food poisoning** is an adverse reaction caused by contaminated food (microorganisms, parasites, or other toxins).

- **Antibodies** are large protein molecules produced by the body's immune system in response to foreign substances.

Nutri-Speak

The word **allergy** comes from the Greek words *allos*, meaning "other," and *ergon*, meaning "working." In other words, the immune system is working other than normally expected.

Diagnosing a True Food Allergy

Many folks view this whole food-sensitivity business as faddism and quackery, and unfortunately, we have earned this mindset. Did you know that out of the gazillions of people who think they have a food allergy, less than 2 percent of the American adult population actually have one? Why does the idea of a food allergy get so recklessly thrown around? One reason may be that people are often quick to blame physical ailments on food. Another aggravating reason for all the misdiagnoses are those so-called "allergy quacks" that grab your hard-earned money and diagnose you with the "allergy of the month."

In today's world, a true food allergy can be properly diagnosed with scientific sound testing. If you think you might suffer from an allergic response to certain foods, get it checked out. The first step is to find a qualified and reputable physician who has been certified by the American Board of Allergy and Immunology. Ask your primary doctor for a referral, *or* call the American Academy of Allergy and Immunology at 1-800-822-2762, and it'll set you up with a physician in your area. Next, schedule an appointment. Here's what you can expect:

- **Thorough medical history.** You'll give a detailed history of both your and your family's medical background. Special attention will be given to the type and frequency of your symptoms, along with when the symptoms occur in relation to eating food.

- **Complete physical examination.** You'll have a routine physical exam, with special focus on the areas where you experience the suspected food-allergy symptoms.

- **Food-elimination diets.** The doctor will probably have you keep a food diary while you eliminate all suspicious foods from your diet. The allergist might then tell you to slowly, one at a time, add these foods back to your diet so you can specifically identify which foods might cause an adverse reaction.

- **Skin tests.** An extract of a particular food is placed on the skin (usually on the arm or back) and then pricked or scratched into the skin to look for a reaction of itching or swelling. This isn't 100 percent reliable because people who aren't allergic can develop skin rashes. On the other hand, some people don't show skin reactions but do have allergic responses when they eat the food.

- **RAST (radioallergosorbent test).** This test involves mixing small samples of your blood with food extracts in a test tube. If you are truly allergic to a particular food, your blood will produce antibodies to fight off the food extract. One advantage is that this test is performed outside your body, so you don't have to deal with the itching and swelling if the test is positive. Note: this test will only foretell an allergy, not the extent of sensitivity to the offending food.

- **Double-blind food-challenge tests.** This type of test must be performed under close supervision, preferably in an allergist's office or hospital, and it is considered the "gold standard" in food-allergy testing. Two capsules of dried food are prepared, one with the real McCoy and another with a nonreactive substance. Neither doctor nor patient knows which is which (a double-blind challenge). These challenges can rule out, as well as detect, allergies or intolerances to foods and other food substances such as additives.

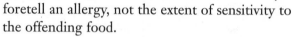

Food for Thought

For further information and a free newsletter on food allergies, send a self-addressed stamped envelope to:

The Food Allergy and Anaphylaxis Network (FAAN)
10400 Eaton Place, Suite 107
Fairfax, VA 22030
1-800-929-4040
www.foodallergy.org

Treating a True Food Allergy

What's the treatment once you're diagnosed with a true food allergy? Avoid the offending food!

Although this list is not a substitute for consulting a registered dietitian, it can provide a pretty good idea of which food ingredients to avoid after you've been diagnosed with one of the following food allergies:

◆ **Cow's milk.** Check labels carefully and avoid all foods with the following ingredients: milk, yogurt, cheese, cottage cheese, custard, casein, whey, ghee, milk solids, curds, sodium caseinate, lactoglobulin, lactalbumin, milk chocolate, buttermilk, cream, sour cream, and butter.

◆ **Wheat.** Avoid all foods with the following ingredients: wheat, wheat germ, all-purpose flour, duram flour, cracker meal, couscous, bulgur, whole-wheat berries, cake flour, gluten flour, pastry flour, graham flour, semolina, bran, cereal or malt extract, modified food starch, farina, and graham.

◆ **Corn.** Avoid all foods with the following ingredients: fresh, canned, or frozen corn (regular and creamed), hominy, corn grits, maize, cornmeal, corn flour, corn sugar, baking powder, corn syrup, cornstarch, modified food starch, dextrin, malto-dextrins, dextrose, fructose, lactic acid, corn alcohol, vegetable gums, sorbitol, vinegar, and popcorn.

◆ **Soy.** Avoid all foods with the following ingredients: soy, lecithin, tofu, textured vegetable protein (TVP), tempeh, modified food starch, soy miso, soy sauce, teriyaki sauce, and soybean flour.

> **CAUTION**
>
> **Overrated-Undercooked**
>
> Some people are diagnosed with allergies to food additives such as sulfites (food preservatives), tartrazine (food colorings), and MSG (flavor enhancer) and therefore must check ingredient labels with extreme care and ask a lot of questions when dining out.

> **Food for Thought**
>
> For a complete resource of specialty foods (wheat-free, egg-free, soy-free, dairy-free, corn-free, nut-free, rice-free), call Miss Roben's at 1-800-891-0083, or visit the website at www.missroben.com.

◆ **Nuts.** Folks who are allergic to peanuts and other types of nuts not only have to avoid the obvious plain nuts and nut butters, but also need to be on the lookout for "hidden" nuts tossed into baked goods, vegetarian dishes, candies, cereals, salads, and stir-fry meals.

◆ **Eggs.** Avoid all foods that indicate the presence of an egg by listing any of the following ingredients: powdered or dry egg, egg white, dried egg yolk, egg substitute, eggnog, albumin, ovalbumin, ovomucin, ovomucoid, vitellin, ovovitellin, livetin, globulin, and ovoglobulin egg albumin.

◆ **Shellfish.** Avoid all shrimp, lobster, prawn, crab, crawfish, crayfish, clams, oysters, scallops, snails, octopus, squid, mussels, and geoducks.

Some people have such severe food allergies that they can even exhibit symptoms from the following:

◆ Kissing the lips of someone who has eaten the offending food

◆ Just smelling and inhaling the offending food while it cooks

◆ Coming into contact with utensils that have touched the offending food—make certain that food companies do *not* have cross-contamination from product to product

What's the Difference Between Allergy and Intolerance?

The difference lies in how your body handles the offending food. A food allergy affects the body's immune system; a food intolerance generally affects the body's metabolism. In other words, the body cannot properly digest a food or food substance, resulting in "intestinal chaos"—a.k.a. the gurgles.

What's Lactose Intolerance All About?

If you can't stomach milk and you experience bloating, nausea, cramping, excessive gas, or a bad case of the runs after eating a dairy food, you are not alone. In fact, an estimated 30 to 50 million Americans suffer from some degree of lactose intolerance, which is the inability to digest the milk sugar *lactose*. In fact, I once had a client tell me he visited so many restrooms while touring through Europe he was ready to write *The Complete Idiot's Guide to European Bathrooms.*

> **Food for Thought**
>
> Don't confuse a lactose intolerance with a milk allergy. A lactose intolerance involves difficulty digesting the milk sugar lactose; a milk allergy involves an allergic reaction from the protein components in cow's milk. Folks who suffer from milk allergies cannot tolerate reduced-lactose products because the part of the milk they are allergic to (milk proteins) is still present.

Why can't some people tolerate dairy foods? People who are lactose intolerant are unable to produce enough of the enzyme *lactase*, which is responsible for the digestion of lactose. Just imagine trying to tear down a skyscraper without a bulldozer; it's not gonna happen! Just like the bulldozer, lactase must break down, digest, and absorb lactose in the bloodstream. What's more, this type of intolerance affects people at different levels. Whereas one person might dash for the bathroom after just one sip of milk, others can tolerate small amounts of dairy without any problem.

Who generally tends to have a problem digesting milk?

♦ Up to 70 percent of the entire world's population does not produce enough of the enzyme lactase and therefore has some degree of lactose intolerance.

♦ In the United States alone, the following groups experience some or all symptoms of lactose intolerance:

More than 80 percent of Asian Americans

79 percent of Native Americans

75 percent of African Americans

51 percent of Hispanic Americans

21 percent of Caucasian Americans

Food for Thought

For further information and a free brochure on lactose intolerance, call 1-800-LACTAID.

♦ In rare cases, some people are born unable to produce the enzyme lactase due to a congenital defect.

♦ Following gastric surgery, people taking chronic antibiotics or anti-inflammatory drugs might also lose their ability (both short-term and long-term) to digest lactose.

♦ People might develop a temporary lactose intolerance during or following a bout of the flu, a stomach virus, or irritable bowel (spastic colon). During these instances, your doctor will probably tell you to avoid all milk and dairy because the enzyme lactase is easily destroyed with any stomach irritation. In these cases, when you recover, so does your ability to produce lactase.

Living with a Lactose Intolerance

The following tips are helpful for people who have difficulty digesting lactose. As mentioned earlier, the degree of lactose intolerance can vary from person to person; therefore, not everyone will be able to handle all of the suggestions. Give them each a shot, but be sure that you're in a comfortable place if some seem a bit risky. Keep in mind that lactose-containing foods are generally your best sources for the mineral calcium, so children and women with increased calcium requirements should load up on the nondairy sources and speak with a registered dietitian about the possibility of calcium supplementation.

♦ Carefully look through the list of food ingredients and check for obvious and disguised lactose, including milk, cheese, cream, margarine, sour cream, milk solids, milk chocolate, whey, curds, malted milk, and skim-milk solids. Remember that people with severe lactose problems might not be able to tolerate even the small amounts in pancakes, biscuits, cookies, cakes, instant potatoes, salad dressings, sauces, gravies, lunch meats, soups, powdered coffee creamers, and whipped toppings.

♦ Be aware that a lot of over-the-counter medications have added lactose. Speak with your pharmacist if you're not completely sure.

♦ Although most lactose-intolerant people can't gulp down a straight glass of milk, some can tolerate smaller amounts of dairy combined with other foods. For instance, try a bowl of cereal with fruit and milk, or a slice of pizza with a lot of veggies (easy on the cheese), or a ham sandwich with one slice of cheese.

> **Food for Thought**
>
> Despite the widespread notion that chocolate, sugar, dairy products, and other fatty foods are responsible for pimples, most dermatologists today rarely identify an underlying relationship between acne and diet.

♦ Some people with lactose intolerance can tolerate yogurt because the bacteria in the yogurt actually metabolizes the milk sugar lactose for you.

♦ Also try cultured buttermilk and sweet acidophilus milk. Some folks find them easier to digest than regular milk.

♦ When real ice cream is a lethal poison, try a nondairy substitute such as Toffuti or Rice Dream.

♦ Stock up on special lactose-reduced products, including Dairy Ease and Lactaid milk, cottage cheese, yogurts, cream cheese, and ice cream.

♦ Try the special tablets and drops that you can add to regular milk; they will almost completely break down the lactose after about 24 hours in the fridge.

♦ Also look for the special lactase enzyme pills in your pharmacy that you can swallow *before* eating or drinking a dairy product. This comes in handy when you think you might encounter a difficult situation.

♦ Try taking probiotic supplements. The term *probiotic* refers to several active cultures that may help promote healthy digestion.

◆ In severe cases, even the lactose-reduced products might not be tolerated. But don't cheat your body of calcium just because you can't stomach the dairy. Buy calcium-fortified juice, calcium-fortified soymilk, and any other calcium-fortified food products you can get. Note: definitely speak with your physician or a registered dietitian about calcium supplementation.

Celiac Disease: Life Without Wheat, Rye, Barley, and Oats

Another food-related condition (less common than lactose intolerance) is *gluten-sensitive enteropathy*, better known as *celiac disease* or *gluten intolerance*. Celiac disease is a chronic disorder found in genetically susceptible individuals who exhibit severe intestinal distress after eating anything made with *gluten*, a protein found in wheat, rye, barley, and oats. People with this condition must follow a lifelong diet, avoiding all offending foods, or suffer the potential for malnourishment from chronic diarrhea and nutrient malabsorption.

As you can imagine, life on this diet is no picnic; a bowl of pasta, a bagel, cereal, crackers, or even a slice of bread can send a celiac's intestines into a sumo-wrestling match. Obviously, with the tremendous amount of food restrictions, members of the gluten-free club should consult a knowledgeable nutritionist. What's more, become best friends with your local health food store. It's celiac-friendly and will generally carry the specialty items you need.

> **Nutri-Speak**
>
> **Gluten intolerance** is an intestinal disorder that involves gluten—a protein component of many grains. Gluten is broken down into two parts; gliadin and glutenin. Gliadin is the portion that can be toxic to the small intestines and may result in malabsorption of vital nutrients.

> **Food for Thought**
>
> For further info on celiac disease, write to ...
>
> Celiac Disease Foundation
> 13251 Ventura Blvd., Suite 3
> Studio City, CA 91604-1838
> 818-990-2354
>
> For further reading on life without gluten or wheat, order ...
>
> *Against the Grain*
> Jax Peters Lowell
> Henry Holt and Company, Inc.
> 1-800-488-5233
>
> *Incredible Edible Gluten-Free Foods for Kids*
> Sheri L. Sanderson
> Woodbine House, 2002
> 1-800-843-7323
> www.woodbinehouse.com
>
> *Kids With Celiac Disease*
> Danna Korn
> Woodbine House, 2002
> 1-800-843-7323
> www.woodbinehouse.com

Irritable Bowel Syndrome

Although not completely understood, irritable bowel syndrome (IBS) seems to be more common these days than the sniffles. With symptoms ranging from excessive gas, cramping, bloating, and intermittent bouts of constipation and diarrhea, IBS (also called a spastic colon) usually has nothing to do with food allergies or intolerances. It's more likely a functional problem with the muscular movement of your intestines. In fact, it's generally diagnosed when the serious gastrointestinal ailments are ruled out. Some doctors say that people can even bring it on with anxiety or nerves.

Dietary treatments that can help alleviate the symptoms include eating slowly, increasing fiber gradually (insoluble and soluble), eating several smaller meals throughout the day, and taking probiotic supplements. Also, you may want to keep a food log for a week or two to see whether any particular foods exacerbate the symptoms. Some common culprits include alcohol, tobacco, caffeine, carbonated beverages, dairy foods, fatty foods, beans, sorbitol, spicy foods, and cruciferous veggies such as cauliflower, cabbage, and broccoli. Also, see whether there's a correlation between your work schedule and the days you're feeling bad; some people find that the symptoms improve on the weekends when they're relaxing.

You can also try alternative remedies such as taking enteric-coated capsules of peppermint oil three times a day between meals (skip this one if you have heartburn), or explore yoga, meditation, or hypnosis to lessen stress and anxiety, which can sometimes wind up in your gut. Also, for women who notice IBS flare-ups around the time of menstruation, take evening primrose oil or black cohosh.

For the Caffeine-Sensitive

Some people are extremely sensitive to caffeine; they become dizzy, shaky, and sometimes nauseous. Here's a list of some beverages and foods to watch:

Caffeine Amounts in Popular Foods/Beverages

Food/Beverage	Caffeine (in Milligrams)
Brewed Coffee (8 fluid ounces)	approx 100–150 mgs
Brewed Decaf (8 fluid ounces)	less than 5 milligrams
Espresso (1 ounce)	40 milligrams

Food/Beverage	Caffeine (in Milligrams)
Brewed Tea, black and green (8 fluid ounces)	approx 50 milligrams
Popular Iced Teas, Snapple and Arizona (8 ounces)	15–20 milligrams
Cocoa Powder (1 TB)	12 milligrams
Chocolate (1.7 oz bar)	12–20 milligrams for popular brands
Red Bull (8.5 ounces)	80 milligrams
Hot Chocolate (8 ounces)	5 milligrams
Popular Soda, diet and regular (8 ounces)	25–45 milligrams
OTC Meds:	
Vivarin	200 milligrams
No Doz	100 milligrams
Excedrin	65 milligrams

Also, some of the "energy" drinks incorporate herbal caffeine that goes under the names guarana seeds, kola nuts, and yerba mate leaves.

If you think you may be suffering from a food sensitivity or intolerance—check it out. Keep a detailed food log for one week and include everything you eat and drink; you may even want to include the times of day that you are eating and drinking. Pay close attention to your body's reaction and see if you can find any correlation to a single food (such as peppers, oranges, and beans) or an entire food group (such as milk, yogurt, and cheese). Also, you can meet with a registered dietitian who can help you determine the foods that are aggravating your system.

Managing Migraines

If you have ever had a migraine headache, you're well aware of the horrific agony. From severe pain to nausea and vomiting, migraines can be incredibly debilitating.

The following list provides you with strategies to lessen the onset and intensity. Keep in mind, different things work for different people. And always check with your physician before starting any supplement (feverfew, omega-3s, calcium, or a multi-vitamin/mineral).

◆ **Feverfew.** This herb inhibits platelet aggregation and may help prevent the vessels from restricting. The recommended dose is 50–125 mg daily.

◆ **Omega-3 fatty acids.** Try one tablespoon per day of flaxseed oil or ground flaxseeds. Also, incorporate fatty fish such as salmon, herring, and mackerel— and cereals fortified with omega-3 fats.

◆ **Multi-vitamin/mineral.** Look for any brand that provides 100 percent of your daily requirements, but make sure it has the USP stamp of approval.

◆ **Calcium.** Consider taking calcium carbonate or calcium citrate supplements— up to 1,200 mg each day.

◆ **Prevent hypoglycemia.** Eat every two hours so your blood sugars remain stable. Also, include foods rich in soluble fiber.

◆ **Foods to avoid.** The following foods seem to be commonly associated with migraines:

  ◆ *Cheese, beer, and wine.* These contain histamines and/or vasoactive compounds that cause blood vessels to expand.

  ◆ *Nitrites.* These are common ingredients in lunch meats and smoked/cured meats; they dilate blood vessels and may trigger migraines.

◆ **Non-nutritional strategies include the following:**

  ◆ Acupuncture.

  ◆ Chiropractic acupressure.

  ◆ During an attack, try submerging your feet in hot water while placing an ice compress on the back of your neck. This helps draw blood away from your feet.

  ◆ Stretching, yoga, facial stretch.

  ◆ A large percentage of migraine headaches may be caused by migraine medications. The "rebound effect" of analgesic and ergotamine compounds has been implicated as a contributing factor for sufferers of daily headaches. Discuss this phenomenon with your prescribing doctor if you are taking a lot of analgesics or if you use ergotamine derivatives. Withdrawal from these products can temporarily make headaches worse but may ultimately provide relief.

Alleviating PMS

Premenstrual syndrome (PMS) is an imbalance of the estrogen and progesterone hormones before a woman's menstrual cycle. This imbalance is believed to be responsible for the lousy side symptoms that cause women to feel anxious and irritable. Progesterone is referred to as the "harmony hormone" and levels are significantly decreased between ovulation and the onset of menstruation. Estrogen, on the other hand, is notably high at that time.

The following suggestions may help to alleviate some of the common discomforts that women experience. These symptoms include irritability, bloating, cramping, fatigue, and more.

- **Increase whole grains.** Eat 4+ servings of whole-grain breads and/or cereals daily. Whole grains are loaded with B-vitamins, which may become depleted due to elevated estrogen levels before the menstrual cycle.

- **Include soluble fiber (and complex carbohydrates).** Oats, lentils, and fruits and vegetables contain soluble fiber which can help stabilize blood sugar levels and curb sugar cravings. Furthermore, soluble fiber-rich foods keep you feeling fuller for longer periods of time and can help with weight-management efforts. Examples include soybeans, sweet potatoes, oatmeal, and vegetarian chili.

  Another bonus from carbohydrates in general: simple and complex carbs are believed to increase serotonin production, a chemical that helps to calm your mood.

- **Limit sugar.** Eating excessive sugar may increase the risk for blood-sugar swings (highs and lows). Sugar swings may then intensify further sugar cravings and dampen your mood. Limit your intake of hard candy, syrups, sweetened beverages, cookies, cakes, and other foods with added sugar.

- **Avoid excessive caffeine.** Limit coffee, tea, chocolate, and other caffeinated products in your diet (no more than 2 cups each day). Caffeine has been shown to increase irritability.

- **Avoid excessive salt.** Salts attract water and increase the risk for uncomfortable water retention. Avoid the salt shaker, salty chips, pickles, soy sauce, teriyaki sauce, soups, canned foods, and sauerkraut.

- **Load up on leafy, green vegetables.** Spinach, kale, bok choy, and dark lettuce contain vitamin E, which may help decrease breast tenderness.

◆ **Include magnesium-rich foods.** Low magnesium is associated with tiredness, headaches, and shakiness. Eating foods rich in this mineral will help to combat these symptoms. Good choices include nuts, whole grains, beans, milk, and seeds.

◆ **Include calcium-rich foods.** Adequate calcium has been shown to significantly decrease some of the common symptoms of PMS. Good sources include low-fat dairy (skim milk, low-fat yogurt, low-fat cheese), sardines (with the bones!), soybeans, black-eyed peas, collard greens, almonds, tofu, broccoli, and other calcium-fortified foods and beverages.

◆ **Include lean protein.** Lean protein helps to regulate normal blood sugar levels (less volatile swings in mood). Select fish, poultry, low-fat dairy, beans, lentils, tofu, and lean red meat—and avoid fatty meats or whole-milk cheese.

◆ **Include omega-3 fatty acids.** Studies have suggested there is a correlation between the consumption of fish oils (rich in omega-3s) and a decrease in the symptoms of PMS. The exact mechanism is not clear, but results were convincing enough to encourage women to increase their omega-3 fatty acid intake to treat symptoms. Opt for fatty fish several times a week (tuna, mackerel, salmon, herring), and include flaxseeds, flaxseed oil, and walnuts in your diet.

◆ **Avoid high-fat foods.** Fried and fatty foods take a long time to digest and can make you feel sluggish. Stay away from French fries, deep-fried vegetables, fried chicken, chips, chocolates, and excessive cakes and cookies.

◆ **Eat sensibly.** Avoid extreme dieting or overeating. Bizarre eating behaviors will worsen your mood and exaggerate the symptoms associated with PMS.

The Least You Need to Know

◆ A food allergy is when your body misinterprets a harmless food as an intruder and produces antibodies to fight off the foreign substance. It affects the immune system, whereas a food intolerance generally affects only the digestive system.

◆ Lactose intolerance is the inability to produce enough of the enzyme lactase, which is responsible for digesting the milk sugar lactose. Symptoms include bloating, cramping, gas, diarrhea, and nausea.

◆ Celiac disease is a condition that causes severe malabsorption after ingesting the protein gluten, which is found in wheat, rye, oats, and barley.

◆ Irritable bowel syndrome is a functional problem with the muscular movement of the intestines, resulting in intermittent bouts of constipation, diarrhea, bloating, and gas.

◆ PMS can be managed through sensible eating and incorporating foods rich in calcium, omega-3s, magnesium, B-vitamins, and soluble fiber.

◆ Migraines may be alleviated by taking feverfew or calcium, avoiding foods with histamines and nitrates, and preventing hypoglycemia.

Going Vegetarian

In This Chapter

- ◆ The reasons people go vegetarian
- ◆ Types of vegetarian diets
- ◆ Great vegetarian protein and iron sources
- ◆ What's soy protein all about?
- ◆ Meatless recipes to tantalize your taste buds

Vegetarian diets are becoming popular, with more and more Americans jumping on the "tofu bandwagon." Like every other prudent diet, people following vegetarian food plans must eat well-balanced, varied meals and include fruits, vegetables, nuts, seeds, low-fat dairy (depending upon your vegetarian restrictions), legumes, and plenty of whole-grain products. Although a typical vegetarian eating plan tends to be super-low in saturated fat and cholesterol, it's not automatically low in *total* fat and sugar. Therefore, veg-heads, like meat-heads, need to limit their intake of fatty foods, oils, spreads, and sweets.

The Various Types of Vegetarians

A vegetarian diet, when properly followed, can be one of the healthiest diets out there. Benefits of the vegetarian diet include:

- **Decreased obesity.** Vegans are rarely obese and, on the average, ovolacto-vegetarians are leaner than those who eat meat. However, being vegetarian doesn't guarantee a slim figure. If you eat foods that are high in fat, you can consume as many or more calories than meat eaters.

- **Less risk of coronary heart disease (CHD).** Vegetarians tend to have lower blood cholesterol levels and diets with lower overall saturated fat content.

- **Lower rates of hypertension.** The reason for this is still unknown, but researchers think it might be related to increased potassium, magnesium, polyunsaturated fat, and fiber intake. All the same, more research is still needed to determine whether the diet itself has anything to do with the lower levels.

Vegetarian eating covers broad territory and can run the gamut from people who avoid *all* animal products to people who simply refrain from eating a few select animal foods. Here's a look at the assortment of vegetarian-style eaters:

- **Vegans.** This is the strictest type of vegetarian (sort of the pope of all vegetarians). Vegans abstain from eating or using *all* animal products, from eating meat, dairy, and eggs, to wearing wool, silk, or leather. If you're a vegan, you'll need to be extra careful about getting adequate protein, iron, calcium, vitamin D, vitamin B-12, and zinc.

- **Lacto-vegetarians.** This group eliminates meat and eggs but includes all dairy products.

- **Ovolacto-vegetarians.** This group eliminates all meat (red meat, poultry, fish, and seafood); however, they do include dairy products and eggs.

- **Semi-vegetarians.** This group does not eat red meat but eats most chicken, turkey, and fish, along with all dairy and eggs.

Food for Thought

Although tofu and other soy proteins contain some fat, they're very low in saturated fat and contain no cholesterol. For more information and free brochures on soy protein, call 1-800-TALK-SOY.

- **Pseudo-vegetarians.** This group will not eat meat on the days they decide they're vegetarian but will, however, inhale hamburgers and steak sandwiches when they get a craving.

- **Raw foodists.** This group claims that heating food over 116 degrees Fahrenheit destroys the food's enzymes, making it harder to digest and preventing nutrients from being absorbed. Raw foodists eat only uncooked, unprocessed vegetables, fruits, nuts, and seeds. Grains and grain products, meat, milk, eggs and other animal foods are *out*, as is alcohol, coffee, tea, and even vitamin supplements.

◆ **Macrobiotics.** This is more a philosophy and lifestyle than a simple diet. Meals revolve around certain types of vegetables (no potatoes, tomatoes, eggplant, peppers, spinach, beets, and zucchini), legumes, sea vegetables, soy foods, soups, spring water (no ice), herbal teas, and small amounts of fish, fruit, and sweeteners.

How to Ensure an Adequate Protein Intake

All vegetarians can easily meet their protein needs. Protein doesn't discriminate; it's found in both animal and plant foods. Low-fat dairy and eggs can provide generous amounts of protein for vegetarians who dare to eat them, and the vegans in the crowd should become close pals with tofu, nuts, seeds, lentils, and tempeh. Flip back to Chapter 3 to refresh your memory on complementary proteins—that is, making a complete protein (a protein containing all of the essential amino acids) by combining two or more incomplete plant proteins.

The Many Faces of Soy Protein

Decades ago, soy foods were one of the world's best kept secrets. Finally out of the closet and raring to jump into just about any recipe, soy protein can boost the protein, calcium, and iron content of almost any dish. Go ahead and experiment by incorporating some of the following varieties into your meals, and remember that unflavored soy will take on any flavor you cook or marinate with:

◆ **Soymilk.** Start your day with a glass of soymilk, or pour it over your cereal for breakfast. Soymilk provides about 4–10 grams of protein per one cup serving and can be found in low-fat and flavored varieties.

◆ **Isolated soy protein.** This powdery substance is literally 90 percent pure protein because most of the fat and carbohydrate has been discarded. It's made from defatted soy flour and can be strategically blended into muffins, pancakes, and cookies to help boost your daily protein. A 1-ounce serving (approximately 4 tablespoons) contains 13–23 grams of protein.

◆ **Soy flour.** Here's another great way to hike up the protein in your baked products. Soy flour can be used for quick breads, muffins, cookies, and brownies, and a ¹/₂ cup serving supplies 22 grams of protein.

◆ **Textured soy protein (TSP).** Also called textured vegetable protein (TVP), this is made from defatted soy flour and takes on a granular, flake, or chunk characteristic. TSP comes both plain and flavored and can be mixed into chili, tacos, veggie burgers, vegetarian casseroles, and stews. When mixed with water, 1 cup prepared provides 22 grams of protein.

◆ **Vegetable-type soybeans.** These dry, mature soybeans are loaded with 14 grams of protein per ¹/₂ cup serving. What's more, they also contain fiber— double bonus. Tasting both sweet and buttery, their flavor makes them a nice addition to stir-fry dishes, salads, and soups.

◆ **Tempeh.** This cultured soyfood has a tender, chewy consistency that makes it a great candidate for grilled sandwiches, chunky soups, salads, casseroles, and chili. A 4-ounce serving provides 17 grams of protein, about 80 milligrams of calcium, and 10 percent of your daily iron.

◆ **Tofu.** Just about anything goes with this soy protein. "I'll have a tofu à la mode!" It's made from soymilk curds and can be blended, scrambled, stir-fried, grilled, baked; you name it, chances are it can be done with tofu. There are three types of tofu:

   ◆ **Firm tofu** is stiff, dense, and perfect for stir-fry dishes, soups, or anywhere that you want tofu to maintain its shape. A 4-ounce serving of firm tofu supplies 13 grams protein, 120 milligrams calcium, and about 40 percent of your daily iron.

   ◆ **Soft tofu** provides 9 grams protein, 130 milligrams calcium, and a little less than 40 percent of your daily iron from a 4-ounce serving. Soft tofu is good for dishes that require blended tofu (commonly used in soups).

   ◆ **Silken tofu** is creamy and custard-like and therefore also works well in pureed or blended recipes such as dips, soups, and pies. Silken tofu doesn't provide as much calcium as the more solid tofu varieties (only 40 milligrams), but it is the lowest in fat and is packed with 9¹/₂ grams of protein per 4-ounce serving.

Ironing Out the Plant Foods

Unfortunately for this less-carnivorous crowd, the *heme iron* found in animal foods is much more absorbable than the *nonheme* iron supplied from plants. But that's okay;

just go out of your way to eat an abundance of iron-rich plant foods and you'll meet your quota. Foods rich in iron include dried beans, spinach, chard, beet greens, black-strap molasses, bulgur, prune juice, and dried fruits. You might also find that your favorite breakfast cereals are fortified with this mineral. Another trick of the trade is to boost the amount of iron absorbed at a meal by including a food rich in vitamin C (tomatoes, orange juice, and so on). For further information on increasing iron, see Chapter 8.

Food for Thought

Vegans who don't eat dairy and aren't regularly out in the sun should buy foods fortified with vitamin D or speak with their doctors about vitamin D supplementation.

Searching for Nondairy Calcium

For the lactos and ovolactos, low-fat dairy is brimming with calcium. On the other hand, for all you vegans, it takes some planning, but you, too, can meet your daily calcium requirements by including collard greens, broccoli, beans, kale, turnip greens, calcium-fortified orange juice, calcium-fortified grains, almonds, and, of course, your calcium-fortified soymilk products (including tofu, soybeans, and tempeh).

Have You Had Enough B-12 Today?

Getting enough vitamin B-12 can also be an obstacle for strict vegans, simply because B-12 is derived primarily from animal foods. Once again, you lactos and ovolactos are off the hook because dairy and eggs provide enough to satisfy your daily requirements. The vegan gang has to dig a little deeper. Buy food products that are B-12–fortified: cereals, breads, some soy-analogs, and possibly tempeh. You might also want to pop a B-12 supplement providing 100 percent of the RDA, just to be safe.

Don't Forget the Kitchen Zinc

Not only do you have to get all of the necessary RDA of calcium, protein, B-12, and other nutrients, yet another concern for the strict vegetarian is getting a fair share of zinc. Although this mineral is found in whole-grain products, tofu, nuts, seeds, and wheat germ, our bodies absorb much less "plant zinc" than "animal zinc." This is because *phytic acid* (a substance in the fiber) combines with the zinc and prevents it from being fully absorbed. Therefore, vegetarians need to pay particular attention to getting an abundance of this mineral.

A Day in the Life of a Vegan

Menu 1

Breakfast

Amaranth flakes with soy milk

Fresh blueberries and raspberries

English muffin topped with apple butter

Lunch

Peanut butter and banana sandwich

Cup of vegetarian chili topped with scallions

Glass of low-fat soymilk

Snack

Mixture of dried fruit and walnuts

Glass of juice or soymilk

Dinner

Vegetable-tempeh stir-fry (carrots, broccoli, cauliflower, and tempeh) with
   brown rice

Sweet potato

Steamed kale sprinkled with sesame seeds

Glass of soymilk

Dessert

Rice Dream (ice cream substitute)

Sliced bananas

Menu 2

Breakfast

Scrambled tofu (see recipe) with whole-wheat toast

Bowl of oatmeal with chopped dates and almonds

Glass of cranberry-orange juice

Lunch

Bowl of lentil soup with sourdough rolls

Carrot sticks with hummus dip

Glass of juice or soymilk

Snack

Piece of banana bread

Glass of soymilk

Dinner
Whole-wheat tortilla stuffed with beans, salsa, and arugula
Spinach salad drizzled with olive oil and red wine vinegar

Dessert
Baked apple with maple syrup and chopped walnuts

Q & A

Help, I'm in love with a meat-eater! What do I do?

Relax; mixed marriages are in! If cooking is a major hassle because you and your partner don't eat the same foods, plan some neutral meals that you'll both enjoy. For example, make a large dish of stir-fry vegetables and brown rice. You take a portion and toss in tofu; he or she takes a portion and throws in chicken or beef.

Tips for the Vegetarian Dining Out

Whether you're dining out to be social or because you just don't feel like cooking, if you're trying to stick to a vegetarian diet, it can be tough to get satisfied, let alone nourished. Here are some tips to get through a night out without starving:

◆ When your dining buddies won't have anything to do with a vegetarian restaurant, suggest Chinese, Vietnamese, Thai, or Italian. There are always a bunch of vegetarian entrees on the menu.

◆ If there aren't any vegetarian entrees, make up a full meal by selecting a few side dishes. For example, have a baked potato or a house salad and ask whether they'll serve a side of beans. Better yet, request a special vegetarian entree. Most restaurants can be pretty accommodating.

◆ Soup can be a great option in any type of restaurant. Remember to ask whether the soup is meat-based or vegetable-based.

◆ Feel free to make substitutions and special requests. For instance, change a bacon, lettuce, and tomato sandwich to a cheese, lettuce, and tomato sandwich, or change an order of chicken fajitas to veggie fajitas.

Food for Thought _____

Pregnant vegetarians need to pay extra attention to their diets. For some further reading, pick up

Vegetarian Pregnancy
by Sharon Yntema
McBooks Press
1-888-BOOKS11

Bringing up kids in a veggie household? For further reading, pick up

Vegetarian Children
by Sharon Yntema
McBooks Press
1-888-BOOKS11

Remarkably "Meatless" Recipes

Order some of these award-winning vegetarian cookbooks:

Skinny Vegetarian Entrees
Phyllis Magida and Sue Spliter
Surrey Books
1-800-326-4430

New Vegetarian Cuisine
Linda Rosensweig, from the pages of *Prevention Magazine*
Rosdale Books
1-800-848-4735

The Enchanted Broccoli Forest
Mollie Katzen
Ten Speed Press
1-800-841-2665

The Vegetarian Times Cookbook
Macmillan Publishers
1-800-428-5331

Cajun Red Beans and Rice

1 cup long-grain white rice

½ onion, peeled and diced
    ¼ inch

2 cups water

Pinch cayenne pepper

1 (15¼-oz.) can kidney beans,
    drained and rinsed

1 green bell pepper, diced
    ¼ inch

2 tsp. paprika

¼ tsp. garlic powder

1 cup canned, crushed tomatoes

2 bay leaves

1 tsp. Worcestershire

4 TB. green onions, chopped

Serves four
Nutrition Information
Calories: 290
Total fat: 1 gram
Saturated fat: 0 gram
Dietary fiber: 7 grams
Protein: 10 grams
Sodium: 170 mg
Cholesterol: 0 mg

Copyright © Food for
Health Newsletter, *1996.*
Reprinted with permission.

Place all ingredients (except for the chopped, green onions) in a large
saucepan; cover and bring to a boil. Reduce heat and simmer 15 to 20
minutes until rice is tender and liquid is evaporated. Top each portion
with 1 tablespoon of chopped green onion. Balance out this meal with
a dark, leafy green salad tossed with nonfat Italian salad dressing.

Vegetarian Spinach Lasagna

Serves eight
Nutrition Information
Calories: 243
Total fat: 7.5 grams
Saturated fat: 3 grams
Dietary fiber: 3 grams
Protein: 19 grams
Sodium: 479 mg
Cholesterol: 43 mg

From the kitchen of Ellen Schloss

2 (10–12 oz.) boxes frozen spinach, chopped

2 lbs. low-fat ricotta cheese

1 whole egg + 2 egg whites

¾ tsp. pepper

Garlic and basil, to taste

¼ TB. oregano

4 cups skim milk mozzarella cheese, shredded

Nonstick cooking spray

1 (32-oz.) jar of tomato/marinara sauce (low-sodium)

1 package lasagna noodles, uncooked

1 cup water (for cooking only)

Cook and drain spinach well, and then set aside. Mix together ricotta cheese, eggs, pepper, garlic, basil, oregano, and only half of the mozzarella cheese. Add in spinach and mix again thoroughly. Coat lasagna pan with nonstick spray and preheat oven to 350°. Cover the bottom of the pan with tomato sauce and then place a layer of uncooked lasagna noodles. Next, spread half of spinach-cheese mixture evenly on top, and repeat the layers (noodles and then remaining spinach-cheese mixture). Place on top one more layer of noodles (total of 3 noodle layers) and pour on remaining tomato sauce. Sprinkle on other half of mozzarella cheese. Last, pour water around the edge of the pan (this will cook the noodles) and cover tightly with tin foil. Bake for 1 hour and 15 minutes, until cheese is bubbling. Let stand and cool for 15 minutes before slicing.

Scrambled Tofu

16 oz. of firm tofu

2 TB. mellow barley
  light miso

Dash of ground cumin

Fresh ground pepper,
  to taste

5 TB. of water

½ tsp. turmeric

Dash of garlic powder

Serves four
Nutrition Information
(Tofu Only)
Calories: 82
Total fat: 4 grams
Saturated fat: 1 gram
Dietary fiber: 0 gram
Protein: 8 grams
Sodium: 32 mg
Cholesterol: 0 mg

From the kitchen of Meredith Gunsberg, M.S., R.D.

Mash tofu in a small saucepan. In a separate bowl, whisk together all remaining ingredients. Heat tofu over medium flame and immediately add in miso mixture. Stir constantly until scrambled tofu mixture is heated through. Serve hot with toast and ketchup if desired.

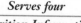

Cucumber Yogurt Dip

1 large cucumber, peeled,
  seeded, and grated

Juice of one small lemon

2 cloves garlic, pressed

1 cup nonfat plain yogurt

1–2 tsp. fresh chives,
  finely chopped

Serves four
Nutrition Information
(¼ of Dip)
Calories: 32
Total fat: 0 gram
Saturated fat: 0 gram
Dietary fiber: 0 gram
Protein: 3 grams
Sodium: 270 mg
Cholesterol: 0 mg

From the kitchen of Meredith Gunsberg M.S., R.D.

Combine all ingredients (except chives) and mix thoroughly. Sprinkle chives on top before serving. Serve with pita bread and plenty of raw vegetables. Yields just over 1 cup.

Chunky Vegetarian Chili

Serves six
Nutrition Information
(Chili Only)
Calories: 330
Total fat: 2.4 grams
Saturated fat: 0 gram
Dietary fiber: 14 grams
Protein: 22 grams
Sodium: 400 mg
Cholesterol: 0 mg

From the kitchen of Meredith Gunsberg M.S., R.D.

½ cup texturized vegetable protein (TVP)

¼ cup boiling water

½ TB. olive oil

1 large onion, diced

3 cloves garlic, minced

2 medium carrots, chopped

2 medium celery stalks, chopped

1 green bell pepper, seeded and chopped

8 oz. mushrooms, quartered

Juice of one lemon

½ tsp. dried basil

2–4 TB. fresh chives and/or parsley (optional)

½ tsp. dried oregano

⅛ tsp. red pepper flakes

1½ tsp. chili powder

1½ tsp. ground cumin

1 (15-oz.) can pinto beans

1 (15-oz.) can kidney beans

1 large tomato, chopped

1 (28-oz.) can crushed tomatoes

½ TB. Marsala wine (optional)

1 TB. tomato paste

Combine the TVP and boiling water in a bowl and set aside. Meanwhile, heat oil in a large stock pot; add onions and sauté until soft (about 3 minutes). Next, add garlic, carrots, celery, green pepper, mushrooms, lemon juice, and spices. Cook over medium heat, covered, for 5 minutes.

Stir in TVP, beans, chopped tomato, and crushed tomatoes. Bring to a simmer. Cook uncovered over low heat for 15 minutes, stirring occasionally. Add Marsala wine and tomato paste and simmer again for an additional 5 minutes. Remove pot from heat and stir in fresh herbs. Ladle chili into bowls and garnish with a dollop of low-fat sour cream and chopped red onion. Serve with a fresh loaf of whole-grain bread.

If you're thinking of becoming a vegetarian, you now know the basics. If you are already a vegetarian, check your food with the guidelines presented in this chapter and see how you stack up. And if you simply read this chapter because it was between Chapters 18 and 20—try substituting some of your meat meals with plant-based meals. Vegetarian entrees can offer food variety, interest, and perhaps a unique experience for your taste buds.

The Least You Need to Know

◆ Vegans are the strictest type of vegetarian and avoid all meats, dairy, and eggs. Lacto-vegetarians eat dairy but avoid all meat and eggs. Ovolacto-vegetarians eat dairy and eggs but avoid all meat.

◆ Vegetarians (especially vegans) need to be extra responsible about getting enough protein, calcium, vitamin D, vitamin B-12, iron, and zinc.

◆ A lot of nonanimal foods provide protein. Nuts, seeds, legumes, and soy-based products are all great sources. The less strict lactos and ovolactos can also obtain protein from dairy products and eggs. The key for the vegetarian is to eat plenty of complementary proteins to get all that are required.

◆ Soy protein can help boost the protein, calcium, and iron content of almost any meal.

23

Herbal Remedies and More

In This Chapter

◆ What herbal medicine is all about

◆ Alternative therapies for a variety of ailments

◆ Finding quality herbal products

Herbal remedies were once considered taboo, something only used by witch doctors. Now, botanical supplements are moving into the mainstream, and even some traditional M.D.s are taking the alternative route.

Although extensive research on herbal medicine has been done, you should always be wary of what you're taking. Do your homework, know your manufacturers, and read the bottles carefully. Some of the herbal remedies out there have not been proven to be safe and effective, and it isn't easy to track problems related to herbal products. If you're looking for an alternative way to relieve a particular ailment, go ahead and get down with the herbal vibe. Just tell your physician what you're taking, especially if you're on other medications. Also, be safe and don't combine several remedies at the same time (which could lead to serious side effects)—and never use them when you're pregnant, breast feeding, or planning to become pregnant.

This chapter provides the lowdown on popular herbs that have been shown to do some pretty impressive things. Read on to see if one of them might be right for you.

Judging the Quality of Herbal Products

It can be quite overwhelming to choose a particular herb—all those bottles tend to look alike in the health food store, vitamin shop, pharmacy, and grocery store. And although herbs have properties that can affect our body's internal functions, there are no regulations on herbal supplements within the United States to date. In fact, this lack of regulation means that different manufacturers use different measures of active ingredients per dose, and some may be unreliable.

If you are seriously interested in the herbal world, find an herb-friendly health professional. You can call the American Herbalists Guild at 435-722-8434 for a list of professional practitioners. For more information on herbs and other supplements, you can also check out the excellent website consumerlabs.com.

Q & A

Are all herbs safe since they are natural?

Most herbs can be quite safe if taken as directed under most circumstances. However, because herbs can potentially have medicinal abilities, you should never take them lightly. Read labels closely, follow dosage directions, and discontinue if you experience any uncomfortable side effects such as throat irritations, upset stomach, diarrhea, and headaches. Also, some people may even experience an allergic reaction to a particular herb.

Nutri-Speak

Tincture is a liquid extract that utilizes a combination of ethyl alcohol and water as the solvent. The advantages of using tinctures are that they have an increased shelf life and do not have to be refrigerated. The disadvantages are that they contain alcohol, which is a problem for people who abstain and for children—and they do not taste pleasant.

For Female Health

Over the centuries, many herbal products have been created for the special needs and health concerns of women. This section will cover black cohosh and evening primrose oil.

Black Cohosh

Use: This herb has traditionally been used to combat menopausal symptoms like hot flashes, vaginal dryness, moodiness, and fatigue. Rigorous human trials are still lacking, but in 2001, the American College of Obstetricians and Gynecologists stated that black cohosh may be helpful for relieving menopausal symptoms in the short term (6 months or less).

Safety and Side Effects: Black cohosh can cause stomach discomfort and headaches, and there are questions about its estrogenicity. If it does turn out to be estrogenic, long-term use may adversely affect uterine or breast tissue in susceptible women.

Evening Primrose Oil

Use: The evening primrose plant is a natural source of an unusual fatty acid called gamma-linolenic acid (GLA), which occurs in only a few other plants, such as borage oil and black currant. GLA is a natural anti-inflammatory that works by modifying the synthesis of *prostaglandins*, which are believed to be involved in a variety of *premenstrual syndrome* (*PMS*) symptoms (as well as arthritis and autoimmune diseases). It also promotes healthy growth of the hair, skin, and nails.

Safety and Side Effects: Lowers the seizure threshold in people taking the drug Phenobarbital.

> **Nutri-Speak**
>
> **Prostaglandins** are hormonelike compounds that were first discovered in the prostate gland (*prosto*-glandins). **Premen-strual syndrome** is a cluster of symptoms, including both physical and emotional pain that some women experience before and during the onset of menstruation.

For Male Health

Like women, men can also benefit from herbs that target their special needs. Although men do not commonly buy and take herbs as often as women, they are becoming more popular. Here are two herbs that cover important male issues: saw palmetto and yohimbe.

Saw Palmetto

Use: This herb is used for BPH (*benign prostatic hyperplasia*). It reduces the size of the prostate in BPH and has a diuretic property. It might also stimulate the appetite and enhance the sex drive. Note: saw palmetto is *not* a treatment for prostate cancer.

Safety and Side Effects: May cause nausea, abdominal pain, and prolonged bleeding time. If you take saw palmetto, you should use a condom while engaging in intercourse because the semen might cause fetal damage.

Yohimbe

Use: This aphrodisiac dilates blood vessels of the skin and mucus membranes (including those of the sexual organs).

Safety and Side Effects: High doses (20 mg or more per day) can cause a rise or fall in blood pressure, anxiety, increased heart rate, and increased urination, among other symptoms. Do not use yohimbe if you are taking tricyclic antidepressants, phenothiazines, blood pressure medication, nasal decongestants, or stimulants. It should also not be taken by anyone suffering from hypotension (low blood pressure), hypertension (high blood pressure), diabetes, or heart, liver, or kidney disease.

For Depression, Sleeping, and Aging

Are you feeling restless, tense, depressed, or having trouble sleeping at night? Or, maybe you simply want to defy some of the signs of aging. Read on—this section examines some herbs that may be worth a try.

Valerian

Use: Valerian is used to treat insomnia, mild anxiety, restlessness, high blood pressure, and symptoms of menstruation and menopause. It does not appear to be habit-forming, and its horrible odor would probably prevent anyone from becoming dependent even if it *were* addictive. (You can get around this unpleasant feature by taking valerian in capsule form).

Side Effects and Drug Interactions: Do not combine valerian with alcohol, and be aware that it may intensify the effect of certain sedatives.

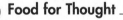

Food for Thought

A few drops of lavender oil in the bath can help you relax. In fact, some say that after massaging your body with the lavender bath water, you are more apt to have a sound sleep.

Gingko Biloba

Use: Derived from the gingko tree and originating in China 200 million years ago, it has been used for centuries as a digestive aid. Tests have shown that it thins the blood and therefore increases circulation in the brain and extremities, making it good for enhancing memory and easing symptoms of age-related cognitive decline and early-stage dementia.

Safety and Side Effects: Large doses may cause restlessness, diarrhea, nausea, and vomiting. Gingko biloba should not be used if you are taking blood thinners, such as aspirin or Coumadin, or thiazides.

DHEA

Use: DHEA is not an herb, but a hormone that is produced by the adrenal glands and converted to testosterone and estrogen in the body. Hormone production declines with age in both men and women (10 percent every 10 years after your mid-20s), so this supplement supports normal sex hormone levels.

Safety and Side Effects: Do not take DHEA unless blood tests indicate your levels are decreased, and then, take only under a doctor's supervision. You should also avoid DHEA if you have had ovarian, adrenal, or thyroid tumors. Side effects that can occur with doses over 50 mg per day include acne, irritability, fatigue, and hirsutism in women (abnormal coarse hair growth, usually on the facial area).

St. John's Wort

Use: This herb is used to treat mild to moderate depression and seasonal affective disorder. Hypericin and pseudohypericin are the active ingredients, which aid in serotonin re-uptake inhibition in the brain. Although this might be one of the most popular and widely used herbs, its action as an antidepressant is not yet fully understood. Therefore, it is not a miracle drug or something that should be used lightly.

Safety and Side Effects: May cause photosensitivity in individuals with fair skin. This herb also interacts with various antidepressants and stimulant medications, anesthetics, MAO inhibitors, and the food substance tyramine (found in aged cheese, wine, fermented soy products, cured meats, and beer). It may also reduce the bioavailability of the drugs Digoxin, Cyclosporine, Theophylline, and Indinavir. Furthermore, a recent small study indicates that it may amplify the effect of the blood-thinner Plavix.

Asian Ginseng (a.k.a. Korean or Chinese)

Use: Ginseng helps alleviate fatigue and stress, enhances cognitive function and physical endurance, and aids in resistance to disease. It is widely used by athletes because of its ability to improve aerobic capacity and recovery time following exertion, but it does contain panaxosides, which have been shown to exert a hypoglycemic effect.

Safety and Side Effects: In rare cases, it can cause over-stimulation, hence insomnia, and it is not recommended for those with high blood pressure. Long-term use might cause menstrual abnormalities and breast tenderness in women. Ginseng may also decrease the effectiveness of the blood-thinning medication Coumadin.

Chamomile

Use: This is known as a "cure-all," like Grandma's chicken soup. It's a cornerstone of European and American herbal medicine that has been used to treat irritable bowel syndrome, infant colic, mouth sores, anxiety, insomnia, menstrual cramps, and digestive problems.

Safety and Side Effects: None reported.

SAM-e

Use: SAM-e (pronounced "Sammy") is the commonly used name for S-Adenosyl-Methionine. SAM-e naturally occurs in every living cell and takes part in several biological reactions in the human body. It is used to help alleviate depression, osteoarthritis, fibromyalgia, and liver disease.

Safety and Side Effects: May occasionally cause nausea and stomach upset (enteric-coated products may reduce these side effects). Do not use SAM-e if you are taking antidepressants such as MAO inhibitors, SSRIs, and tricyclics. Use of SAM-e may also result in a deep hole in your pocket because it is a *very* expensive product!

Heart Disease

Heart disease remains a leading cause of death in both men and women. The following section provides information on two herbs that may help to fight heart disease—garlic and hawthorne.

Garlic

Use: Garlic may help prevent atherosclerosis (hardening of the arteries); however, reports that it reduces cholesterol and blood pressure are overblown. It is also used to help prevent colds and certain types of cancer.

Safety and Side Effects: Garlic is a natural blood thinner, and therefore should not be taken prior to surgery or with blood-thinning medications and supplements.

Hawthorne

Use: Hawthorne is taken for cardiovascular ailments, including high blood pressure, hardening of the arteries, angina, and, potentially, early stages of congestive heart failure. It is not for acute attacks because the action is slow. This herb dilates the blood vessels, especially the coronary vessels, reducing peripheral resistance and thus lowering the blood pressure. It has a direct effect on the heart itself, which is especially noticeable in cases of heart damage.

Safety and Side Effects: None reported.

Liver Disease

The liver is one of the major organs impacted by alcohol and pharmaceutical drugs. This section reviews milk thistle—an impressive herb that has been shown to protect and regenerate the liver.

Milk Thistle

Use: Milk thistle is taken for chronic inflammatory liver disease, such as cirrhosis and hepatitis, as well as more acute conditions. It protects healthy liver cells, as well as ones that have not yet been damaged by toxic substances.

Safety and Side Effects: May have a mild laxative effect in some people.

Respiratory Ailments

One of the top-selling herbs in the United States, echinacea has become an everyday household name. From fighting colds to ear infections, this section will run through everything you'll need to know.

Echinacea

Use: Echinacea is popular for the prevention and treatment of the common cold and flu and adjunctive treatment in recent infections (middle ear, respiratory tract, urinary tract, and vaginal candidiasis). It is also an immunity booster. A "rest" period is recommended after eight weeks because its effects might diminish if used longer.

Safety and Side Effects: Do not take echinacea if you have an autoimmune disease or if you are taking immune-suppressing drugs.

Arthritis

Arthritis involves the painful inflammation of joints and can be caused by various conditions. If you are suffering from a form of arthritis, you may want to try one of these two supplements: boswellia and glucosamine chondroitin.

Boswellia

Use: This is intended for the treatment of rheumatoid arthritis, osteoarthritis, and possibly Crohn's disease. It is an anti-inflammatory agent that improves mobility and decreases joint pain and stiffness. At this point, it is still unclear whether long-term use will reduce joint destruction.

Glucosamine and Chondroitin

Although this supplement is not an herb, it's still considered "alternative" and is definitely worth mentioning in this chapter.

Use: The combination of glucosamine and chondroitin has been shown to slow the progression and substantially reduce the symptoms of osteoarthritis in many patients. *Glucosamine* stimulates the production of collagen—a protein that helps hold the joints together and acts as a shock-absorbing cushion between the joints. Chondroitin acts as a "liquid magnet"—helping to attract fluid to the cartilage, which acts as a buffer. Chondroitin might also protect existing cartilage from premature breakdown by inhibiting certain enzymes that can destroy the cartilage.

Safety and Side Effects: Glucosamine can cause gastrointestinal discomfort, skin reactions, drowsiness, and headache. Chondroitin can also cause stomach upset, and since it is similar in structure to the blood-thinning drug Heparin, you should not use it in conjunction with blood-thinning drugs or supplements without your doctor's approval.

Migraines

Migraines are characterized by severe head pain, plus one or more of a range of symptoms including nausea, vomiting, and sensitivity to light. A migraine attack can last up to 72 hours and leave a person completely immobile. This section provides information on feverfew—an herb that may help to alleviate these debilitating headaches.

Feverfew

Use: This herb inhibits platelet aggregation and also helps prevent the vessels from constricting. The result is a reduction in the severity, duration, and frequency of migraines and an improvement in blood-vessel tone.

Safety and Side Effects: Feverfew enhances the effectiveness of the blood thinner Coumadin, so it may increase bleeding.

Cancer

The incidence of cancer is quite low in the Asian countries. Therefore, scientists constantly conduct research to investigate which of their cultural practices may help ward off this horrific illness. This section will provide you with some exciting news about green tea—and then you can read more in Chapter 18.

Green Tea

Use: Green tea is rich in polyphenols—substances that have strong antioxidant, anti-carcinogenic, antitumorigenic, and antibiotic properties. That's a lot of "antis" for something that is so good for you!

Safety and Side Effects: The caffeine in green tea may be a problem for some people—especially those taking MAO inhibitors. And if you're taking blood-thinning medications, you should avoid drinking too much green tea because it contains vitamin K, which is a natural coagulant.

More Herbal Remedies Worth Mentioning

Yes, there are even more herbs to talk about. Find out how ginger can settle your stomach, bilberry can help your eyes, rosemary can get your blood pumping, peppermint can aid in indigestion, and aloe can heal your wounds.

Ginger

Use: Ginger helps relieve motion sickness, nausea from morning sickness, and indigestion or an upset stomach. It has an overall calming effect on the digestive system because it increases the secretion of digestive juices, including saliva, thereby neutralizing stomach acids and toxins.

Safety and Side Effects: Ginger increases the effectiveness of the blood thinner Coumadin.

Bilberry

Use: Bilberry is used to help combat retinopathy, cataracts and macular degeneration, peripheral vascular disease, varicose veins, and hemorrhoids. It promotes the formation of normal connective tissue, and protects this tissue from damage caused by inflammation.

Safety and Side Effects: None reported.

Rosemary

Use: It'll spice up more than just that roast chicken—in fact, your entire circulatory system! Recommended for its tonic, astringent, and diaphoretic effects (it increases perspiration), rosemary is said to aid in digestion and can be made into a hair tonic that will prevent baldness. It is also great for those with low blood pressure and can be used to stimulate menstruation.

Safety and Side Effects: Large quantities of the oil are needed for therapeutic purposes, and it's not safe when taken internally. (It can irritate the stomach, intestines, and kidneys.)

Peppermint

Use: Peppermint has served as a treatment for indigestion, flatulence, colic, and even menstrual cramping. Menthol, the active ingredient, can aid in digestion because it reduces the tonus of the lower esophageal sphincter and facilitates belching for relief.

Safety and Side Effects: Excessive intake of peppermint oil can cause nausea, loss of appetite, heart problems, loss of balance, and other nervous system problems. At the extreme, it can also lead to kidney failure. Peppermint oil may increase levels of the drug cyclosporine in the body.

Aloe

Aloe is an ingredient in two products that are completely different in terms of usage and chemical composition.

Aloe vera gel or mucilage is a thin, clear, jellylike substance that is used externally to treat wounds and sunburn. Although there is controversy about whether aloe gel retains its properties in preparation, fluid from a fresh leaf has been shown to promote attachment and growth of normal human cells. This type of aloe is recommended as an external wound healer.

Aloe latex or juice is quite different. In fact, it acts as a laxative and is clearly not recommended.

Safety and Side Effects: Aloe vera gel appears to be safe, but some people may experience an allergic reaction.

Using herbs can be a convenient way to alleviate everything from headaches to upset stomachs. Use this chapter as a reference guide, and look things up when you are searching for a cure to a particular ache or ailment. Once again, I cannot stress too much the importance of checking things out with your physician—especially if you are taking medication and/or have a serious illness.

The Least You Need to Know

- In the last decade, herbal remedies have become popular treatments for a variety of ailments. If you want to get into herbal culture, do it slowly and monitor yourself as you go along.

- Never indulge in herbal remedies when you're pregnant, planning on becoming pregnant, or lactating.

- Always consult with a physician before using herbs, especially if you're already taking other prescription drugs.

- Do some research: know your manufacturers, be aware of what you're taking, read the bottles, and follow the instructions carefully. Adverse reactions are not uncommon.

Part **5**

Pregnancy and Parenting

Let the cravings begin! Being pregnant is both exciting and overwhelming, and the importance of good nutrition (and exercise) for mothers-to-be can't be stressed enough. This section contains essential information on how to eat right and stay fit during your nine months of growing girth.

This part of the book is also dedicated to the younger folks. As a mother and nutritionist, I understand all too well the challenge of getting your kids to eat healthfully. If we could only mold carrots and spinach into bar shapes and pop a "Snickers" wrapper on top, life would be so much simpler! Read on for creative suggestions on how to sneak veggies into meals, make lower-fat snacks taste great, and encourage more physical activity.

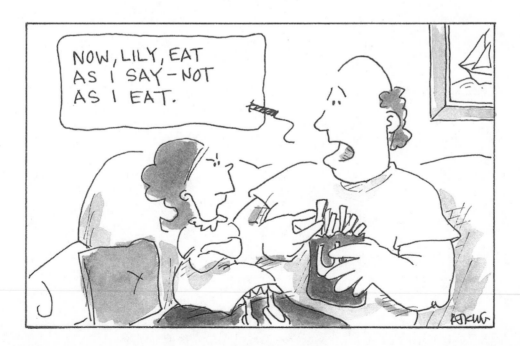

Chapter 24

Eating Your Way Through Pregnancy

In This Chapter

- Eating for a healthy pregnancy
- How much weight should you gain?
- Boosting your protein, dairy, iron, and fluid intake
- Strategies to reduce constipation, nausea, heartburn, and water retention
- The full story on fish and mercury
- A comprehensive five-day meal plan—with recipes and nutritional information

Yippee, you're pregnant—congratulations on your exciting news! This chapter provides all the info you'll need to properly nourish yourself *and* your growing baby.

Are You Really Eating for Two?

Has anyone ever said, "Go ahead and pack it in; you're eating for two"? Well, that's both true and false. *True* because your food selections will directly affect your growing baby. In other words, eat plenty of quality foods, loaded with nutrients, and you'll shower that growing bambino with all the right ingredients—and if you eat junk, your baby gets junk!

On the other hand, this statement is also *false* because you're clearly *not* eating for two adults. In fact, your growing baby is only a fraction of your size—so it's not the time to win a gold medal in the food Olympics.

Increased Calories and Protein

It's true that you do require more calories. In fact, over the course of your pregnancy, you'll need to consume about an extra 70,000 calories. Obviously, this caloric increase is spread out over nine months: it ends up being approximately 150 extra calories a day during the first trimester (the first three months) and around 300 extra calories a day during the second and third trimesters (the last six months).

You'll also need an additional 10 grams of protein within those extra daily calories. Your daily dose goes from 50 to 60 grams when you're pregnant, for the development of your precious fetus. Getting this increased protein is *not* typically a problem. Most women already overshoot their needs, and consuming extra dairy and larger servings of lean meat, fish, poultry, eggs, and legumes will ensure that you get enough. For a more detailed description on how much protein you'll need, see the section "Adjusting Your Eating Plan," later in this chapter.

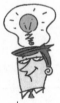

Food for Thought

You don't need to gain that much weight during the first trimester of your pregnancy. In fact, aim for a total of 2–5 pounds.

A Weighty Issue: How Many Pounds Should You Gain?

It always seems like the first thing everyone asks when you return from your doctor's office is "How much weight did you gain?" None of their business! Understand that all women are different—and the rate and speed will vary from person to person. Some gain a lot in the second trimester, and then it drastically slows down in the third—whereas others have a nice, even gain throughout. Here's what's recommended for most healthy women:

Pre-Pregnancy Weight	Suggested Gain	Weekly Gain in Second and Third Trimesters
Underweight (below 90% of desirable weight)	28–40 pounds	>1 pound
Normal weight (see range in Chapter 26)	25–35 pounds	.8–1 pound
Moderately overweight (more than 120–135% of desirable weight)	15–25 pounds	.7 pound
Very overweight (more than 135% of desirable weight)	15–20 pounds	.5 pound

Keep in mind that "desirable" weights fall within a range. You can see where you stand "pre-pregnancy" by comparing your weight in pounds with the height/weight chart in Chapter 26. Also, understand that there are special circumstances where some women will *need* to gain more, some less. For instance, women carrying twins will need to gain about 35–45 pounds, and although women with triplets almost *never* carry full term (they typically deliver around 33 weeks), if they did, they would need to gain in the vicinity of 50–70 pounds—*and hire three full-time nannies and a massage therapist.* Rap with your doctor and listen to his or her advice on this weighty issue.

> **Q & A**
>
> **Where does the extra weight go?**
> Baby: 7–8 pounds
> Placenta: 1–2 pounds
> Amniotic fluid: 1½–2 pounds
> Uterine tissue: 2 pounds
> Breast tissue: 1–2 pounds
> Fluid volume: 6–10 pounds
> Fat: 6+ pounds
> Total: 25–35 pounds

Adjusting Your Eating Plan

Let's ensure that you're gaining weight with the proper foods. Although individual requirements vary depending on calorie needs, the following chart gives some guidance in determining the basics of your diet:

Food Group	Daily Servings	Sample Servings
Breads/grains	6+	1 slice bread, or ½ small bagel, 1 serving cereal, or ½ cup cooked rice or pasta
Fruits	3+	1 medium fruit, or 1 cup berries or melon, or ½ cup fruit juice

continues

continues

Food Group	Daily Servings	Sample Servings
Vegetables	3+	1 cup raw leafy veggies, or $^1\!/_2$ cup cooked veggies
Milk/yogurt/cheese	3–4	1 cup milk, or 1 cup yogurt, or $^3\!/_4$ cup cottage cheese, or $1^1\!/_2$ oz. of hard cheese
Meat/poultry/fish	2–3	2–3 oz. lean meat, or 2 eggs (limit 2 per week), or $^2\!/_3$ cup tofu, or 2–3 oz. fish or poultry
Fluids	8+	8 oz. of water, seltzer, and other beverages
Fats/sweets	Moderation	Try your best to keep these foods to a minimum

Why All the Hype on Calcium?

Although calcium is needed throughout life, it is particularly important during pregnancy. (At last, you finally learn why everyone pesters you to drink your milk.) Your daily requirements remain at 1,000 milligrams—but some experts recommend up to 1,500 milligrams. That's approximately 3–4 servings of dairy (for example, 1 cup of milk + 1 cup pudding + 1 cup fruit yogurt + $1^1\!/_2$ ounces of hard cheese).

As you learned in Chapter 8, calcium is responsible for strong bones and teeth and for the proper functioning of blood vessels, nerves, and muscles, as well as maintaining healthy connective tissue. During pregnancy, calcium is especially critical because you have to worry about your own bones *and* your growing baby's bones, tissues, and teeth as well. In fact, your baby counts on *your* calcium for normal development. Therefore, when you skimp on the calcium-rich foods (and don't take supplementation), the calcium in your bones will be supplied to meet the increased demands of the growing fetus. In other words, you'll be placing yourself at a much greater risk for osteoporosis. See Chapter 8 for the calcium content of various foods, both dairy and nondairy.

> **Q & A**
>
> Won't the prenatal vitamins cover all the calcium my baby will need?
>
> Definitely not! Prenatal supplements supply about 200–250 milligrams per pill; that's not even one serving from the dairy group.

CAUTION **Overrated-Undercooked** _____

Don't think, "Hey, I'm pregnant; I can eat *whatever* and *whenever* I want!" With pregnancy comes increased caloric and nutrient requirements, but you can meet these needs without putting on 20 pounds of flub. Don't deprive yourself of cravings; that's one of the fun things about pregnancy. (Chocolate was definitely one of mine.) Just don't go overboard. Extra weight gained during your pregnancy is extra weight you'll be wearing *after* the baby is born.

Hiking Up the Iron

Ever wonder why the prenatal vitamins are loaded with iron? It's because during pregnancy, your body requires about double the amount of this mineral than usual. In fact, you go from normally needing 15 milligrams to requiring a daily dose of 30 milligrams when you're expecting.

Why do pregnant women require more iron? Remember, iron is found in your blood and is responsible for carrying and delivering oxygen to every cell in your body. Pregnant women have an *expanded* blood volume, so it makes sense that more blood requires more iron. Also, you have to supply oxygen to both your cells *and* the cells of your growing baby. Once again, this greater demand for oxygen requires greater amounts of iron.

Because nursing your baby *also* requires an increase in a variety of nutrients, nursing women will also benefit from following the same general eating guidelines discussed in this chapter. Take a look:

	Before	**Pregnant**	**Lactating**
Calories	Varies	+300	+500
Protein (g)	50	60	65 for first six months 62 for second six months
Calcium (mg)	1,000	1,000	1,000
Folic acid (mg)	400	600	500
Iron (mg)	15	30	15

These requirements are for healthy women 19–50 years of age.

Just because the prenatal vitamins are brimming with the stuff, don't think you can slack off in the food department. Understand that prenatal supplements (providing around 30–60 milligrams) are merely "just in case"—you still need to eat a lot of iron-rich foods. On the eating plan, you require 2–3 servings of protein foods each day. This will help satisfy your body's extra demand for *both* protein and iron because the best absorbable iron is found in the foods within this group. For further tips on boosting your iron, flip back to Chapter 8.

Food for Thought

Pregnant women with lactose intolerance should eat plenty of *nondairy* calcium-fortified foods, along with the special lactose-reduced products. Also, speak with your physician about calcium supplementation. (For further information on lactose intolerance, see Chapter 20.)

- **Best sources of heme iron:** Animal foods such as liver, beef, pork, lamb, veal, chicken, turkey, and eggs.

- **Good sources of nonheme iron:** Nonanimal foods such as enriched breads and cereals, beans, dried fruits, seeds, nuts, broccoli, spinach, collard greens, barley, chickpeas, and blackstrap molasses.

Blast Your Baby with Vitamins!

During pregnancy you want to provide your growing baby with plenty of nutrients—including the antioxidants: vitamin C and beta-carotene. Read on and learn which fruits and vegetables supply the biggest bang for your buck.

- **Fruits rich in vitamin C:** Oranges, grapefruit, mango, strawberries, papaya, raspberries, tangerines, kiwis, cantaloupe, guava, lemons, orange juice, grapefruit juice, and other vitamin C–fortified juices.

- **Vegetables rich in vitamin C:** Broccoli, tomato, sweet potato, pepper, kale, cabbage, brussels sprouts, rutabaga, cauliflower, and spinach.

- **Fruits rich in beta-carotene:** Apricots, cantaloupe, papaya, mango, prunes, peaches, nectarines, tangerines, watermelon, and guava.

- **Vegetables rich in beta-carotene:** Broccoli, brussels sprouts, carrots, collard greens, escarole, dark green lettuce, spinach, sweet potatoes, kale, butternut squash, chicory, red peppers, and tomato juice.

Keep on Drinkin', Sippin', Gulpin', and Guzzlin'!

Proper hydration is another vital component for a healthy pregnancy. Did you know that the average female is about 55–65 percent water, and the average newborn is about 85 percent water? During this nine-month period of bodily change, shift, and growth (to put it mildly), your fluid demands skyrocket for the following reasons:

- You need to maintain your *expanded* blood supply and fluid volume. You see, through the blood and lymphatic system, water helps deliver oxygen and other nutrients all over your body.

- Like always, fluids are needed to help wash down your food and assist in nutrient absorption.

- Extra fluids, along with fiber, can help to alleviate some of the bothersome plumbing problems (alias "mom-to-be" constipation).

- Fluid provides a cushion for the developing fetus and also helps lubricate your joints.

- Lastly, fluid is needed for the normal functioning of *every* cell in your body.

"Favorable fluids" you should be guzzling down include water, club soda, bottled water, vegetable juice, seltzer, calcium-fortified fruit juice, and skim or 1% low-fat milk.

Liquids you should steer clear of are alcohol, coffee, tea, soft drinks, diet cola (and other artificially sweetened drinks), and questionable herbal teas.

Also realize that in some instances, you might need even *more* than the already increased amount: for example, if you're perspiring in hot weather, or when you're exercising, or if you have any type of fever, vomiting, or diarrhea. (Obviously, in the last cases, contact your doctor immediately.)

Foods to Forget!

The following is a suggested list of foods to *avoid* (or moderate) until after the baby is born:

- **Raw foods:** This includes sushi and other raw seafood, beef tartar, undercooked poultry, raw or unpasteurized milk, soft-cooked and poached eggs, cookie dough, and Caesar salad. These foods increase your risk of bacterial infection.

- **Alcohol:** Avoid all beer, wine, and liquor.

- **Caffeine:** This includes tea, coffee, and any other highly caffeinated beverages. If you must include regular coffee or tea, try to do so in moderation (1–2 cups per day).

- **Nitrates, nitrites, and nitrosamines:** These are found in hot dogs, bacon, bologna, ham, deli turkey, and any other processed cold cuts.

- **Herbal teas:** Some have medicinal properties. Check with your physician before consuming teas other than mint teas or raspberry leaf.

- **Monosodium glutamate (MSG):** Commonly found in Chinese food, soups, and frozen convenience meals, it can cause headaches, dizziness, and nausea.

- **Artificial sweeteners:** Since the safety of these sweeteners is controversial, it may be best to use in moderation:

  - Aspartame (NutraSweet)

  - Saccharine (Sweet N' Low)

  - Sucralose (Splenda)

- **High-mercury fish:** King mackerel, swordfish, shark, and tilefish. (See the explanation for this in the next section.)

- **Cheeses:** This includes soft, unpasteurized cheeses such as Brie, Camembert, feta, goat, Limburger, Montrachet, Neufchâtel, queso fresco, Point-Leveque, and ricotta. Also avoid unpasteurized semi-soft cheeses such as Gorgonzola, Muenster, and Roquefort. These cheeses carry a bacteria called listeria monocytogenes, which has the potential to be dangerous. Hard cheeses and pasteurized cheeses do not contain listeria. Additionally, all American cheeses are made with pasteurized milk and are therefore safe to eat during pregnancy. Imported cheeses, however, are not pasteurized and should be carefully considered.

  At cocktail parties, if you don't know what types of cheeses are being served, avoid them completely.

- **Olestra:** Because it is a fat malabsorber, it's not appropriate to consume olestra during pregnancy. It can cause abdominal cramping, diarrhea, and malabsorption of fat-soluble vitamins.

Overrated-Undercooked

Fish with the highest levels of mercury to avoid are:

- Shark
- Swordfish
- King mackerel
- Tilefish

Check out the *Natural Resources Defense Council*'s website: http://www.nrdc.org. There you'll find a "mercury calculator," which will help you determine how much mercury from fish you typically consume.

The Story on Mercury and Fish

Mercury occurs naturally in the environment and can also be released into the air through industrial pollution. This mercury then falls into surface water, streams, and oceans, creating a potentially toxic substance called methylmercury. Fish absorb the methylmercury from water as they feed on aquatic organisms.

Nearly all fish contain trace amounts of methylmercury, but it is not harmful in such low levels. Long-lived, larger fish feed on other fish and accumulate the highest levels of methylmercury. These fish include shark, tilefish, swordfish, and king mackerel, and pose the greatest risk to people who eat them regularly.

The primary danger from methylmercury in fish is to the developing nervous system of the unborn child. Thus, pregnant women and women who may become pregnant should completely avoid these high-mercury fish. Additionally, it is important for nursing mothers and young children to avoid eating these fish as well.

Recommendation for Tuna

It is okay for pregnant women and women who may become pregnant to eat *other* fish as long as they limit total fish consumption to no more than twelve ounces total per week. As for tuna, the EPA (Environmental Protection Agency) recommends that you eat only *6 ounces or less* of albacore tuna per week. Albacore is the white kind, and it contains more mercury than chunk light tuna.

For updates on the latest information in your area, contact the EPA for current advice on fish consumption from fresh lakes and streams. Also check with your state or local health department to see if there are special advisories on fish caught from waters in your local area. Furthermore, you can contact "Risks of Mercury in Seafood" by calling 1-888-safefood #9.

Q & A

What is gestational diabetes?

Gestational diabetes is the onset of high blood sugar (or carbohydrate intolerance) that is generally detected around the twenty-eighth week of pregnancy. Because this condition is caused by the placenta putting out large doses of anti-insulin hormones, as soon as the placenta is removed (during the baby's delivery), the condition disappears in almost all cases. Women diagnosed with gestational diabetes have very specific dietary concerns and should work with a qualified nutritionist (registered dietitian) on appropriate meal planning.

The Many Trials and Tribulations of Having a Baby

When embarking on the road to motherly bliss, some women glow and others, shall I say, turn green. I was one of the unlucky green women. Although agonizing and uncomfortable (to put it *mildly*), these lousy side effects, including constipation, nausea, water retention, and heartburn, are merely normal pregnancy occurrences and most certainly worth the beautiful end product.

Food for Thought

Getting enough folic acid can *drastically* reduce the risk for babies developing neural tube defects such as spina bifida. So fill up on the green leafy veggies and get precautionary backup from a prenatal vitamin that supplies folic acid.

The "Uh-Oh, Better Get Drano" Feeling

Most pregnant women experience the constipation blues at one time or another during the nine-month haul. Why does food tend to stop dead in its tracks before reaching its final destination anyway? Unfortunately, there are a bunch of explanations:

♦ Hormonal changes

♦ The increased pressure on your intestinal tract as your baby grows

♦ All of the extra iron in your prenatal supplements

- ◆ Not enough fiber in your diet

- ◆ Not drinking enough fluids

- ◆ Plain old lack of exercise

Yes, it's true that the first three circumstances are completely uncontrollable, but let's focus on the last three: fiber, fluid, and exercise, which are quite controllable and can *dramatically* decrease your plumbing problems.

First, increase your dietary fiber by eating more fresh fruit, veggies, and whole-grain foods. Better yet, flip back to Chapter 6 and read the tips for boosting your daily intake of fiber. Next, drink a ton of fluids. Stay tuned for Chapter 25, which provides exercise guidelines during pregnancy.

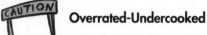

Overrated-Undercooked

Sometimes, the increased iron can cause constipation, diarrhea, dark-colored stools, and abdominal discomfort. Don't be alarmed; it's just par for the course. Be sure to increase your fiber and fluids and move around as much as possible.

Ugh! That Nagging Nausea

Commonly known as "morning sickness," the awful nausea and vomiting can occur at *any* time of the day, so don't be misled. One bit of reassuring news: although horridly unpleasant, it's *normal* and thought to simply be a side effect from the hormonal changes that take place during pregnancy. If you're on a first-name basis with your toilet, hang in there; the nausea usually disappears by week 14.

Here are some tips to help reduce the nausea:

- ◆ Nibble on carbohydrate-rich foods throughout the day. They are easy to digest and will provide your body with some energy (calories). For example, bagels, pretzels, crackers, cereal, and rice cakes are all primo snacks.

- ◆ If you tend to be nauseated in the early morning, keep some of the preceding carbs by your bed. Pop something into your mouth *before* getting up; this will start the digestive process and get rid of excess stomach acid.

- ◆ Most women find cold foods easier to tolerate than hot foods; however, everyone is unique. What makes one woman sick might be soothing to another. In other words, listen to your own body and go ahead with whatever works best for you.

- Avoid any sharp cooking odors, and open the windows for some fresh air.

- When you just can't take solid foods, suck on an ice pop or frozen fruit bars or sip on lemonade and fruit juice.

- Avoid high-fat foods because they sit in your stomach longer and can exacerbate the nausea.

- Sometimes, iron supplements can intensify nausea. If you are taking iron pills, take them with a snack or two hours after a meal with some ginger ale. If the nausea persists, you might also want to speak with your doctor about possibly holding off on the iron until you feel better.

- Do *not* take prenatal vitamins on an empty stomach; take them with a meal or snack.

Contact your doctor immediately if you have persistent vomiting, are losing weight, or are too nauseated to take in fluids.

What's All the Swelling About?

Edema is the uncomfortable swelling, or retention of water, that occurs primarily in your feet, ankles, and hands during pregnancy. As long as there's no increase in blood pressure or protein in the urine, edema is normal and unfortunately tends to get worse in the last trimester. However, there is no need to panic; most of this bother-some fluid will be lost during and shortly after your baby's delivery.

Get some relief from the effects of edema:

- Lie down with your feet elevated on a pillow.

- Remove all of your tight rings.

- Wear loose, comfortable shoes.

- Ease up on the salty stuff such as sauerkraut, pickles, soy sauce, salty pretzels, and chips.

- *Never* restrict your fluid intake; always continue to drink plenty of fluids.

Oh, My Aching Heart

Contrary to the name, *heartburn* is actually a burning sensation in your lower esophagus that is usually accompanied by a sour taste. Although this dreadful feeling can happen at any time during your pregnancy, it's most common toward the last few months, when your baby is rapidly growing and exerting pressure on your stomach and uterus. What's more, during pregnancy, the valve between your stomach and esophagus can become relaxed, making it easy for the food to occasionally reverse directions.

Some simple remedies to ease heartburn:

◆ Relax and eat your food slowly.

◆ Instead of eating a lot at one sitting, eat several smaller meals throughout the day.

◆ Limit fluids *with* meals, but increase fluids *between* meals.

◆ Chew gum or suck candy. Of course, your dentist will hate me, but it can help to neutralize the acid.

◆ Never lie flat after you have eaten. In fact, keep your head elevated when you sleep with the help of extra pillows and by placing a couple of books underneath the mattress to help tilt it slightly upward.

◆ Avoid wearing tight clothing. Stick with items that are loose and comfortable.

◆ Stand up and walk around. This can help encourage your gastric juices to flow in the right direction.

◆ Keep a log and track some foods that might be triggering your heartburn. Some common culprits include regular and decaf coffee, colas, spicy foods, greasy fried foods, chocolate, citrus fruits and juices, and tomato-based products.

◆ Do not take any antacids without your doctor's approval.

Five-Day Pregnancy Meal Plan

Here's a five-day meal plan to get you started on your healthy eating track. You'll notice the adjustments for the first trimester at the bottom of each menu; this is because your body requires fewer calories during the first three months and more during the last six months.

Menu 1

Breakfast
1 cup whole-grain cereal topped with
1 cup 1% low-fat milk and 1 TB. of chopped nuts
$^1/_2$ cantaloupe (or 1 cup berries)
8 oz. grapefruit juice

Lunch
Turkey/cheese sandwich (2 oz. turkey, 1$^1/_2$ oz. cheese, with roasted peppers on
  2 slices whole-wheat bread)
1 cup vegetable soup
Glass of seltzer water with 4 oz. cranberry juice

Snack
Yogurt/fruit shake (blend 1 cup low-fat frozen yogurt, 1 banana, and $^1/_2$–1 cup
strawberries or blueberries)

Dinner
Tossed salad with 2 TB. dressing
5 oz. grilled chicken breast, cut into chunks and stir-fried with 1 cup assorted
veggies (with 1 TB. olive oil and 1 tsp. of low-sodium soy sauce)
1 cup brown rice
Seltzer or water with fresh lemon

Snack
1 cup 1% low-fat milk
4 graham crackers topped with 1 TB. of peanut butter

Nutrition Information:

Calories: 2,544	Iron: 25 mg
Fat: 26% (74 grams)	Calcium: 1,645 mg
Carbohydrate: 53%	Folic acid: 465 mcg
Fiber: 38 grams	B-6: 4.7 mg
Protein: 21%	Zinc: 18 mg

For the first trimester, skip the midnight snack of milk, graham crackers, and
peanut butter, and you'll have the following nutrition information:

Calories: 2,288	Iron: 24 mg
Fat: 24% (62 grams)	Calcium: 1,335 mg
Carbohydrate: 54%	Folic acid: 438 mcg

Fiber: 37 grams

Protein: 22%

B-6: 4.5 mg

Zinc: 16 mg

Menu 2

Breakfast
1 cup oatmeal with $^1/_4$ cup raisins
Whole-wheat pita bread
2 tsp. reduced-fat margarine and 1 TB. jam
1 cup 1% low-fat milk

Lunch
Open-faced tuna melt (recipe in Chapter 11)
Carrot sticks with 2 TB. of low-fat dressing
8 oz. orange juice
Apple

Snack
1 cup low-fat fruit yogurt
2 oatmeal raisin cookies
Seltzer with lemon

Dinner
4 oz. broiled beef sirloin
$1^1/_2$ cups linguini with $^1/_2$ cup marinara sauce
1 cup steamed spinach with garlic and 1 tsp. olive oil
1 cup fruit salad with 1 TB. of chopped walnuts
Water or seltzer

Snack
Frozen yogurt pop
6 mini flavored rice cakes

Nutrition Information:
Calories: 2,517

Fat: 24% (67 grams)

Carbohydrate: 55%

Fiber: 34 grams

Protein: 21%

Iron: 20 mg

Calcium: 1,772 mg

Folic acid: 406 mcg

B-6: 2.5 mg

Zinc: 19 mg

For the first trimester, skip the night-time snack of frozen yogurt and rice cakes, and you'll have the following nutrition information:

Calories: 2,342	Iron: 20 mg
Fat: 24% (63 grams)	Calcium: 1,667 mg
Carbohydrate: 54%	Folic acid: 402 mcg
Fiber: 34 grams	B-6: 2.4 mg
Protein: 22%	Zinc: 19 mg

Menu 3

Breakfast
2 whole-grain waffles
1 TB. margarine
1 cup strawberries (or small banana)
1 cup low-fat fruit yogurt
1 cup 1% low-fat milk

Lunch
Egg white–veggie omelet (recipe in Chapter 11)
Toasted bagel with 2 TB. cream cheese and 1 TB. jam
1 serving canned peaches in light syrup
Seltzer water or club soda

Snack
Granola bar
1 cup frozen seedless grapes
8 oz. orange juice

Dinner
Tossed salad with 2 TB. dressing
4–5 oz. grilled fish
$1\frac{1}{2}$ cups couscous
Steamed carrots
Frozen fruit bar
Water or seltzer with lemon

Snack
1 slice of whole-grain toast
$1\frac{1}{2}$ oz. low-fat cheese

Nutrition Information:

Calories: 2,554	Iron: 15 mg
Fat: 25% (70 grams)	Calcium: 1,827 mg
Carbohydrate: 55%	Folic acid: 457 mcg
Fiber: 30 grams	B-6: 2.1 mg
Protein: 20%	Zinc: 10 mg

For the first trimester, skip the night-time snack of whole-grain toast and cheese, and you'll have the following nutrition information:

Calories: 2,322
Fat: 24% (63 grams)
Carbohydrate: 57%
Fiber: 27 grams
Protein: 19%

Iron: 13 mg
Calcium: 1,363 mg
Folic acid: 435 mcg
B-6: 2.0 mg
Zinc: 8 mg

Menu 4

Breakfast
French Toast á la Mode (recipe in Chapter 11)
8 oz. grapefruit juice

Lunch
Chef salad with lettuce, tomato, carrots, and 1 oz. roast beef
2 oz. turkey breast
1½ oz. Swiss cheese
2 TB. vinaigrette dressing
Whole-grain roll
½ cup dried apricots mixed with 2 TB. of almonds
Club soda

Snack
1 cup frozen yogurt topped with granola
Nectarine

Dinner
1½ cups cooked pasta with 3 oz. tofu
1 cup cooked broccoli (or peapods and carrots)
½ cup marinara sauce
1 cup fresh strawberries with 3 TB. whipped cream
Club soda with lemon

Snack
Slice of angel food cake
1 cup low-fat milk

Nutrition Information:
Calories: 2,550
Fat: 25% (71 grams)
Carbohydrate: 55%
Fiber: 32 grams
Protein: 20%

Iron: 23 mg
Calcium: 1,764 mg
Folic acid: 446 mcg
B-6: 2.3 mg
Zinc: 14 mg

For the first trimester, skip the night-time snack of angel food cake and milk plus the granola on the frozen yogurt at midday, and you'll have the following nutrition information:

Calories: 2,232
Fat: 25% (61 grams)
Carbohydrate: 55%
Fiber: 29 grams
Protein: 20%

Iron: 21 mg
Calcium: 1,400 mg
Folic acid: 406 mcg
B-6: 2.0 mg
Zinc: 12 mg

Menu 5

Breakfast
1 cup whole-grain cereal
1 cup 1% low-fat milk
1 cup raspberries
1 slice raisin bread with 1 TB. of peanut butter
8 oz. orange juice (calcium-fortified)

Lunch
1½ cups rice and 1 cup black beans
1 cup fresh fruit salad topped with 2 TB. of granola and 1 TB. of chopped walnuts
Club soda

Snack
Yogurt/fruit shake
1 chocolate-chip cookie

Dinner
5 oz. grilled chicken breast
1 cup steamed kale with 1 tsp. olive oil and garlic
Baked sweet potato with 2 tsp. of margarine
Baked apple with cinnamon
Water

Snack
1 cup frozen seedless grapes or a frozen fruit bar
1 cup 1% low-fat milk

Nutrition Information:
Calories: 2,485
Fat: 25% (69 grams)
Carbohydrate: 58%
Fiber: 53 grams
Protein: 17%

Iron: 26 mg
Calcium: 1,443 mg
Folic acid: 642 mcg
B-6: 3.4 mg
Zinc: 16 mg

For the first trimester, skip the night-time snack of milk and grapes *plus* the chocolate chip cookie at midday, and you'll have the following nutrition information:

Calories: 2,246

Fat: 25% (62 grams)

Carbohydrate: 58%

Fiber: 51 grams

Protein: 17%

Iron: 26 mg

Calcium: 1,100 mg

Folic acid: 625 mcg

B-6: 3.2 mg

Zinc: 15 mg

Eating a balanced and varied diet will provide you and your baby with the 40 or so nutrients important for good health. Pay extra attention to folate, iron, calcium, and protein—and take good care of yourself by monitoring your weight gain and being physically active. Pregnancy is one of the most exciting times in a woman's life, so enjoy!

The Least You Need to Know

◆ You'll need about an extra 70,000 calories during the entire nine-month haul! That's about 150 extra calories each day during the first trimester and around 300 extra calories each day during the second and third trimesters.

◆ Adequate protein, calcium, iron, folic acid, and a variety of other nutrients are required throughout your pregnancy to cover the increased demands of the growing fetus.

◆ Healthy, normal-weight women should aim for a 25–35 pound weight gain.

◆ Although nausea, constipation, water retention, and heartburn can be quite unpleasant, rest assured they are generally normal side effects of pregnancy.

Chapter 25

Exercising Your Way Through Pregnancy

In This Chapter

- ◆ The pros of exercising through pregnancy
- ◆ How much and how hard
- ◆ Important tips for safety
- ◆ Appropriate exercise programs

Way back in the olden days (you know, when our parents had us), pregnancy was a time for rest—not exercise. *You're pregnant? Relax, put your feet up and have a few bon bons.* Today, we know better. In fact, research shows that pregnant women who regularly exercise have fewer aches and pains, better self-esteem, more stamina, strength, and energy, and perhaps less fear of the delivery room.

Naturally, pregnancy is not the time to beat the world record in the high jump or place in the New York City marathon, but you can certainly continue with a modified version of your regular exercise regimen. You can even begin a prenatal exercise program if you're a newcomer to the world of fitness. Compare delivering a baby to participating in an Olympic event: the nine-month pregnancy is your chance to train for the big day.

Most Doctors Give the Green Light for Exercise

Most obstetricians today are keen on the idea of pregnant women exercising their way to the delivery room—within the limits of common sense, of course. However, because certain medical instances rule out exercise, and nobody knows you better medically than your obstetrician, never begin exercising without first discussing it with your personal physician.

Q & A

Can you start exercising for the first time when you're pregnant—even if you're totally out of shape?

Yes! In fact, studies report that beginners can safely reap the benefits from exercise as long as they take it easy, appropriately warm up and cool down, keep their heart rates within a safe range, and have appropriate supervision for at least the first few sessions. Naturally, fitness novices must get the okay from their docs before jumping in.

What Do the Experts Say?

This is a summary of the appropriate guidelines and recommendations from the American College of Obstetricians and Gynecologists (ACOG) on exercise during pregnancy and postpartum.

For healthy pregnant women who have no additional risk factors, ACOG recommends the following:

1. During pregnancy, women can continue to exercise and derive health benefits even from mild to moderate exercise routines. Regular exercise—at least three times per week—is preferable to intermittent activity.

2. Avoid exercise in the supine position (lying on your back) after the first trimester. This position can decrease the cardiac output (blood flow) to the uterus. Also avoid prolonged periods of motionless standing.

3. Pregnant women have less oxygen available for aerobic activity and therefore should not expect to be able to do what they did pre-pregnancy. Pay close attention to your body, and modify your exercise intensity according to how you feel. Always stop exercising when you feel fatigued and *never* push your body to exhaustion.

Although some women might be able to continue with their regular weight-bearing exercises at the same intensity as they did pre-pregnancy, non–weight-bearing exercises such as swimming and biking might be easier to do and present less risk of injury.

4. Your changing size, shape, and weight can make certain exercises difficult. Avoid activities that can throw off your balance and possibly cause you to fall. Further, avoid any exercise with the potential for even mild abdominal trauma.

5. Pregnancy requires an additional 300 calories a day. Thus, women who exercise during pregnancy should be particularly careful to eat an adequate diet.

6. Pregnant women who exercise in the first trimester should stay cool by drinking plenty of water, wearing appropriate clothing, and avoiding very humid or hot environments.

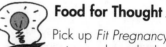

Food for Thought

Pick up *Fit Pregnancy* magazine and get the latest scoop on keeping fit while you're expecting. From the folks over at *Shape* magazine, it hits the newsstands three to four times each year.

7. Resume your pre-pregnancy exercise routines gradually after giving birth. Many of the physical changes that take place during pregnancy persist for four to six weeks.

You should not exercise during pregnancy if you have any of the following conditions:

◆ Pregnancy-induced hypertension (high blood pressure)

◆ Preterm rupture of membranes

◆ Preterm labor during the prior or current pregnancy

◆ Incompetent cervix/cerclage (a surgical procedure to close the cervix to keep the fetus intact in utero)

◆ Persistent second- or third-trimester bleeding

◆ Intrauterine growth retardation

In addition, women with certain other medical or obstetric conditions, including chronic hypertension or active thyroid, cardiac, vascular, or pulmonary disease, should be evaluated carefully in order to determine whether an exercise program is appropriate.

Q & A

Do fit women have easier deliveries than unfit women?

I hate to say it, but probably not. An easy delivery has more to do with genetics, the positioning of the baby, and a lot of luck. I've heard of "super-fit" women who had labors from hell, and I've heard of sedentary women who popped out babies with just four pushes. Go figure.

However, one thing is for sure: fit moms can better handle prolonged, agonizing labor and bounce back with a quicker recuperation period than unfit moms.

Warming Up, Cooling Down, and All the Stuff in the Middle

Pregnant or not, the ABCs of exercise remain the same. Be sure to begin each session with an appropriate warm-up—some light aerobic activity that will rev up your system and prepare your body for the exercise to follow. Next, continue with a low- to moderate-intensity aerobic segment and pay close attention to your body's cues. During pregnancy, work at a comfortable pace, stop when you feel fatigued, and never push yourself to exhaustion. Lastly, always end your aerobic session with a proper cool-down; gradually slow down the pace to bring your heart rate back to a resting level. See Chapter 14 for further details on exercise programs.

Food for Thought

The mysterious art of yoga involves breathing, relaxation, stretching, and body awareness. Therefore, yoga can play a magical role in making you feel terrific during and after your pregnancy.

Stretch Your Bod—Carefully

Regular, consistent stretching can help to maintain your flexibility and prevent some of the muscle tightness that typically sneaks up on you during the last trimester. As always, stretching must be preceded by some type of warm-up activity to increase your circulation and internal body temperature. Also, be sure to ease into each stretch gradually and hold for 10–30 seconds; never bounce! During pregnancy, the object is to stretch nice and easy. Don't ever push a stretch past the point of your pain-free range of motion.

Keep a Check on the Intensity

As of 1994, the American College of Obstetricians and Gynecologists (ACOG) lifted the rule that limited pregnant exercisers to a heart rate of 140 beats per minute or less. Today, there are no limitations on heart rate: you can monitor your own intensity as long as you exercise common sense. Keep in mind, you should *always* be able to comfortably carry on a conversation to ensure you are working in a safe aerobic range, and never push through fatigue, cramping, or any other discomfort. (Review the section on checking your heart rate in Chapter 14.)

Understand that being pregnant means you will typically fatigue more easily. Therefore, be cautious in the gym and modify your pre-pregnancy routine by decreasing both workout intensity and length. Also, don't expect to keep up with those nonpregnant jocks; find some less competitive opponents.

Q & A

What should I expect during the first, second, and third trimesters?

During the first trimester, size is not the issue; your raging hormones are! Because some women feel incredibly tired and queasy, listen to your body and do whatever activity you can manage until you feel better.

During the second trimester, most women bounce back and feel like themselves again. If you feel up to it, this is a terrific time to incorporate regular exercise into your weekly schedule.

During the last trimester, your growing waistline and weight might affect your stamina, agility, and balance. Think about switching to gentler activities that won't strain your joints and muscles (for instance, swimming and walking).

"Energize" Without All the Slamming and Jamming!

When it comes to selecting the type of exercise, every woman is different. One woman might be perfectly okay with modifying her usual sport (for instance, a runner might continue to jog at a slower pace), but other women

Food for Thought

Don't wait to get thirsty: keep a water bottle close by and drink before, during, and after your workouts to ensure that you and your baby are adequately hydrated.

are uncomfortable with the jarring and jolting on the joints—especially in the last trimester, when weight begins to climb. Think about switching to gentler activities, such as walking instead of running, swimming instead of high-impact aerobics, or pedaling on a stationary bike.

Take a Walk with Your Baby

Some of the great things about walking include that there's no crashing impact, you can select your own pace and distance, you get quality "think time" (a precious commodity after the baby arrives), and you can do it just about anywhere. For some fresh air, go for a trek around the neighborhood or hit a scenic trail. If the weather doesn't suit you, try a treadmill or wander about your local shopping mall. Anything goes; just remember these key points:

- You need to keep a strong, upright posture; lead with your chest.

- Rhythmically move your arms forward and back from the shoulders. Do not swing them higher than your chest or across your midline.

- Do not walk outdoors when the ground is icy. Remember, your balance is not as keen as it used to be.

- Don't try to conquer steep hills that can send your heart rate soaring or place a lot of stress on your back.

- Do not walk in steamy, hot, or humid weather.

CAUTION **Overrated-Undercooked** _____

Reduce your risk for injury by avoiding activities that require a lot of balance and coordination because as your body shifts, so does your center of gravity due to your enlarged belly, breasts, and uterus. Back off from things that might land you on the ground: skiing, horseback riding, biking, and skating. Avoid sports that involve sharp, jerky movements such as swinging a tennis racket, volleyball, bowling, and so on.

- Keep your body and baby well hydrated. Drink before, during, and after your walk.

- Eat a snack before you start your walk to prevent a drop in your blood sugar.

- Wear comfortable shoes with good support. Some women's feet swell during pregnancy, so you might need shoes or sneaks at least one half size bigger.

◆ Wear appropriate clothing. On cold days, wear layers that can be shed and tied around your waist as you heat up.

Sign Up for a Prenatal Exercise Class

Prenatal exercise classes are specially designed for expectant moms and take into consideration your shifting center of gravity, reduced stamina, and ever-changing bod. Generally, these specialty classes focus on thorough warm-ups, cool-downs, aerobic workouts, and stretching. In some instances, they might also include strength training and yoga. All exercises are carefully choreographed to keep you energized, but in a comfortable and appropriate fashion. Furthermore, you won't feel self-conscious because everyone in the class is in the same boat—give or take a few inches (or yards) around the waist. In other words, it's highly unlikely that the woman standing next to you will be wearing a thong leotard (and if she is, more power to her*)*. It's also a nice place to bond, swap pregnancy war stories, and meet other women who are soon to have kids the same age as your own.

You can typically find out what's available in your area by checking with the local health clubs, hospitals, birthing centers, or even your obstetrician's office.

Q & A

What the heck are kegals?

Kegals are exercises to strengthen the muscles within the pelvic floor (sort of deep inside, between your vagina and belly button). To figure out where these muscles are, stop and start your urine flow when you're sitting on the toilet. Once you find them, regularly strengthen your pelvic-floor muscles with tightening and relaxing exercises. Pull upward and inward toward the body's midline, hold for about 5–10 seconds, and then relax. Repeat them for as many times as you can, as often as you are willing. Kegal exercises can be done sitting, standing, or lying down and can drastically help to increase genital circulation, strengthen and maintain the pelvic floor muscles, and prevent incontinence after the baby is born.

Yes, "Moms-to-Be" Can Lift Weights

Being pregnant doesn't necessarily mean passing up the weight room. In fact, some light weight training might cut back on some of the back and shoulder pain associated with enlarged breasts, extra weight, and a growing uterus. It might also reduce the leg cramps and neck strain that some women experience toward the last trimester. Personally, my favorite benefit from prenatal lifting is that your muscles will be primed for the "baby *aftermath.*" That is, you'll be ready to lug around your pocketbook, diaper bag, and stroller on one arm, while carrying your baby on the other. To this day, I still amaze my sister Debra with the amount of equipment I can juggle with just two arms!

If you're experienced with weights, you can continue with a modified version of your regular routine. (Adjust the amount of weight and number of reps to how you feel.) However, if you are a novice with the dumbbells and machines, this is definitely not the time to lift anything unsupervised. You can ask a qualified trainer who is experienced with pregnant women to show you the ropes.

Some things to consider:

- Regroup your weight-training goals. Instead of focusing on intense workouts that will increase strength and define your muscles, relax, take it easy, and simply concentrate on strength maintenance.

- Because you might become less agile and coordinated due to the extra weight you are carrying, consider sticking with the machines. They offer much more support and require less balance than the free weights.

- Be aware that some machines require inappropriate positioning, and as your belly expands in front, you literally might not be able to fit on some of the machines comfortably. (Ah, isn't pregnancy fun?) But don't let that halt the workout: ask a trainer to show you some safe (perhaps nonmachine) exercises. Or simply forget about that exercise until you're back to your pre-pregnancy routine.

- The amount of weight you should lift depends on your pre-pregnancy strength and how you feel during your pregnancy. Lift what feels slightly challenging during the last few reps, not an amount that really pushes your limit.

- Pay close attention to your form and concentrate on smooth and steady breathing.

- Don't be discouraged if you have to cut back on the weights as you get further into your pregnancy. In fact, expect to cut back. Remember, you're pregnant—not Wonder Woman. Women typically get more tired and have less agility and balance toward the end of the nine-month term.

- If at any point you feel nauseous, dizzy, overly fatigued, or any other uncomfortable sensation (cramping, knotting, tingling), stop exercising immediately and speak with your doctor before continuing.

Q & A

Can I lie on my back and do sit-ups?

Yes, but only during the first trimester. After the fourth month, you risk pinching off the inferior vena cava, an important large vein that carries blood back to the heart. During pregnancy, the weight of your growing uterus might compress this vein and cause you to feel faint. Instead of stomach exercises on your back, ask a trainer to show you how to work your abdominals on your side or standing up.

Bouncing Back After the Baby Arrives

Generally, five to six weeks after delivering your bundle of joy, your doctor will give you the okay to resume all exercise—which is easier said than done. Between the sleep deprivation and feeling like your body's been through a war, merely scheduling in the time and getting the motivation is a feat in itself. Take a deep breath and round up some energy because exercise can do wonders for both your mind and body. Start slow, go at your own pace, and gradually ease back into your pre-pregnancy routine.

The Least You Need to Know

- Women who regularly exercise during pregnancy tend to have fewer aches and pains, better self-esteem, and more stamina, strength, and energy.

- Because some medical instances rule out exercise, always get the okay from your doctor before beginning an exercise program.

- Because pregnancy generally reduces your stamina, speed, and agility, expect to modify your pre-pregnancy routines by decreasing your workout intensity and length. Also, always keep your heart rate within a comfortable working range and never push your body to exhaustion.

- Most pregnant women prefer gentler activities that do not strain the joints, such as swimming, walking, and stationary bikes—especially during the last trimester when your girth and weight start to climb.

- Drink plenty of water before, during, and after exercise to ensure that you and your baby are well hydrated.

26

Feeding the Younger Folks

In This Chapter

◆ Foods for the first year of life

◆ Nutrition guidelines for growing kids

◆ Involving your kids in the kitchen

◆ Healthy snack attacks

◆ Getting your couch potato to exercise

Being a kid these days is a pretty demanding job. Between homework, after-school activities, sports, being popular, and keeping up with fashion, it's especially important that the younger folks learn to keep their bodies fit and healthy so that they're better-equipped to take on the world.

As a mother, as well as a nutritionist, I understand that nobody knows your children better than you. Therefore, this chapter is not about telling you what you should and shouldn't feed your kids, but merely offers suggestions and guidelines to help you in this endeavor. Read on to learn how to encourage your kids to eat nutritious foods and get plenty of physical activity. Bear in mind that healthy kids grow up to be healthy adults.

Your Very First Food Decision: Breast Milk or Formula?

Most pediatricians and nutritionists across the board agree that breast milk is the food of choice for growing babies. First, nursing is a beautiful mother-baby bonding experience, and it's economically savvy. In other words, it's cheap! But most importantly, breast milk has the capability to protect your baby from several infections because it is believed to carry immunities (protective substances) from mother to infant. *Colostrum*, the yellowish pre-milk substance secreted in the first few days after delivery, might carry even more antibodies—plus it's loaded with protein and zinc.

Nutri-Speak

Colostrum is a yellowish pre-milk substance that is secreted in the first few days after delivery. Colostrum is rich in protein and zinc—and may carry antibodies from mom to baby.

For all you women who choose not to nurse, or aren't able to nurse, don't lose any sleep. Companies today make sophisticated baby formulas that closely mimic the components in human milk. What's more, babies that are formula-fed can receive just as much "snuggling time" and form close bonds with mom as babies that are breast-fed. Whatever you decide (the bottle or the breast), rest assured all kids have a shot at Harvard University and the Olympic soccer team!

When and How to Start Solids

Although you might choose to nurse past six months, at this point your growing baby will need more calories and iron than breast milk or formulas alone can supply. Generally, pediatricians recommend beginning solid foods between four and six months. Here are some strategies for getting started:

Overrated-Undercooked

Don't be overzealous about buying "low-fat" foods for your infant. Although it's a good practice for older children, the first two years of life require extra calories and fat for proper growth and development. Stick with the whole-fat dairy until your child turns two years old or your pediatrician says otherwise.

♦ A general rule of thumb is to introduce only one new food at a time (over three to five days) to rule out food allergies and intolerances. If your baby tolerates a food, and you don't notice any adverse reactions (skin rashes, wheezing, diarrhea, stomachaches), you can graduate on to the next food item.

As your baby moves up in age and food variety, keep a watchful eye on items known to cause allergies such as wheat, egg white, nut butters, and cow's milk. In fact, avoid giving egg whites and regular dairy until after the first year. Completely hold off on peanuts and peanut butter for the first two years ... and three years if there's a family history.

◆ Rice cereal is usually recommended for the first food introduction because it is the least allergenic. Follow the directions on the box (usually 3–5 tablespoons of dry cereal is mixed with breast milk, formula, or water). Although it might seem bland to you, don't add anything else (sugar, salt, honey). Your baby will find it perfectly fine, and it's really the texture that you want him or her to get used to.

◆ After cereal has passed the test, try some pureed fruit and pureed veggies. (I recommend that you start with the veggies.) Watch how your baby starts to master the art of pushing the food back into the mouth with the tongue; what a genius!

◆ By age 6 to 10 months, your baby's digestive system is maturing and it's time to introduce all sorts of mashed concoctions. Try strained meats, chicken, turkey, egg yolks (continue to avoid egg whites), and mashed lentils and beans.

Food for Thought

It's a good idea to start with vegetables before fruit. After introducing the sweetness of fruit, some infants are not so willing to eat the vegetables.

◆ By 12 months, you can go ahead and substitute regular cow's milk for formula, with your pediatrician's okay. Encourage at least two to three full cups of milk per day, but not so much that your child will be too full for the solid foods that supply the necessary calories and iron. You can also go ahead and add cheese and plain yogurts.

◆ Go at your own pace, and listen to what your pediatrician has to say about the growth and development of your little one—clearly the best indication of your baby's nutritional status.

Popular first-year foods:

◆ Rice cereals

◆ Squash

◆ Green beans

◆ Yogurt, plain

◆ Peaches

◆ Chicken

◆ Turkey

◆ Barley cereals

◆ Sweet potato

◆ Peas

◆ Applesauce

◆ Plums

◆ Beef

◆ Oat cereals

◆ Carrots

◆ Avocado

◆ Bananas

◆ Pears

◆ Lamb

The Wrong Stuff

Watch out for certain foods. During the first year, avoid foods that are difficult to chew and could cause choking, such as nuts, popcorn, hard candy, and raw baby carrots. Also avoid foods that have tough outer skins, such as grapes and hot dogs.

Food for Thought

Until the age of 24 years, kids are laying down the foundation for a lifetime of strong, healthy bones, so discourage all the sugary beverages and encourage them to drink milk and calcium-fortified juice (diluted with water).

Honey should definitely be avoided in children under one year of age because it can cause infant botulism. Honey is sometimes contaminated with spores of clostridium botulinum, and in an infant's intestines these spores can grow and produce a toxin that can make a baby sick and—in extreme cases—cause death. Adults need not worry because "friendly" bacteria present in their intestines prevent these spores from growing.

Be extra cautious when introducing foods that tend to be highly allergenic, such as egg whites, wheat, corn, nuts, seafood, citrus fruits, cow's milk, chocolate, cocoa, seafood, pork, berries, soy, and tomatoes.

The Right Stuff for Growing Kids

These are the basic guidelines for children three years and older. Keep in mind that this chart represents the minimum requirements. Obviously, active kids who participate in after-school sports (or kids who just plain run around a lot) will need more food than the average couch potato. Also, expect the portion sizes to vary; younger children generally eat much smaller portions than older kids.

Food Group	Suggested Servings/Day	Key Nutrients
Bread and grain group	6+	Carbohydrates, B-vitamins, iron
Vegetable group	3+	Vitamin C, vitamin A, folic acid, magnesium, fiber
Fruit group	2+	Vitamin C, vitamin A, potassium, fiber
Milk, yogurt, and cheese group	3+	Calcium, riboflavin, protein
Meat, poultry, dried beans, eggs, and nuts group	2	Protein, B-vitamins, iron, zinc

---

Q & A

Should I worry if my kids aren't getting enough food?

Probably not. Children generally eat when they are hungry and stop when they are full. You might, however, want to pay attention to daily food choices among various food groups. If certain foods are consistently left out, brainstorm on ways to work them into the day.

Be a Healthy Role Model

Monkey see, monkey do! As your children grow, they observe and copy everything you do—eating habits included. Remember, actions speak much louder than words, so start munching on produce and don't skip breakfast!

Cook with Your Kids, Not for Them!

Introduce your kids to healthy eating and the kitchen! I've found that children are more interested and willing to eat unfamiliar foods when they participate in the preparation. Try some of the following suggestions:

♦ Select a few nights each week and involve your kids with dinner planning and preparation. Designate different jobs for each child.

♦ You might prefer to single out one child at a time. For instance, Tuesday night might be the night you and your son whip up a creative dinner concoction for the family. Thursday night might be a special night for just you and your daughter to plan the evening spread.

Food for Thought

Typically, the more color on your plate, the more vitamin content. For example, a plate of noodles with broccoli, tomato sauce, and parmesan cheese will have a lot more color and vitamin content than a plate of plain noodles with butter.

♦ How about an entire "theme night?" For example, one night might be Japanese. Make chicken teriyaki over rice; you can set up a table on the floor, sit on pillows, and use chopsticks instead of forks. Or make it Greek night and serve Greek salads while wearing togas.

Healthy after-school snacks include the following:

- Fresh fruit
- Frozen bananas and grapes
- Red peppers and cherry tomatoes
- Celery and light cream cheese
- Low-fat yogurt topped with whole-grain cereal
- Soy crisps
- Natural, unsweetened applesauce
- Fruit cocktail in light syrup
- Bananas and apple slices with peanut butter
- Whole-grain crackers with apple butter
- Bowl of whole grain cereal with skim low-fat milk
- English muffin pizzas (part skim mozzarella)
- Frozen fruit, low-fat yogurt, and ice cream pops
- Blender smoothies (skim milk, frozen yogurt, and fresh fruit)
- Granola bars
- Pretzels (preferably oat bran)
- Flavored rice cakes
- Whole-wheat pita triangles and hummus
- Air crisp crackers
- Light microwave popcorn
- String cheese (part skim)
- Banana-Berry Frosty (see recipe)
- Peanut Butter Yogurt Milkshake (see recipe)
- Jazzed-Up Popcorn (see recipe)

Fun and Easy Recipes

Here are a few recipes that will help your kids enjoy cooking.

Breakfast Berry Crepes

2 cups whole grain flour

1 egg, beaten

2$\frac{1}{2}$ cups low-fat milk

Nonstick vegetable spray

$\frac{1}{2}$ cup blueberries

$\frac{1}{2}$ cup raspberries

$\frac{1}{2}$ cup sliced strawberries

> *Serves four*

*From the kitchen of
Andrea Mendonca*

Place flour in a bowl and add egg plus 2 cups milk (save $\frac{1}{2}$ cup). Beat with a wire whisk until all lumps are gone and mixture is completely smooth. Gradually add remaining $\frac{1}{2}$ cup milk to make a thin batter. Use nonstick cooking spray on hot skillet (medium-high temperature) and pour enough batter in the pan to make a large circle. Sprinkle desired amount of fruit on top and press down into crepe. Cook for approximately 2–3 more minutes and then flip crepe and cook the other side. Carefully lift onto a plate and roll it all the way up.

Jazzed-Up Popcorn

Parmesan cheese

Ground cinnamon

Chili powder and garlic

Low-sodium soy sauce

> *Serves four*

*From the kitchen of
Andrea Mendonca*

Make air-popped popcorn, spray on some nonstick cooking spray, and then jazz it up with one of the above ingredients.

Tuna Salad Cones

Serves four

From the kitchen of Mia, Jason, and Harley Bauer

1 (5-oz.) can water-packed tuna

1 large grated carrot

¹/₂ chopped tomato

1 oz. shredded low-fat cheddar cheese (optional)

1 TB reduced fat mayo (any brand 25 cal per TB) or optional low-fat Italian dressing

Open can of tuna and drain off liquid. Mash up tuna and mix in grated carrot, chopped tomato, and some shredded low-fat cheddar cheese (if using). Lightly mix with low-fat mayonnaise or Italian salad dressing and scoop into flat-bottomed ice cream cones (not the sugar kind). Serve for lunch or at a party; your kids will love them!

Banana-Berry Frosty

Serves two

From the kitchen of Jesse, Cole, and Ayden

1 cup low-fat milk

3–4 ice cubes

2 tsp. vanilla

¹/₂ banana

¹/₂ cup fresh strawberries

Place all the ingredients into the blender and mix until smooth and fluffy.

Peanut Butter Yogurt Milkshake

Serves two

From the kitchen of Haley and Mike Simon

4 big scoops of vanilla frozen yogurt

1 cup low-fat milk

1–2 TB. peanut butter

Mix all ingredients in the blender until thick and smooth.

Food for Thought

More than one in five children and adolescents ages 6-17 are overweight. Strategies to help an overweight child:

♦ **Encourage breakfast.** A balanced breakfast helps to jumpstart the metabolism and regulates the appetite throughout the rest of the day.

♦ **Increase fiber.** Fiber-rich foods can increase fullness and help stabilize blood sugar levels for better appetite regulation.

♦ **Buy low-fat dairy.** Low-fat milk, cheese, and yogurt contain significantly fewer calories and less saturated fat than the whole-milk counterparts. Stock the fridge!

♦ **Moderate starch.** Try to minimize the starch with meals, and stick with one to two servings at each. This helps moderate overall calories.

♦ **Discourage liquid calories.** Always encourage solid food versus liquid calories. Limit or avoid soda, fruit juice, and other sugary beverages.

♦ **Encourage physical activity.** Every day, anything goes! Active kids burn calories, increase muscle and bone density, and are out of the kitchen.

♦ **When appropriate, recruit outside help.** If your child's weight and food are becoming a family battleground, seek the help of a pediatric or adolescent nutritionist. It's often less stressful (and more productive) to have an outside expert try to empower your son or daughter.

What About Sweets?

Clearly, some foods are healthier than others, but there's room in every meal plan for all foods, even the junky stuff. Develop a positive attitude about food by emphasizing healthy choices and limiting—but not eliminating—the not-so-healthy cakes, cookies, and candy. In fact, forbidding your kids to eat certain foods doesn't work; it only makes the high-fat stuff that much more enticing.

Have a limit of 1–2 dessertlike foods each day—and keep the serving sizes relatively small (2 cookies, small slice of cake, 1 scoop of ice cream). You can also serve healthier dessert alternatives such as chocolate fondue (orange segments, banana slices, and berries dipped in chocolate syrup) or an angel food cake topped with strawberries or chocolate pudding made with skim milk. Each can satisfy a sweet craving with a lot less fat and sugar.

Q & A

How can you get your finicky child to eat healthier?

Education is an important tool. Children as young as two years old can begin to understand the importance of certain food groups. Make it simple and fun by incorporating games, taste tests, and color drawings. A great idea is to hang a sticker chart on the fridge and reward your child each time he or she tastes a new food at a meal—or eats a vegetable at dinner. Don't get hung up on the portion sizes; remember, kids have small capacities and the idea is to create a willingness toward new food (not a clean plate award).

What about your teenagers? As your kids grow up, you tend to have much less control over what they eat. Continue to encourage healthy food choices and certainly downplay the unhealthy stuff—but be careful not to create an obsessive environment of "bad food/good food." It can backfire into a serious eating disorder.

The Sneaky Gourmet: Fifteen Ways to Disguise Vegetables

Your kid won't go near vegetables? See if you can sneak in a few here and there with some of these suggestions:

1. Add a mixed vegetable medley to your meatloaf recipe.

2. Scatter cooked vegetables throughout pasta and then cover with marinara sauce.

3. Grate carrots into tuna or chicken salad and stuff in a pita pocket.

4. Make homemade pizza. Toss on sliced mushrooms and chopped broccoli *before* spreading on the cheese.

5. Make vegetable lasagna. You can stick with a single vegetable such as spinach (see the Spinach Lasagna recipe in Chapter 19) or mix in a variety of chopped, cooked vegetables, such as zucchini, cauliflower, broccoli, carrots, mushrooms, green beans, and so on.

6. Add cooked peas, corn, and carrots to mashed potatoes.

7. Serve vegetable soup with crackers.

8. Puree cooked squash and carrots and then add small amounts into your ground beef or ground turkey. Shape into hamburgers or turkey-burgers and cook on the grill.

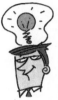

Food for Thought _____

Teach your kids about nutrition through music!

Groovin' Foods is a collection of exciting songs that will entertain and instruct your children on healthy eating. Kids will dance & sing along—while learning about the foods that keep them healthy, fit, and strong. Parents will also love these tunes, which run the gamut from rock & roll, Latin, blues, reggae, pop, and more!

9. Top a baked potato with chopped broccoli and low-fat melted cheese.

10. Make low-fat zucchini and carrot muffins.

11. Serve "make-your-own tacos" and have different stations set up with lean ground beef (or ground turkey), sliced tomatoes, shredded lettuce, and carrots.

12. Make chicken-vegetable kabobs. Alternate chunks of grilled chicken, peppers, tomatoes, onions, zucchini, and mushrooms on metal skewers. Set up a variety of dips that your kids can have fun experimenting with, such as barbecue sauce, honey mustard sauce, sweet and sour sauce, and low-fat salad dressings. Of course, maybe you'll get lucky and your kids will simply like the original marinade.

13. Finely chop cooked broccoli and thoroughly mix into your rice.

14. Turn your kids on to wok cooking and have them assist with washing and cutting up the vegetables. Try chicken-vegetable stir-fry, beef-vegetable stir-fry, or seafood-vegetable stir-fry. Pour them all over rice or linguini and hand out the chopsticks.

15. Make a spinach dip with low-fat plain yogurt, low-fat sour cream, and pureed cooked spinach. Have them dip carrots, celery, peppers, and zucchini slices. If they don't want to dip with raw veggies, give them some crackers; at least they'll get the spinach from the dip.

Food for Thought _____

Have your kids log their exercise for a week so that they understand the importance of regular physical activity and feel proud about the accomplishment.

Monday: Rode my bike for 1 hour

Tuesday: Dance class for 45 minutes

Wednesday: Walked the dog for 20 minutes

Turn Off That Tube!

Too much television generally means too much sitting around. Put a two-hour limit on TV watching and encourage your kids to get up and move. Teach them about the importance of exercise and have them do something physical for at least 30 minutes every day. Have them walk the dog, jump rope, skate, throw a ball around, swim, play tag, play basketball, sign up for an after-school class, or join a sports team.

The Least You Need to Know

◆ Most health experts recommend breast milk over formula because breast milk is believed to pass protective substances from mother to baby.

◆ Typically between four and six months, your pediatrician will give you the okay to start your baby on solids. Stick with one food at a time to rule out food allergies.

◆ All growing kids should eat a daily total of at least six servings of breads and grains, two servings of fruit, three servings of veggies, three servings of dairy, and two servings of meat, poultry, dried beans, fish, eggs, or nuts. Expect younger kids to eat much smaller serving sizes than older children.

◆ Let kids be kids and occasionally eat junk food. Understand that an obsessive environment of denial can backfire.

◆ Put a two-hour limit on television watching and encourage your kids to become physically active.

Part 6

Weight Management 101

Weight control seems to be a full-time job for some people; they're on and off every diet on the planet. My friend Joan once told me her biggest fear of death was that her weight would be printed in her obituary for all to see! Needless to say, she's alive and well and on another crazy diet.

It's finally time to *stop* your weight from going up and down like a yo-yo, and to *start* sticking with a sensible eating plan for life. Whether you want to lose weight, gain weight, or quit obsessing over every bite of food, this final section covers it all. There's an easy-to-use weight loss program for those who want to knock off (and keep off) those extra, unwanted pounds, as well as a bunch of calorie-cramming tips to help you skinny folks beef up your bods. There's also a section devoted to life-threatening eating disorders that includes information about where to find help when food and exercise spiral out of control.

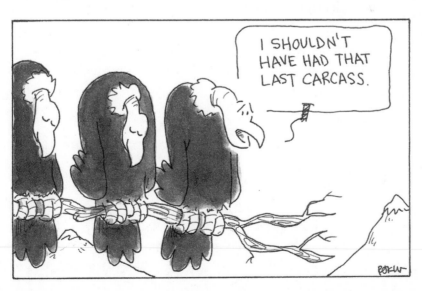

27

Come On, Knock It Off

In This Chapter

- Why crash dieting *doesn't* work
- Identifying your ideal body weight
- Lose weight on a well-balanced program
- Understanding the language of "bubbles"
- Making sense of diet pills
- Maintaining your weight after you've lost

Let's take a walk down memory lane. We've had the Scarsdale Diet, the Grapefruit Diet, the Banana–Cottage Cheese Diet, the Cabbage Soup Diet, the High-Protein Diet, and even the "Lose 10 Pounds in a Week Eating Rice & Mashed Potatoes" Diet (obviously developed by a constipated psychopath).

Unfortunately, crash dieting is an American sport that just won't go away. They're sort of like trick candles on a birthday cake: every time you blow one out, another one pops up to taunt you. But with all these blubber-blasting gimmicks, our national waistline continues to bulge! In fact, most people who lose weight on these crazy programs wind up gaining it all back—plus some extra pounds to boot. What's more, the fad diets usually leave you deprived and irritable.

What's the Best Diet, Anyway?

If you're looking for a quick fix, this chapter is *not* going to help you. The bottom line is that people should lose weight eating the very same healthy foods that they will continue to eat *after* they have lost the weight—that is, moderate amounts of carbs coming from whole grains, fruits and vegetables, low-fat dairy, and lean sources of protein foods. Makes perfect sense, right? To lose weight *forever,* you must work on changing your eating behavior forever. Read through and try my bubble plan. You've got nothing to lose except some unwanted pounds—and perhaps a lifetime of professional dieting.

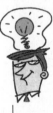

Food for Thought

Now that low-carb diets have been around for a while, we can finally compare how they stack up against the popular low-fat diets of the '90s. Drum roll please … Research from the famed National Weight Registry indicates that no matter how you lost those pounds initially, you have a better chance of keeping them off if you limit your fat intake—not your carbs.

What Should You Weigh?

First, figure out a realistic weight to strive for. Here's a quick way to estimate your healthy weight range:

♦ **For men:** Start with 106 pounds for 5 feet, and then add 6 pounds for every inch over 5 feet (or subtract 6 pounds for every inch under 5 feet).

Then, calculate the weight range for your frame by subtracting or adding 10 percent of the sum to your number.

Example: A man standing 5'10" will calculate 106 + 60 = 166 pounds. If he is small-framed, he *subtracts* 10 percent of that from 166 pounds to get 150 pounds. If he is large-framed, he *adds* 10 percent to 166 to get 182 pounds. Therefore, a man who is 5'10" has a healthy weight range between 150 and 182 pounds.

♦ **For women:** Start with 100 pounds for 5 feet, and then add 5 pounds for every inch over 5 feet (or subtract 5 pounds for every inch under 5 feet). Then, calculate your weight range by subtracting and adding 10 percent of that sum to your number.

Example: A woman standing 5'5'' will calculate 100 + 25 = 125 pounds. If she is small-framed, she *subtracts* 10 percent of that from 125 pounds to get 112.5 pounds. If she is large-framed, she *adds* 10 percent to 125 to get 137.5 pounds. Therefore, a woman who is 5'5'' has a healthy weight range between 112.5 and 137.5 pounds.

Here's another quick way to get a visual of your weight range. Simply use it as a guideline because the numbers seem to slightly vary from chart to chart.

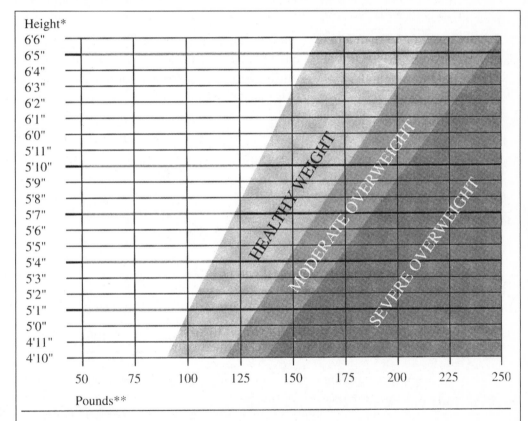

*Without shoes.
**Without clothes. The higher weights apply to people with more muscle and bone, such as many men.

Source: *Report of the Dietary Guidelines Advisory Committee on the Dietary Guidelines for Americans, 1995,* pages 23-24.

Testing Your Body Fat: Getting Pinched, Dunked, and Zapped

Although your weight indicates the sum total of *all* your body parts, it doesn't take into consideration your body composition (the amount of body fat versus lean body mass), which is important to know because muscle weighs more than fat. In fact, some people might appear a bit high on the weight chart *but* have very little body fat, indicating that the weight is coming from muscle mass and *not* blubber mass. (Of course, *you* know whether that extra weight is solid muscle or just … extra weight.)

To get a more accurate idea about where you stand in terms of fat, check out your body fat percentage by getting pinched, dunked, or zapped—especially if you regularly work out. Compare your results with the normative ranges in the following chart:

Ideal Body Fat Percentage for Men

Age (yr)	Excellent	Good	Fair	Risky
20–24	10.8	14.9	19.0	23.3
25–29	12.8	16.5	20.3	24.3
30–34	14.5	18.0	21.5	25.2
35–39	16.1	19.3	22.6	26.1
40–44	17.5	20.5	23.6	26.9
45–49	18.6	21.5	24.5	27.6
50–54	19.5	22.3	25.2	28.3
55–59	20.0	22.9	25.9	28.9
60+	20.3	23.4	26.4	29.5

Ideal Body Fat Percentage for Women

Age (yr)	Excellent	Good	Fair	Risky
20–24	18.9	22.0	25.0	29.6
25–29	18.9	22.1	25.4	29.8
30–34	19.7	22.7	26.4	30.5
35–39	21.0	24.0	27.7	31.5
40–44	22.6	25.6	29.3	32.8

Age (yr)	Excellent	Good	Fair	Risky
45–49	24.3	27.3	30.9	34.1
50–54	25.8	28.9	32.3	35.5
55–59	27.0	30.2	33.5	36.7
60+	27.6	30.9	34.2	37.7

Skin-Fold Calipers

Getting "pinched" involves what are called *calipers*, a contraption that looks like a handgun with salad tongs. A tester positions the gun on certain parts of your body and grabs your fat so that it is pulled away from your muscle and bone. (Sounds painful, but it's not.) After gathering a few different measurements, typically from the back of your arm, your thigh, your abdomen, your shoulder, and your hip, the tester will plug each number into a formula to calibrate your overall body fat percentage.

Although the calipers are quick, simple, and convenient, the test results can sometimes be skewed if a tester pinches some muscle along with the fat *or* does not pinch enough of the fat. You will also need to have this type of test performed *before* a workout; during exercise, your skin slightly swells, which can make you appear fatter than you are.

Food for Thought

Take a trained athlete and a couch potato of the same height and weight: the athlete looks healthier and leaner and most likely wears a smaller clothing size than the couch spud. This is because muscle weighs more than fat, even though it takes up less space.

Underwater Weighing

Getting "dunked" is actually the most accurate of the classic methods of body-fat testing. Basically, you sit on a scale in a small pool of warm water. Next, you blow *all* the air out of your lungs and dunk underneath until you are completely submerged for about five seconds. Your underwater weight will then register on a digital scale; a tester plugs that number into a formula to determine the percentage of body fat.

Bio-Electrical Impedance

Getting "zapped" requires you to lie on your back with one electrode attached to your hand and another to your foot. A signal is then sent from one electrode to the other. The faster the signal travels, the more muscle you have. On the other hand, the slower the signal moves, the more fat you have because fat impedes, or blocks, the signal.

How Many Calories Should You Eat for Weight Loss and Weight Maintenance?

Counting the calories in each morsel of food that you eat is *not* the way to go. But you can get a general idea of how many total calories you should eat each day, to either maintain *or* lose weight, with the following formula:

1. First find your BMR (basal metabolic rate: the amount of calories needed to perform your normal bodily functions at rest).

   BMR = your current weight × 10

2. Next, multiply your BMR by an activity factor.

   BMR × 0.30 (for average daily activities)

3. Last, add your BMR to your activity factor.

Food for Thought

If you decide to work with a nutritionist, remember: you want a food partner, not a food dictator! Find a qualified registered dietitian (R.D.) who will move at your pace and make you feel completely comfortable. For a registered dietitian in your area, call the American Dietetic Association at 1-800-366-1655, or visit their website at www.eatright.org.

Here's an example of a 130-pound woman:

130 pounds × 10 = BMR of 1,300 calories

1,300 calories × .30 = 390 activity factor

1,300 + 390 = 1,690 calories per day

People who participate in regular physical activity more than three times a week will need to raise the activity factor to .40–.60.

The example shows that an average 130-pound woman can maintain her weight on 1,690 calories per day. Now, let's say she wants to lose a few pounds. To lose weight, she needs to create a negative balance by reducing the amount of daily calories and increasing her exercise to burn even more calories. For instance, she needs to get on a 1,400-calorie food plan, plus work out aerobically 4–5 days per week. She'd have no problem shedding some weight safely and efficiently.

Plug your own stats into the formula, and figure out what it will take calorically to melt away those unwanted pounds. Understand that no one should ever eat less than 1,200 calories per day; you will slow down your metabolism and set yourself up to gain all the weight back. Even if you are very petite, and the math works out to be less than 1,200—stick with 1,200 calories and jack up your exercise.

The "Bubble Game" and Your Personal Weight-Loss Plan

Now that you've done the math, roll up your sleeves and get ready to learn about bubbles. On the following pages you'll be provided with several plans that use bubbles to represent serving sizes (OOO). Each bubble plan is designed to provide a specific caloric level—1,200 calories, 1,400 calories, 1,600 calories, or 1,800 calories. You'll select one of the balanced weight-loss plans and experiment and create an in-between plan of your own. Make it into a game and simply follow the bubble sheets by focusing on the number of total daily servings from each of the five food groups. Notice that all the calculations have been done for you, so there's no need to count a single calorie. In fact, calorie counting from here on in is off-limits.

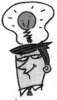

Food for Thought

People are different and lose weight at different speeds on different plans. For instance, you and your friend might do the math and come up with the same 1,400-calorie weight-loss plan, but she might lose 1–2 pounds each week, and you might only lose half a pound each week. In this case, assume that you have a slower metabolism and need to step up your exercise and use the lower 1,200-calorie plan.

Understanding the Bubbles

A bubble is simply a serving size; therefore, the number of bubbles in each food group is the total number of servings in your plan for each day. For example, if you are following the 1,200-calorie plan, you have two fruit bubbles and three grain/bread bubbles, which represents two servings of fruit and three servings of grain. Browse the various items under each food category, and learn exactly what counts as one serving so that you know how to plan your foods for the day.

It's *not* necessary to weigh or measure; an eyeball guesstimation will work just fine. Here's how to guesstimate your serving sizes, and remember, this is only a general list; there are a gazillion other foods that can fit perfectly into each category, so go ahead and plug in your favorites.

One Grain/Bread Bubble = Approximately 80 Calories

- 1 medium slice of *any* type of bread
- ¹/₂ small bagel or English muffin
- Small pita bread (or ¹/₂ large)
- 1 serving cereal (hot or cold)
- ¹/₂ cup cooked pasta, rice, barley, or couscous

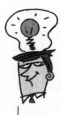

Food for Thought

A sensible weight-loss plan should shed pounds slowly but steadily—approximately one to two pounds per week.

- Small baked potato or sweet potato (size of your fist)
- ¹/₂ cup peas or corn
- 1 oz. (small bag) pretzels
- Low-fat granola bar
- 2 fig cookies

Note: Some vegetables are included in this group because they are very starchy.

Here are some common grains and how they can count:

- Pasta entree = five grain bubbles
- Side of pasta or rice = two grain bubbles
- Medium baked potato = two grain bubbles
- Large, hot pretzel = three grain bubbles
- Potato knish = three grain bubbles
- Large New York bagel = four to five grain bubbles

One Vegetable Bubble = Approximately 25 Calories

Most vegetables are unlimited; just make sure to eat your *minimal* quota!

- 1 cup raw vegetables
- ¹/₂ cup cooked vegetables
- 1 cup vegetable juice

The only exceptions are the starchy potatoes, peas, and corn, which get counted as grains.

One Fruit Bubble = Approximately 60–90 Calories

- Any medium piece of fruit (apple, small banana, pear, and so on)
- ¹/₂ small cantaloupe
- Large wedge of watermelon or honeydew
- 1 cup fresh fruit salad or berries
- Small glass fruit juice (about ¹/₂ cup)
- Large scoop of fruit sorbet
- Noncreamy frozen fruit bar
- Small handful of dried fruit

One Milk Bubble = Approximately 90–150 Calories

- 1 cup low-fat milk (skim or 1%)
- 1 (8-oz.) container of nonfat (flavored) yogurt
- Small low-fat frozen yogurt
- 2–3 slices of low-fat hard cheese (or 1¹/₂ oz.)
- ³/₄ cup (big scoop) low-fat cottage cheese
- 1 cup low-fat pudding
- Skim milk cappuccino, cafe latte, or hot cocoa
- 3–4 TB. Parmesan cheese

One Milk Plus One Fat = Approximately 150–200 Calories

- 1 cup whole milk

- Regular cheese on anything

- One scoop real ice cream

- Regular hot chocolate, cappuccino, or cafe latte

- 1 cup chocolate pudding

- *Anything* else made with whole milk

One Protein Bubble = Approximately 225 Calories per 3 Ounces

- Approximately 3 oz. of lean meat, poultry, or fish (the size of a deck of cards), unless otherwise indicated

- Chicken breast (3 oz.)

- Turkey breast (3 oz.)

- Lean red meats (3 oz.)

- Turkey burger or veggie burger (3 oz.)

- All seafood and fish (3 oz.)

- Tofu (6 oz.)

- Egg whites (approximately 4)

- Whole eggs (2)—but eat occasionally

- Beans ($^{1}/_{2}$–1 cup cooked)

One Fat Bubble = Approximately 45 Calories

- Any time you *think* something is prepared with fat: for example, sautéed vegetables, a sauce on your fish, fried chicken cutlet, and so on.

- Any time you use 1 tsp. butter, oil, margarine, or mayonnaise

- 1 TB. cream cheese, peanut butter, or salad dressing

- 2 TB. of sour cream

For reduced-calorie spreads, double the serving size; you do *not* need to count fat-free spreads at all.

"Free Foods" That Don't Count as Anything!

- Mustard
- Cocktail sauce
- Catsup
- Salsa
- Soy sauce*
- Tomato sauce
- Teriyaki sauce*
- Bouillon*
- Worcestershire sauce
- Sugar
- All spices and seasonings
- Sugar substitutes
- Jams and jellies
- Hard candies (3 per day)
- Pancake syrup (a circle only)
- Chewing gum (1 pack per day)
- Fat-free salad dressings and spreads (in moderation)
- Coffee/tea
- Horseradish
- Sugar-free beverages

These foods are extremely high in salt; when they're available, choose the low-sodium versions.

Tracking Your Food on the Daily Bubble Sheets

Make 20 or more copies of the food plan on the following pages that's right for you, and chart your daily food intake for the first few weeks, just to get the hang of it. After eating each meal or snack, check off the appropriate bubbles at the bottom. This will help you to keep an eye on exactly how much food you've eaten and how much is left for the rest of the day.

Approximately 1,200-Calorie Food Plan

Breakfast

Lunch

Snack

Dinner

Snack

Grains and breads: ○○○

Vegetables: ○○○

Fruits: ○○

Milks: ○○

Protein foods: ○○

Fats: ○○

Water: ○○○○○○○

Sample Day of 1,200-Calorie Food Plan

Breakfast
1 serving of dry, high-fiber cereal
1 cup skim milk
1 banana

Lunch
Large salad with 3 oz. grilled chicken with 1 TB. of dressing (or 2 TB. of low-fat Italian salad dressing)
Small whole-wheat pita bread

Snack
Low-fat frozen yogurt

Dinner
Lean steak, 3 oz.
A lot of steamed broccoli
Small baked potato with 1 tsp. of margarine
1 cup fresh strawberries

Grains and breads: ○○○

Vegetables: ○○○

Fruit: ○○

Milk: ○○

Protein foods: ○○

Fat: ○○

Water: ○○○○○○○

Approximately 1,400-Calorie Food Plan

Breakfast

Lunch

Snack

Dinner

Snack

Grains and breads: ○○○○

Vegetables: ○○○

Fruits: ○○○

Milks: ○○

Protein foods: ○○

Fats: ○○○

Water: ○○○○○○○

Sample Day of 1,400-Food Calorie Plan

Breakfast

Toasted whole-grain English muffin with 1 TB. cream cheese
1 cup low-fat milk plus 1 cup blueberries in a blender with ice

Lunch

3 oz. turkey breast on a spinach tortilla wrap
Lettuce, tomato slices, and mustard
An apple

Snack

A pear

Dinner

Tossed green salad with 1 oz. of grated low-fat cheese and fat-free dressing
4 oz. grilled fish in lemon
Medium baked potato with 2 TB. sour cream
Steamed spinach

Grains and breads: ○○○○

Vegetables: ○○○

Fruits: ○○○

Milks: ○○

Protein foods: ○○

Fats: ○○○

Water: ○○○○○○○

Approximately 1,600-Calorie Food Plan

Breakfast

Lunch

Snack

Dinner

Snack

Grains and breads: ○○○○○○

Vegetables: ○○○

Fruits: ○○○

Milks: ○○

Protein foods: ○○

Fats: ○○○

Water: ○○○○○○○

Sample Day of 1,600-Calorie Food Plan

Breakfast
Bowl of oatmeal with some skim milk
Container of nonfat flavored yogurt
Small glass orange juice

Lunch
Hamburger on bun
Side salad with 1 TB. dressing
Fresh fruit salad

Snack
Frozen fruit bar

Dinner
Stir-fry chicken and a lot of veggies (use only 1–2 tsp. oil and
   low sodium soy sauce)
1 cup brown rice
Small frozen yogurt

Grains and breads: ○○○○○○

Vegetables: ○○○

Fruits: ○○○

Milk: ○○

Protein foods: ○○

Fats: ○○○

Water: ○○○○○○○

Approximately 1,800-Calorie Food Plan

Breakfast

Lunch

Snack

Dinner

Snack

Grains and breads: ○○○○○○○

Vegetables: ○○○○○○

Fruits: ○○○○

Milk: ○○○

Protein foods: ○○

Fats: ○○○

Water: ○○○○○○○

Sample Day of 1,800-Calorie Food Plan

Breakfast
Egg-white omelet with veggies (use 1 whole egg plus 2 egg whites and nonstick cooking spray)

2 slices whole-wheat toast with 2 tsp. reduced-fat margarine
Sliced bananas and strawberries, ¹/₂ cup
1 cup of skim milk

Lunch
1 slice vegetable cheese pizza
Tossed salad with low-fat dressing

Snack
Peach
2 fig cookies

Dinner
Grilled salmon (3–4 oz.),
Marinate in lemon and 1 tsp. olive oil
1¹/₂ cups pasta with marinara sauce
Grated low-fat mozzarella cheese (1¹/₂ oz.)
Cooked carrots and green beans
A baked apple

Grains and breads: ○○○○○○○

Vegetables: ○○○○○○

Fruits: ○○○○

Milk: ○○○

Protein foods: ○○

Fats: ○○○

Water: ○○○○○○○

No More "I've Blown It" Syndrome; All Foods Are Allowed

Are you guilty of the "all-or-nothing" mentality? Do you place all your faves "off limits" when you diet, and then, the second you eat anything on the "bad list," you go whole hog and eat the house? ("I've already blown it—might as well polish off the rest of the chips and cookies. I'll start fresh on Monday.")

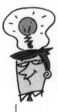

Food for Thought

Did you know that six pieces of broken cookie equals an entire cookie that you could have enjoyed?

Diets fail when you're deprived of your favorite foods—even if they aren't healthy. You *don't* gain weight from occasionally eating moderate amounts of high-fat foods. In fact, you *lose* weight because in the end, you don't feel deprived, and you're not tempted to bag your whole weight-loss program.

The following list shows you that almost *anything* can fit in: you just have to cross off the appropriate bubbles and account for the food items during that day. Try your best to stick with healthier choices most of the time, but go ahead and occasionally splurge on pizza, cookies, cake, or anything else that tempts your palate; I encourage it! Simply stay within your daily bubble limit by shifting other meals around to compensate, and you'll still lose weight.

Fat-combo foods have fat built in. In other words, they are not straight oil, dressing, or butter—but fat combos such as pizza, chocolate, and so on.

- Cookies (2 medium) = 1 grain, 1 fat
- Cake (medium slice, *any* type) = 2 grains, 2 fats
- Donut = 2 grains, 2 fats
- Large bakery cookie = 2 grains, 2 fats
- Scone (medium) = 2 grains, 2 fats
- Danish/pastry = 2 grains, 2 fats
- Bakery muffin (large) = 3 grains, 2 fats
- Potato chips (small bag) = 1 grain, 1 fat
- Corn chips (small bag) = 1 grain, 1 fat
- Chocolate bar (Kit-Kat, Snickers, and so on) = 1 grain, 3 fats

- Coleslaw ($\frac{1}{2}$ cup) = 1 vegetable, 1 fat

- Potato salad ($\frac{1}{2}$ cup) = 1 grain, 1 fat

- Real ice cream (2 scoops) = 2 milks, 2 fats

- French fries (about 20) = 2 grains, 2 fats

- Chinese lo mein (1 cup) = 2 grains, 2 fats

- Cornbread (medium piece) = 1 grain, 1 fat

- Cream soups (1 cup) = 1 grain, 1 fat, 1 vegetable

- Macaroni and cheese (1 cup) = 2 grains, 1 milk (or protein), 1 fat

- Pizza (1 medium slice) = 2 grains, 1 milk (or protein), 1 vegetable, 1 fat

Notice that for macaroni and cheese and pizza, the cheese can either be counted as milk or protein.

Q & A

Where do you carry your excess padding, on your belly or butt?

Studies have shown that people carrying excess fat on the upper body and stomach suffer more health risks than people carrying fat on the hips and buttocks. Weight that is carried in the abdominal region is closer to the heart and the larger coronary arteries—versus weight on the hips. Therefore, it poses a greater risk for heart disease.

Making Sense of Diet Pills

With so many over-the-counter diet remedies promoting weight loss, it's no wonder that desperate folks continue to throw away their hard-earned money. This section presents ammunition for making a more rational decision the next time you find yourself searching the shelves at your local pharmacy or health food store. Remember to always read every ingredient listed on a brand name label; chances are you'll find one or more of the following substances. If it sounds too good to be true ...

- **Ephedra (Ma Huang, Ephedrine):** Ephedra is the botanical form from the plant ma huang. The synthetic alkaloids, ephedrine and pseudoephedrine, are found in many over-the-counter cold and asthma medications and dietary supplements. Ephedra alkaloids are powerful central nervous system stimulants and cause vasoconstriction and cardiac stimulation. According to a review study in 1995, several studies suggested that ephedrine *plus* caffeine act by centrally suppressing appetite and peripherally stimulating fat oxidation. Ephedra alone did not show any significant effect on weight loss. That's why you'll generally find caffeine (or guarana) coupled with ephedra in the over-the-counter diet remedies.

Unfortunately, the side effects are extremely dangerous and outweigh any weight-loss advantage: rapid heartbeat, hypertension, arteriole constriction, heart attack, stroke, tremors, insomnia, and death in individuals in otherwise good health.

◆ **Guarana:** Guarana, not recommended, is a caffeine alkaloid. What's more, it is a natural diuretic and laxative, and that's what causes the weight loss. Unfortunately, it also speeds up your pulse rate, increases blood pressure, and increases the heart rate. Not worth the risk!

◆ **Chitosan:** Found in a few popular diet supplements, chitosan (KITE-oh-san) is a dietary fiberlike substance made from chitin, which forms the hard shells of crabs, lobsters, and other shellfish. Chitosan works by binding to fat and other fat-soluble substances. According to the manufacturers, this undigested fat is then excreted in our bowel movements. By reducing the amount of fat we absorb, these pills hope to make it easier to lose weight. However, there is *no* clear evidence to suggest that these weight-loss pills have any sort of lasting effect on weight loss. Moreover, some pill manufacturers themselves have stated that there are no guarantees as to their effectiveness.

Chitosan can block the absorption of certain medications and fat-soluble vitamins. For example, drugs such as estrogen and contraceptives are fat-soluble and therefore subject to interference from chitosan. Also, shellfish-allergic folks should stay clear of it.

◆ **Carnitine (L-Carnitine):** Carnitine is synthesized in the body from lysine and methionine, two essential amino acids. It plays a central role in transporting long-chain fatty acids into the mitochondria for oxidation. It also affects the metabolism of acetyl-coenzyme-A. However, supplemental carnitine only "provides extra energy" if a true clinical carnitine deficiency exists. There is no evidence that carnitine supplementation in healthy individuals improves energy, or enhances weight loss.

◆ **Chromium:** Chromium is an essential trace mineral. In its biologically active form, chromium influences insulin and therefore plays a role in carbohydrate, lipid, and protein metabolism. Because of its potential effect on metabolism, chromium has been used as a weight-loss aid and muscle builder for years. Chromium supplements come in the form of picolinate, chloride, and nicotinate. As expected, many studies have shown that chromium in supplemental form does *not* enhance weight loss. Furthermore, some of the lousy side effects may include headaches, sleep disturbances, and mood swings. Forget it.

◆ **DHEA (dehydroepiandosterone):** DHEA is the most abundant hormone secreted by the adrenal glands and it naturally declines with age. In the tissues, DHEA is converted into active androgens and estrogens and these hormone levels may be connected with body fat, body composition, and waist-to-hip ratio. A 2004 study showed that 52 elderly, DHEA-*deficient* individuals who were given DHEA supplements had significant decreases in abdominal fat. That doesn't mean everyone should run out and buy DHEA supplements, however, because DHEA may increase the risk for hormone-related cancers such as prostate, breast, and endometrial. If you really want to try DHEA, have your physician measure your blood levels first.

◆ **CLA (Conjugated Linoleic Acid):** CLA is a fatty acid processed from sunflower or safflower oil. The fatty acid is also naturally found in beef and dairy products. Preliminary evidence suggests it may have an anti-carcinogenic effect, but only in animal studies—human studies have yet to come. What's more, preliminary animal studies show that CLA may decrease body fat and increase lean body mass, while reducing appetite. This may be an interesting future supplement, but for now, human research is lacking and the long-term safety has not yet been established.

◆ **Yohimbine:** Yohimbine is the major alkaloid present in the bark of the yohimbe tree found in West Africa. Yohimbine stimulates norepinephrine release and has been used for weight loss and as an aphrodisiac. Studies have shown some success with weight loss in obese patients who are also on low-calorie diets; however, sample sizes were small and food was restricted. Side effects include nervousness, insomnia, anxiety, frequent urination, dizziness, tremors, headache, joint soreness, and blood pressure swings. To date, there is insufficient evidence regarding the safety and efficacy of yohimbine with weight loss.

◆ **Citrus Aurantium:** This herb is better known as bitter orange and—like ephedra—high doses can cause hypertension. It also has the potential to affect the metabolism of other drugs you may be taking. Oh—and did I mention that it probably has no effect on weight?

The Scoop on Prescription Diet Pills

Other approved diet prescription drugs available on the market include Xenical and Phentermine.

- ◆ **Xenical:** Xenical is the first in a new class of diet pills that decrease the body's fat absorption by 30 percent. This drug can create urgent bowel movements and should only be taken in conjunction with a well-balanced food plan. The side effects are obviously uncomfortable and may also involve the malabsorption of vitamins A, D, E, and K—along with decreasing the effectiveness of certain medications.

- ◆ **Phentermine:** Phentermine is the phen in Fen/Phen and was widely used in conjunction with another drug called Fenfluramine Hydrochloride (Fen), which has been taken off the market at the request of the FDA for possibly causing heart valve damage. Prescribed by a doctor, Phentermine is an amphetaminelike substance that may help suppress appetite and slightly increase the metabolism. However, the overall effectiveness of this drug is still very questionable and tolerance builds up quickly after the first few weeks. Phentermine should always be taken while following a calorie-controlled diet plan. Also, you should avoid Phentermine if you have high blood pressure, a hyperactive thyroid, glaucoma, diabetes, or emotional problems. Side effects of this drug include sleeplessness, irritability, headaches, increased blood pressure, stomach upset, and constipation.

- ◆ **Meridia:** This drug increases your sense of fullness, helping you eat less food while still being satisfied. Like Phentermine, Meridia can raise blood pressure and therefore should be used with caution by people who have hypertension.

- ◆ **Topamax:** Topamax was designed as an anti-seizure medication, but it also turns out to help binge-eaters control their eating. Side effects of Topamax include sleep problems, mood changes, and difficulty with memory, concentration, and attention.

- ◆ **Wellbutrin:** Wellbutrin is an antidepressant that has been shown to help some people lose weight. Side effects include headache, insomnia, dry mouth, dizziness, and skin rash.

- ◆ **Metformin/Glucophage:** This is a drug designed to control insulin and glucose levels in people with diabetes. It also helps nondiabetics control food cravings—thereby facilitating weight loss. Metformin's most serious side effect is lactic acidosis, which occurs mainly in people with kidney or liver problems.

Setting Realistic Goals

Don't overwhelm yourself trying to lose a tremendous amount of weight. Instead, break it into smaller, more achievable short-term goals. For example, if you have your heart set on losing, say, 40 pounds, aim for 10 pounds at a time. Even with a mere eight pounds to lose, strive for knocking off two pounds at a time.

Also, understand that genetics play a key role in determining your body makeup, so don't dream about that "Barbie-doll body"; it's not gonna happen. Take a look at your mom, dad, and other relatives. Biology isn't destiny, but heredity does play an integral part in shaping your shape.

The most important thing is to learn to love the body you have and keep your focus on ways to make it healthy. You might never be a size six or have bulging muscles, but you can learn to be happy with the body you have by taking care of it.

Food for Thought

Don't obsess over the scale; it can drive you nuts! Limit the times you weigh yourself to no more than once or twice a week. In fact, avoid hopping on the scale each time you hit the bathroom by packing it away in the closet between weigh-ins, or simply weigh yourself outside your home (at the gym, your doctor's office, and so on).

Get Moving and Keep Moving

Following a healthy food plan is only half of the weight-loss equation: you've gotta move to lose! Numerous studies have shown that exercise helps promote weight loss *and* weight maintenance by revving up your metabolism (that is, burning more calories). What's more, exercise relieves stress and can even psych up your state of mind so that you're motivated to make smart food choices during the day.

Maintaining Your Weight After You've Lost It

So you have reached your goal—now what? "Hooray!" on one hand, "Eek!" on the other! Maintaining your weight is actually harder than losing weight because there's no goal to strive for; you're already there. Hang tight and read the following tips. This time, your shapely physique is here to stay.

◆ The trick is to loosen the diet reins, but not too much. Continue with a *modified* version of your bubble plan (in your head only) because it's wel-balanced and encourages you to eat healthfully.

◆ Figure out a five-pound weight range with your present weight in the middle. For example, if your weight is 130 pounds, give yourself a range of 128–132 pounds. Continue to weigh in once every week or so, and if you go over the range, get back on the bubble sheets.

◆ Plan one meal "off" each week—in other words, a meal that doesn't fit or calculate into your plan (anything you'd like). If your weight continues to stay put, add a second meal off, or possibly a dessert. Experiment and see what your body can handle; everyone is different.

◆ You might prefer to simply add a few more grains to your plan (or a fruit and milk). See what your weekly weigh-ins reveal (or if your clothes seem to "shrink" or "grow") and never panic if you think you've gained. Just take away some of the additions the following week. Remember, the key to maintaining is to find out how much food your body can handle.

◆ Absolutely continue with your regular exercise program. Exercise allows you to eat more food because it burns mega-calories and keeps you tight and toned and because it zaps body fat and increases your lean body mass.

The Least You Need to Know

◆ Fad diets don't work. People should lose weight eating the very same healthy foods they will continue to eat after the weight is lost.

◆ Avoid over-the-counter diet aids that promise quick weight loss. Although the majority of these supplements are nothing more than a waste of money, certain supplements such as ephedra (also known as Ma Huang) can be downright dangerous.

◆ Your weight on the scale is the sum total of all your body parts (fat mass and lean mass); therefore, it's also helpful to test your body-fat percentage because this identifies how much of your body is actually fat.

◆ Don't set your heart on a Barbie/Ken-doll body. Plan realistic weight-loss goals by understanding that genetics play a key role in body make-up.

◆ Learn to love the body you have, and focus on making it healthy, not necessarily perfect.

Chapter 28

Adding Some Padding

In This Chapter

◆ Strategies to help you gain weight

◆ High-calorie meals and snacks

◆ Refreshing shakes and supplemental beverages to boost your calories

Is your metabolism so speedy that you burn calories quicker than you can pack 'em in? Maybe you're one of those "uninterested in food" people, who look down at their watches and think, "Oops, I forgot to eat lunch." Whatever the reasons for your thin physique, fear not. With some attention and determination, you can start an upward trend on your bathroom scale.

Is Being Underweight a Health Concern?

For some people, being too thin can be a health concern—specifically for people who are underweight because they undereat. When your body does not receive adequate food energy (calories), it basically runs out of gas and leaves you feeling fatigued, irritable, and with decreased concentration. Also, with an inadequate food intake you run the risk of developing vitamin and mineral deficiencies that may cause serious long-term problems (e.g., too little calcium and vitamin D = bone loss).

On the other hand, being underweight may not pose a health risk and might merely be about improving appearance. Some people are born with fast metabolisms that burn calories quicker than they can eat them. In this case, your caloric intake is most probably providing your daily requirements for nutrition, and you'll have to learn to eat more, more often, and eat more calorically dense foods to try to defy your genetics.

To check if you are underweight, flip back to Chapter 26, and look at the height/weight charts provided (or follow the equation provided).

Seven Tips to Help You Pack in the Calories

Gaining weight requires devouring more calories than you burn. In fact, to gain one pound, you need an extra 3,500 calories coming from food. Naturally, that's not at one sitting, but by simply eating an extra 500 calories a day, you can gain a pound per week—because 500 calories × 7 = 3,500 calories.

Stick with the basic food principles and concentrate on the following tips:

♦ Eat larger portions at your three main meals; even consider adding an extra meal to your day.

♦ Snacks are important! Plan at least three snacks a day. Tote along some trail mix, dried fruits, crackers, sports bars, fig bars, and nuts, or keep them in your desk at work.

> **Nutri-Speak**
>
> **Calorically dense foods** provide a lot of calories and fat in a relatively small portion size. (Nuts, seeds, and avocadoes are examples.)

♦ Add *calorically dense foods* to your meals. For example, toss beans, seeds, nuts, peas, avocado, cheese, and dressings into salads. Add shrimp, fish, chunks of chicken, and a lot of Parmesan cheese to pastas. Add crackers, rice, corn, noodles, and beans to your soups. Don't forget the bread basket—spread on the margarine and dig in!

♦ Guzzle tons of pure fruit juice or milk (preferably 1-percent or 2-percent) with and between your meals; it's a great way to painlessly add calories.

♦ Add powdered dry milk to your soups and casseroles.

◆ Try a calorically dense supplement, such as Ensure Plus, Sustacal, Boost, Carnation Instant Breakfast, and Nutriment. Just make sure you drink them between meals or with meals—not instead of meals.

◆ Consult a qualified exercise trainer about embarking on a weight-lifting program. It can help you build muscles and put on some pounds.

Adding More of the Good Stuff

Although the idea is to increase your calories, you also want to keep your diet well balanced and nutritious. The last thing you want to do is shovel in chocolate bars, donuts, cakes, cookies, and other "nutrient-less" stuff that will pad you with fat and supply zippo in the nutrition department. Instead, eat more of the good stuff and stick with foods that are calorically dense. Here are some examples:

Basic, Healthy Meal	To Add Some Calories
Vegetable omelet	Add cheese and a bagel with margarine
Salads	Add shredded cheese, avocado, olives, and plenty of dressing
Pizza	Add extra cheese and vegetables
Pasta	Add olive oil, olives, and Parmesan cheese
Chicken stir-fry	Add peanuts or cashews
Burritos	Add guacamole or sour cream

Here are some high-calorie and nutritional snack ideas:

◆ Frozen-yogurt milkshake (anything goes)

◆ Bowl of cereal with fruit and low-fat milk

◆ Tortilla chips with salsa and guacamole

◆ Peanut butter and jelly on crackers

◆ Bran, corn, or blueberry muffins

◆ Peanut butter on apple slices or bananas

◆ Cheese and crackers

- Cereal mixed with yogurt

- Dried fruit and nut mixture

- Fruit bars and granola bars

Shake It Up Baby

Shakes can be a refreshing, filling alternative to snacks and can add a significant amount of calories to your day. Try these ideas:

- Process in a blender: 4 ice cubes, $1/2$ cup orange juice, $1/2$ cup melon chunks, 1 banana or $1/2$ cup strawberries, and wheat germ (optional). Add more or less juice and fruit to achieve the desired consistency.

- Mix Carnation Instant Breakfast or Ovaltine with 1 cup of low-fat milk.

- Purée 10 oz. silken tofu, $3/4$ cup apple juice, 1 banana, or $1/2$ cup blueberries in a blender and top with walnuts or almonds.

- For a thick smoothie, purée 1 cup yogurt, 2 tsp. honey, 1 banana, and $3/4$ cup fruit juice. (Pineapple or orange juice works well.) Mix in wheat germ if desired.

Wanna gain some weight? Try this sample menu:

Breakfast
Grapenuts cereal (large bowl) with low-fat milk
2 handfuls of raisins
Large glass of orange juice
Bagel with margarine

Lunch
Chicken-salad sandwich on whole-wheat bread
Bowl of vegetable soup with crackers
Apple
Large glass of fruit juice

Dinner
Vegetable cheese pizza
Italian bread dipped in olive oil
Salad with olive oil and vinegar
Flavored fruit drink

Snack 1
8 oz. low-fat milk with Carnation Instant Breakfast
Large blueberry muffin

Snack 2
Peanut butter on crackers with low-fat milk
Dried fruit and nuts
Glass of juice

Bedtime snack
Frozen yogurt cone with sprinkles

Supplements—Extra Calories and Nutrition

Many people do well with the extra calories in a supplemental beverage. These supplements are easy, dense with calories, and—depending upon the brand and flavor—taste pretty good.

The following table is a comprehensive list of the popular supplemental beverages on the market. Read the specifics and decide which one fits your personal needs.

Produce	Manufacturer	Form	Kosher	Size	Cal.	Protein in grams	Carbs. in grams	Fat in grams	Available
Boost High Protein Powder*	Mead Johnson Nutritionals	Powder	Kosher	8 oz.	340	21	48	9	Kmart Pharmacy Home delivery: 1-800-831-3959
Carnation Instant Breakfast [No added sugar]*	Nestlé Clinical Nutrition	Powder	Kosher	8 oz.	220	12	24	8	Food stores everywhere Home delivery: 1-800-776-5446 Information no: 1-800-422-2752 Online ordering: www.nestle clinicalnutrition.com
Carnation Instant Breakfast*	Nestlé Clinical Nutrition	Powder	Kosher	8 oz.	280	12	39	8	Food stores everywhere Home delivery: 1-800-776-5446 Information no: 1-800-422-2752 Online ordering: www.nestle clinicalnutrition.com
Ensure [Lactose-free, gluten-free]	Ross Products	Liquid	Kosher	8 oz.	250	9	40	6	Duane Reade Food Stores/Supermarkets Home delivery: 1-800-986-8502 Online ordering: www.ensure.com
Ensure High Protein	Ross Products	Liquid	Kosher	8 oz.	230	12	31	6	Duane Reade Food Stores/Supermarkets Home delivery: 1-800-986-8502 Online ordering: www.ensure.com
Ensure Light	Ross Products	Liquid	Kosher	8 oz.	200	10	33	3	Duane Reade Food Stores/Supermarkets Home delivery: 1-800-986-8502 Online ordering: www.ensure.com

Produce	Manufacturer	Form	Kosher	Size	Cal.	Protein in grams	Carbs. in grams	Fat in grams	Available
Ensure Plus [Lactose-free, gluten-free]	Ross Products	Liquid	Kosher	8 oz.	360	13	50	11	Duane Reade Food Stores/Supermarkets Home delivery: 1-800-986-8502 Online ordering: www.ensure.com
Ensure with Fiber	Ross Products	Liquid	Kosher	8 oz.	250	9	42	6	Duane Reade Food Stores/Supermarkets Home delivery: 1-800-986-8502 Online ordering: www.ensure.com
Forta Shake*	Ross Products	Powder	Kosher	8 oz.	285	17	35	8	Pharmacy Home delivery: 1-800-986-8502
Meritene*	Novartis Nutrition	Powder		8 oz.	280	18	31	9	Home delivery: 1-800-446-6380
Modulen for IBD [Lactose-free, gluten-free, low-residue]	Nestlé Clinical Nutrition	Powder	Kosher	8 oz.	250	9	2	11.5	Food stores everywhere Home delivery: 1-800-776-5446 Information no: 1-800-422-2752 Online ordering: www.nestle clinicalnutrition.com or www.ModulenIBD.com
Ovaltine*	Himmel Nutrition	Powder		8 oz.	230	10	30	8	Pharmacy Home delivery: 1-800-828-9194
Resource No Added Sugar Health-Shake [Aspartame-sweetened, gluten free]	Novartis Nutrition	Liquid Frozen	Kosher	6 oz.	300	12	34	13	Home delivery: 877-493-2633 Online ordering: www. novartisnutrition.com

continues

continued

Produce	Manufacturer	Form	Kosher	Size	Cal.	Protein in grams	Carbs. in grams	Fat in grams	Available
Resource Diabetic	Novartis Nutrition	Liquid	Kosher	8 oz.	250	15	23	11.1	Home delivery: 1-800-828-9194 Online ordering: www.novartis-nutrition.com
Resource Health-Shake [Gluten-free, low-lactose, low-residue]	Novartis Nutrition	Liquid Frozen	Kosher	6 oz.	300	9	53	6	Home delivery: 877-493-2633 Online ordering: www.novartisnutrition.com
Resource Plus	Novartis Nutrition	Liquid	Kosher	8 oz.	360	13	52	11	Home delivery: 1-800-828-9194 Online ordering: www.novartisnutrition.com
Resource Standard	Novartis Nutrition	Liquid	Kosher	8 oz.	250	9	40	6	Home delivery: 1-800-828-9194 Online ordering: www.novartisnutrition.com
Scandi-Shake Sugar-free*	Scandi-Pharm	Powder		9 oz.	600	15	67	29	Home delivery: 1-800-472-2634 Online ordering: scandipharm.com
Scandi-Shake*	Scandi-Pharm	Powder		9 oz.	600	12	70	29	Home delivery: 1-800-472-2634 Online ordering: www.scandipharm.com

Prepared with 8 oz. whole milk

By following these tips and becoming consistent with larger meals and frequent snacks, you should be able to gain some weight. Remember to focus on more servings of the five major food groups—grains, fruits, vegetables, meats and other protein foods, and dairy—and not try to gain weight by overdoing foods from the food pyramid's tip, which includes high-fat foods.

The Least You Need to Know

- ◆ To gain weight, you must take in more calories than your body burns.

- ◆ Increase your daily calories by eating bigger portions in your meals and by snacking on calorically dense foods that also offer nutrition.

- ◆ Guzzle tons of fruit juice, make creative shakes, or drink the popular supplements that are on the market.

- ◆ Embark on a weight-lifting program. It can help beef up your muscles and your weight.

Chapter 29

Understanding Eating Disorders

In This Chapter

- All about anorexia nervosa and bulimia

- What is compulsive overeating?

- Real-life stories from people with eating issues

- How to help a friend with an eating disorder

The ideal of beauty has become more and more slender—a bone-thin slender, in fact, that most people are not capable of achieving through healthy, normal eating. Surrounded by skinny-minnies on TV, movies, and magazines, it's no wonder that millions of Americans each year suffer from serious eating disorders. More than 90 percent of those afflicted with eating disorders are adolescents and young adult women, who are at a time in their lives when the quest for that "ideal bod" is overwhelming.

Many psychological theories about eating disorders have been proposed, and today there are numerous comprehensive treatment centers to help people who struggle with anorexia nervosa, bulimia, and compulsive overeating. As a society, we need to overcome this obsession with unreasonably low weights and learn to accept and love the healthy genetic shapes we were given. This chapter provides you with the basics on eating disorders so that you can better understand the world of dieting gone haywire—and perhaps help a friend, a relative, or even yourself.

I would also like to extend a very special thanks to three of my clients, who have allowed me to share their struggles with food.

Anorexia Nervosa: The Relentless Pursuit of Thinness

Anorexia nervosa is a complex psychological disorder that literally involves self-starvation. People who suffer from this illness eat next to nothing, refuse to maintain a healthy body weight for their corresponding height, and frequently claim to "feel fat" even though they are obviously emaciated. Because anorexics are severely malnourished, they often experience symptoms of starvation: brittle nails and hair; dry skin; extreme sensitivity to the cold; anemia (low iron); lanugo (fine hair growth on the body surface); loss of bone; swollen joints; and dangerously low blood pressure, heart rates, and potassium levels. If not caught and treated in time, victims of anorexia nervosa can literally "diet themselves to death."

It is estimated that approximately 7 million Americans suffer with anorexia nervosa. 90 percent of the sufferers are women and roughly 10 percent are boys and young men. Although any personality can fall victim to this life-threatening illness, most anorexics tend to be perfectionists who keep their feelings bottled up inside, straight-A students, good athletes, and people who always do the right thing. For anorexics, restricting and controlling food becomes a way to cope with just about anything.

Here are some of the warning signs of anorexia nervosa:

- Abnormal loss of 15 percent (or more) of normal body weight with no medical reason for the loss. It can also be a failure to gain an expected amount of weight during a period of growth for younger children and adolescents.

- An intense fear of becoming fat or gaining weight, along with strict dieting and severe caloric restriction—despite a rail-thin appearance.

- In females, absence of at least three consecutive menstrual cycles otherwise expected to be normal.

- Always moving the diet "finish line." ("Just five more pounds and then I'll stop.")

- Constant preoccupation with food. Anorexics will often cook and prepare food for others but refuse to eat anything themselves.

- Distorted body image. For example, claiming to "have fat hips" even though scales and mirrors show that they are severely emaciated.

- Strange eating rituals such as cutting food into tiny pieces, taking an unusually long time to eat a meal, and constantly preferring to eat alone.

Nutri-Speak

Anorexia nervosa means "appetite loss of nervous origins." **Bulimia** means "ox-like hunger."

- Obsessively over-exercising despite fatigue and weakness.

- Becoming socially withdrawn, isolated, and depressed.

"Weighting to Be Normal"

At 13 years of age and 172 pounds, I wasn't very involved in the world around me. Sure, I saw the fried chicken, mashed potatoes, cakes, and cookies, but boys, clothing, and beaches eluded me. Don't get me wrong, I wasn't miserable all the time; I just wasn't particularly happy. In fact, most of the time I was nothing; I was just FAT!

Like most perfectionists, I seemed to do everything to extremes. Initially, I ate to the fullest, and later, when my doctor told me I needed to lose weight, I dieted to the skinniest. Three hundred sixty-five days later and 52 pounds lighter, the new Jane emerged. I had exercised and dieted my way to health. Burgers and taxis were out, low-fat foods and biking were in.

Not surprisingly, my doctor was ecstatic with my success, and my family was beaming with pride. My friends, on the other hand, were filled with that strange combination of jealousy and admiration, and finally, for the first time in my life, guys noticed me. They whistled when I walked down the street and approached me at school. "Wow," I thought. "If I can get this much attention at 120 pounds, imagine how great life could be at 110."

At 100 pounds, I thought I had found bliss: I could count my ribs, pull down my pants without unbuttoning them, and most importantly, I could go an entire day on just a small fat-free frozen yogurt.

Months flew by, and my weight continued to plummet. Exhausted, freezing, and wearing size-0 clothing, I had propelled myself into a lonely abyss. Summer nights felt like the dead of winter, and the urge to sleep was unstoppable. I knew I was sick—everyone knew I was sick—and I was ultimately diagnosed with anorexia nervosa.

Although I rejected the notion of having a disease, I struggled both mentally and physically with solid foods and decreasing my amount of exercise. Gradually over the course of a year, I regained both my body and my life. I admit, low-fat foods and exercising are still entrenched in my life, but this time in a healthy manner, not as a destructive disaster. I must push myself to eat a risky meal (a "scary" meal with fat) every other day and allow myself to indulge in a dessert treat twice a week. Although I still obsess about my weight, it's no longer about losing; instead, it's about maintaining. I have been at my current healthy, thin weight of 112 pounds for the last year, and I guess you can say I have finally found an ideal way to exercise my "control." I "control" what I eat and how much I exercise, not in a freezing abyss, but in a hot, sweaty gym.

—*Jane Stern, a 20-year-old recovered anorexic*

Bulimia Nervosa

The eating disorder termed *bulimia* is at least two or three times more prevalent than anorexia nervosa. In fact, recent surveys report that about 1 percent of the general population and 4 percent of women aged 18–30 suffer from this troublesome disease. People with bulimia have repeated episodes of *binge eating*—rapidly consuming large quantities of food and then ridding their bodies of the excess calories by vomiting, abusing laxatives or diuretics, and/or exercising obsessively. In most cases, this binge/purge syndrome is an outlet for anxiety, frustration, depression, loneliness, boredom, or sadness. Because most bulimics are typically normal weight, they can keep this a secret and go undetected for years. Although some researchers think the problem is getting worse, others believe that people are just more willing to seek help, and therefore, it's noticed and treated more often.

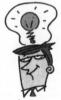

Food for Thought

For further reading, order *The Eating Disorder Catalog*, Gurze Books, 1-800-756-7533, www.gurze.com.

Here are some of the warning signs of bulimia:

♦ Dissatisfaction with body shape and constant preoccupation with becoming thin.

♦ Recurrent mood swings and depression.

♦ Frequent episodes of rapidly consuming large amounts of food (binge eating), followed by attempts to purge (get rid of food) through self-induced vomiting, use of laxatives or diuretics, prolonged exercise, or by following severe low-calorie diets between binges.

◆ Serious physical complications from chronic vomiting, including the erosion of dental enamel from acidic vomit, scars on the hands from sticking fingers down the throat, swollen glands, sore throat, irritation of the esophagus, and poor digestion (heartburn, gas, diarrhea, constipation, bloating). The more serious physical dangers include severe dehydration, loss of potassium (because potassium controls the heartbeat), and rupture of the esophagus.

◆ Awareness that their eating pattern is abnormal.

◆ Fear of not being able to control eating voluntarily.

◆ Light-headedness and dizziness or fainting.

◆ Frequent weight fluctuations of 10 pounds in either direction from the constant bingeing and purging.

Food for Thought

Many people aren't diagnosed with anorexia or bulimia but suffer from less serious "food issues" that nonetheless control and hinder their lives.

Remember that you only have one life to live. Get help and live it to the fullest!

"My Vicious Cycle of Starving-Stuffing"

It all started when I was preparing to go off to college. My anxiety stemmed from separating from my family and manifested itself in a body-image and eating problem. Up until this time, I was a "normal" eater, eating when I was hungry, stopping when I was full, and occasionally overeating during special occasions. I ate chocolate bars, pizza, and movie popcorn without as much as a blink. What was it like then?

Suddenly, it was as if my body wasn't mine anymore. It became this "thing" separate from myself. I became hyper-aware and mentally obsessed with how to control my shape through obsessive exercise and restrictive eating patterns. Skipping two meals in a row and exercising two hours a day became normal to me. I used to stand in front of my dorm room mirror naked, poking and scrutinizing myself out loud. My self-esteem was so low that I actually needed someone to validate all of my insecurities. My overweight roommate would look on in disgust, reassuring me that I wasn't fat. A lot of people in my life got tired of reassuring me of this.

I did not allow myself to enjoy "forbidden foods" for a long time through college. I felt proud of this control but ironically continued with my dissatisfaction over my "chunky body" (which has always been very thin, so I'm told). But after a while of rigid restriction, my body rebelled and my disordered eating took on a new twist: a few days of restricting (sometimes as low as 500 calories a day) and then bam—I would "sabotage" all of my efforts by stuffing myself until I was uncomfortably full! Feeling disgusted, depressed, and ENORMOUS, I would get rid of the calories by making myself vomit, and then struggle back to my extremely low-cal, restrictive diet, and the vicious cycle continued. My weight could fluctuate 10 pounds depending upon the day of the week, but to the outside world, I still remained a "normal" little person.

I also developed strange idiosyncrasies. Certain colors had to be eaten together, and certain foods had to "match" each other, for no particular reason except that they made sense to me. I would also weigh myself up to 25 times each day. There was no room for error, spontaneity, or change.

Finally, coming to terms with the fact that this obsession with food and exercise was ruining my life, I started to see a psychotherapist. For the first time, I realized that my "food thing" was only a symptom of unlimited emotions that I had bottled up inside. I needed to work hard to break free from my extremist attitudes and my belief that being less than perfect was not worth being. (What is "perfect" anyway?)

Today, I allow myself to feel entitled to my words and actions and realize that a middle ground is healthier in relation to feeling, thinking, and eating. I've also worked with a nutritionist for the past year. She has taught me that restricting inevitably leads to bingeing, and I'm desperately trying to do away with black/white days (restricting or bingeing) and instead focusing on the "gray."

I no longer let one M&M dictate my self-esteem, and I have learned that normal eating is flexible and always changing. It's okay to eat a big piece of cake on my birthday, chocolate when I have PMS, and movie popcorn once in a while. "Normal eating" means eating healthy most of the time, while allowing yourself to indulge when you feel like it. It's feeding yourself when you're hungry and sometimes when you're not—even just for the fun of it! It's feeding your mind as well as your body and realizing that weight fluctuations are normal. It is seeing life as more than what you put in your mouth and enjoying social situations for the conversation and laughter. It is learning to accept our bodies, our strengths, and our limitations as well. I admit, every day is a struggle right now, but at least I finally believe that I am worth it.

—A 27-year-old recovering bulimic

Compulsive Overeating

People who compulsively overeat repeatedly consume excessive amounts of food, sometimes to the point of abdominal discomfort. However, unlike bulimics, they do not get rid of the food with any of the methods mentioned earlier. In fact, most people with this type of eating disorder are overweight from the constant bingeing and have a long history of weight fluctuations.

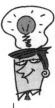

Food for Thought

Eating disorders can sometimes run in families. In fact, the rate of anorexia among sisters has been estimated at 2–10 percent.

Because compulsive overeaters feel out of control with their food (and often eat in secret), there seems to be a high incidence of depression, in addition to the serious medical complications that go hand in hand with being overweight.

"Dieting My Way to Obesity"

The cycle began when I was 11 or 12. I wore a size 7 and thought I looked fat. I dieted, starved, exercised, overate, and ended up a size 9. I did the size 7–9 dance several times until I finally graduated to the 9–11 routine. This continued until I ultimately reached size 13.

The turning point from "eating problem" to "life-threatening disorder" happened in my adult years after the break-up of a serious relationship. I just couldn't face the anxiety of the dating world again! It was also right after my grandmother passed away and my father had a heart attack. Starting a high-powered, senior-level job, my binges became out of control. Suddenly, walking home from work, I felt an urgent need to eat; I stopped at a grocery store, a deli, and a restaurant, buying chips, cakes, ice cream, and cookies. I reached my apartment and rushed into the kitchen, still wearing my heavy winter coat and hat, and started shoveling cake into my mouth. My hands were shaking and not able to get the cake in fast enough. I finished the entire cake, a pint of ice cream, and 20 Oreos before I was finally calm enough to take off my coat and order Chinese take-out.

This routine went on night after night for months. Within six months, I was up 85 pounds, and for the first time in my life, I topped 200 pounds on the scale. I was depressed, desperate, and terrified. I cried on and off all day long—in the shower, on the train, and in my office, frantically searching for help from diet centers, obesity researchers, and hospital programs. I frequently and seriously contemplated suicide.

I was humiliated and weighed 250 pounds. I felt like a heroin addict, only I was addicted to food.

With the understanding, support, and guidance from trusting, caring, and knowledge-able practitioners, a psychiatrist, a nutritionist, group therapy, and anti-depression medication, I am presently working my way out of this perpetual hell. I now follow a nondeprivational approach—all foods in moderation. Believe me, it took a lot for me to be willing to try this because all I've ever known is either 750-calorie diets or 20,000-calorie binges. Today, I allow myself a chocolate bar if I really crave one, and if I need to overeat (not binge) because of a heavy, stressful workload—I give myself permission.

I presently weigh 185 pounds, eat normally, and, at 45, have a rebirth of hope.

—A 45-year-old compulsive overeater

How to Help a Friend or Relative with an Eating Disorder

Combating an eating disorder is huge and generally involves a collaborative team of specialists, including a psychiatrist (or psychologist) to work through the psychologi-cal dynamics, a physician to monitor physical status, and a nutritionist (or dietitian) to reintroduce food as an ally—not an enemy. Here are some things you can do if you suspect a friend or family member has an eating disorder:

◆ Call your local hospital (or some of the treatment centers listed later in this chapter) and gather information on the various programs in your area. Ask about individual therapists, group therapy sessions, and nutritionists that spe-cialize in food issues.

◆ In a very caring and gentle way, discuss your concerns with your friend or rela-tive, and provide some of the professional resources and phone numbers that you've found. Be very supportive and patient; even offer to go along for any initial consults.

◆ If the person is a minor and refuses to get help, you might need to speak with a family member.

Where to Go for Help

The following organizations can provide information, literature, and qualified referrals for the treatment of eating disorders:

National Eating Disorders Association

603 Stewart St., Suite 803
Seattle, WA 98101
Tel: 206-382-3587
Help line and treatment referral line: 1-800-931-2237
www.nationaleatingdisorders.org

National Association of Anorexia Nervosa and Associated Disorders (ANAD)
PO Box 7
Highland Park, IL 60035
Tel: 847-831-3438
Fax: 847-433-4632
www.anad.org
E-mail: anad20@aol.com

Some of the comprehensive treatment centers available include:

Eating Disorders Research Clinic
The New York State Psychiatric Institute
Columbia-Presbyterian Medical Center
1051 Riverside Drive, Unit 98
New York, NY 10032
212-543-5739
www.eatingdisordersclinic.org

*Treatment is free for individuals who meet the criteria for this research program.

Eating Disorders Program
The New York Hospital—Cornell Medical Center
21 Bloomingdale Road
White Plains, NY 10605
914-997-5875

The Renfrew Center
475 Spring Lane
Philadelphia, PA 19128
1-800-736-3739
215-482-5353
www.renfrewcenter.com

The Least You Need to Know

◆ Anorexia nervosa is a life-threatening eating disorder that involves self-induced starvation and refusal to maintain a normal healthy weight.

◆ Bulimia nervosa is a serious eating disorder that involves repeated episodes of rapidly consuming large quantities of food and then ridding the body of the excess calories by self-induced vomiting, laxatives or diuretic abuse, and/or prolonged exercising.

◆ Compulsive overeating is repeatedly eating excessive amounts of food. Unlike bulimics, compulsive overeaters do not purge and therefore tend to be extremely overweight.

◆ Treating an eating disorder generally requires a collaborative approach from a psychiatrist or psychologist, a physician, and a nutritionist.

Recipes for Your Health

Breakfast Berry Crepes

2 cups whole-grain flour

1 egg, beaten

2½ cups low-fat milk

Nonstick vegetable spray

½ cup blueberries

½ cup sliced strawberries

½ cup raspberries

Serves four
Nutrition Information
Calories: 325
Protein: 15 grams
Sodium: 95 mg
Total fat: 4 grams
Saturated fat: 1.6 grams
Cholesterol: 59 mg
Dietary fiber: 5 grams

From the kitchen of Cynthia Williams and Jesse and Cole Bauer

Place flour in a bowl and add egg plus 2 cups of milk. (Save ½ cup.) Beat with a wire whisk until all lumps are gone and the mixture is completely smooth. Gradually add remaining ½ cup milk to make a thin batter. Use nonstick cooking spray on a hot skillet (medium-high temp) and pour enough batter in the pan just to make a large circle. Sprinkle desired amount of fruit on top and press down into crepe. Cook for approximately 2–3 more minutes and then flip crepe and cook the other side. Carefully lift onto a plate and roll it up.

Greek "Village" Salad

4 large tomatoes, cut into chunks

2 green peppers, cut up into rings

1 large red onion, cut into rings

1 large cucumber, peeled and sliced

½ lb. feta cheese, sliced and crumbled

½ cup light Greek salad dressing

Black pepper, to taste

Dried oregano, to taste

Place cut tomatoes in a salad bowl with green pepper, onion, cucumber, and half of crumbled feta cheese. Mix in light Greek salad dressing and black pepper to taste. On top, arrange rest of feta in neat slices and sprinkle with oregano and a bit more dressing.

Garden Tostada

8 corn tortillas

¼ cup nonfat mozzarella

¼ cup nonfat sour cream

Salad

½ red bell pepper, chopped medium

¼ cup chopped scallions

1 Anaheim chili pepper, seeded and chopped medium

4 TB. prepared salsa

2 ripe tomatoes, chopped medium

2 TB. vinegar

2 cups black beans, drained

3 cups shredded dark-green lettuce

Serves four
Nutrition Information
Calories: 300
Protein: 15 grams
Sodium: 200 mg
Total fat: 2 grams
Saturated fat: 0 gram
Cholesterol: 0 mg
Dietary fiber: 9 grams

Preheat oven to 375°. Place corn tortillas on cookie trays; do not overlap. Bake 5 minutes and turn over. Bake 10 more minutes or until curled and golden brown. Combine salad ingredients in large mixing bowl. To serve: Place 2 corn tortillas on each plate. Place salad mixture on top of each tortilla. Place 1 tablespoon nonfat mozzarella and 1 tablespoon sour cream over each tortilla.

Curried Chicken and Rice

1½ cups water

1 cup chicken broth

1 cup canned crushed tomatoes

¼ cup dark, seedless raisins

1 tsp. curry powder

½ tsp. cumin

1¼ cups uncooked basmati rice

12 oz. chicken breasts, boneless, skinless, cut into ½-inch cubes

2 cups broccoli florets

4 TB. nonfat plain yogurt

Serves four
Nutrition Information
Calories: 370
Protein: 28 grams
Sodium: 230 mg
Total fat: 1 gram
Saturated fat: 0 gram
Cholesterol: 50 mg
Dietary fiber: 4 grams

In a large saucepan, combine all ingredients except chicken, broccoli, and nonfat yogurt. Bring to a boil, reduce to a simmer (turn stove to medium or medium-low), and cook covered for 8 minutes or until liquid is almost evaporated. Add chicken breast and broccoli florets and cook an additional 5 minutes or until chicken is done and rice is tender. It might be necessary to add more water. Serve with nonfat yogurt spooned over the top of each portion.

Eggplant Parmigiana

1 large eggplant

2 cups corn-flake crumbs

Pinch cayenne pepper

¼ tsp. garlic powder

1 cup nonfat plain yogurt

Olive oil cooking spray

1 cup grated nonfat
    mozzarella cheese

16 oz. pasta sauce

Preheat oven to 350°. Slice eggplant lengthwise into ¼-inch-thick slices. (It is optimal to get 6 or 8 slices; that way, you have 1½ to 2 slices per person.) Combine corn-flake crumbs, cayenne pepper, and garlic powder in a large mixing bowl. Coat eggplant slices with yogurt on both sides and then press both sides into corn-flake crumb mixture.

Set coated eggplant on a cookie tray sprayed with olive oil cooking spray and spray top of eggplant lightly with olive oil spray. Bake 15 minutes or until crisp and golden brown. Top with grated nonfat mozzarella and bake an additional 3–5 minutes until cheese melts. Serve each portion over ¼ cup hot pasta sauce.

Chicken Teriyaki over Linguine

8 oz. dried linguine noodles

Vegetable oil cooking spray

12 oz. chicken breast strips
(skinless)

1 TB. low-sodium soy sauce

2 TB. orange juice

1¼ cups water

3 cups fresh mixed stir-fry
vegetables

1 cup snow peas

½ cup sliced green onion
(scallions)

1 TB. cornstarch

Serves four
Nutrition Information
Calories: 220
Protein: 25 grams
Sodium: 260 mg
Total fat: 1 gram
Saturated fat: 0 gram
Cholesterol: 50 mg
Dietary fiber: 9 grams

*Copyright © Food for
Health Newsletter, 1996.
Reprinted with permission.*

Cook linguine in 2 quarts of rapidly boiling water. Follow package directions for cooking times. Pasta is done when tender but slightly firm in center. Drain in colander.

Make the sauce: Heat a large 12-inch nonstick skillet and spray with vegetable oil cooking spray. Cook chicken strips just until done, approximately 5–7 minutes; set chicken aside. In the same skillet, add the soy sauce, orange juice, and 1 cup water. Bring to a simmer. Add all vegetables and cook until tender, approximately 6 minutes. Dilute cornstarch in ¼ cup water and stir into vegetable mixture. Broth should form a light glaze. Add chicken and serve over pasta.

Asparagus with Dijon Sauce

Serves four
Nutrition Information
Calories: 20
Protein: 3 grams
Sodium: 51 mg
Total fat: 0.7 gram
Saturated fat: 0.4 gram
Cholesterol: 1 mg
Dietary Fiber: 1.4 grams

¾ lb. fresh asparagus spears

¼ cup reduced-sodium chicken broth

2 tsp. Dijon mustard or tarragon Dijon mustard

1 TB. grated Romano or Asiago cheese

Break woody ends off asparagus and place in skillet. Pour broth over asparagus and then cover and steam over medium heat until crisp-tender (about 4 minutes). Remove asparagus to warm serving plate with slotted spatula and keep warm. Add mustard to skillet; increase heat to high and bring to a boil, stirring constantly. Pour over asparagus and sprinkle with cheese.

Microwave Method

Break woody ends off asparagus and place in 2-quart rectangular microwave-safe dish. Pour broth over asparagus; cover with vented plastic wrap and cook on high power 3–4 minutes or until crisp-tender. Pour off liquid into 1-cup glass measuring cup. Keep asparagus covered. Whisk mustard into juices. Cook uncovered at high power until boiling, about 30 seconds. Pour over asparagus; sprinkle with cheese.

Spaghetti and Turkey Meatballs

Spaghetti, ½ box uncooked
(preferably whole-wheat)

1 lb. lean, ground turkey
breast meat (all ground
white meat)

Black pepper, to taste

Garlic powder, to taste

Parsley, to taste

Paprika, to taste

Chopped, dehydrated onion
flakes, to taste

1½ (26-oz.) jars marinara
sauce*

Cook spaghetti as directed on box. Drain and set aside. Season
ground turkey breast with black pepper, garlic powder, parsley,
paprika, and chopped dehydrated onion flakes. Shape meat into
1-inch balls and place into a large pot with marinara sauce. Cook
on low flame for approximately 50–60 minutes.

(*Choose any brand with 60 calories or less per serving; for
example, Healthy Choice, Ragu Light, Classico Tomato and
Garlic, and the like.)

Serves six
Nutrition Information
(1 cup cooked pasta with 3 turkey meatballs) Calories: 350 Protein: 24 grams Sodium: 630 mg Total fat: 8 grams Saturated fat: 2 grams Cholesterol: 72 mg Dietary fiber: 4 grams

*From the kitchen of Carol
Bauer*

Chicken Cacciatore

Serves six
Nutrition Information
Calories: 310
Protein: 38 grams
Sodium: 841 mg
Total fat: 5 grams
Saturated fat: 1 gram
Cholesterol: 106 mg
Dietary fiber: 5.5 grams

From the kitchen of Ellen Schloss

2 (26-oz.) jars marinara sauce*

½ large green pepper

½ large red pepper

½ large yellow pepper

2 cups sliced mushrooms

6 large chicken cutlets, skinless/boneless—2 lbs. (approx. 5 oz. each breast), cut into thirds

(*Choose any brand with 60 calories or less per serving; for example, Healthy Choice, Ragu Light, Classico Tomato and Basil, and the like.)

Heat marinara sauce in a large pot over stove until boiling. Add peppers and mushrooms and simmer 5 minutes. Add all chicken pieces and mix thoroughly. Cover pot and cook on low heat for 45 minutes.

Bouillabaisse

Serves six
Nutrition Information
Calories: 350
Protein: 44 grams
Sodium: 970 mg
Total fat: 13 grams
Saturated fat: 2 grams
Cholesterol: 187 mg
Dietary fiber: 2.5 grams

From the kitchen of Herbie Schloss

1 cup chopped white onion

2 TB. chopped garlic

2 celery stalks, chopped

¼ cup olive oil

2 cups water

2 (14½-oz.) cans whole tomatoes, chopped with liquid

2 cups sliced mushrooms

1 tsp. dried thyme

1 tsp. bay leaves

2 lbs. crab (fresh crab or seafood salad meat)

½ lb. bay scallops

½ lb. peeled shrimp

¼ cup parsley, chopped

In a large frying pan, over medium-high flame, sauté onion, garlic, celery, and olive oil until tender (approximately 10 minutes). In a separate large pot, pour in water, chopped tomatoes with liquid, mushrooms, thyme, bay leaves, and the onion/celery/garlic mixture; bring to a boil. Stir in crab, bay scallops, and peeled shrimp; bring to a boil, reduce heat, and simmer for 10–15 minutes. Stir in chopped parsley.

Pork Tenderloin

2 TB. low-sodium soy sauce

¼ cup bourbon (or other liquor)

1 TB. brown sugar

1½ lbs. pork tenderloin

Sauce

¼ cup reduced-fat sour cream

¼ cup low-fat mayonnaise

1 TB. scallions

1 TB. mustard, dried

1 TB. vinegar

Serves four
Nutrition Information
Calories: 340
Protein: 39 grams
Sodium: 485 mg
Total fat: 16 grams
Saturated fat: 4.5 grams
Cholesterol: 99 mg
Dietary fiber: 0 gram

From the kitchen of Michelle P.

Preheat oven to 325°. Make marinade: Mix soy sauce, liquor, and brown sugar. In a plastic bag, marinate pork tenderloin for 2–3 hours. Cook for 1 hour. Make sauce by mixing sour cream, mayonnaise, scallions, mustard, and vinegar. Serve sauce on the side or pour over the pork tenderloin.

Caribbean Rice Salad

Serves four
Nutrition Information

Calories: 340
Protein: 11 grams
Sodium: 230 mg
Total fat: 1 gram
Saturated fat: 0 gram
Cholesterol: 0 mg
Dietary fiber: 8 grams

Copyright © Food for
Health Newsletter, *1996.*
Reprinted with permission.

Rice

1½ cups white long-grain rice

Dressing

2 TB. cider vinegar

2 TB. orange juice

4 TB. nonfat Italian salad dressing

Salad

1 (15¼-oz.) can black beans, drained and rinsed

1 orange, peeled, diced into ½-inch cubes, and seeds removed

1 mango, peeled, chopped into ½-inch cubes, and pit removed

1 fresh tomato, diced into ½-inch cubes

½ jalapeño pepper, minced fine, seeds and veins removed

½ red bell pepper, sliced into thin strips and seeds removed

¼ cup sliced green onions

6 cups shredded dark-green lettuce

Prepare long-grain rice according to package directions. If you are in a hurry, use instant rice instead. Allow to cool to room temperature. (This process can be hurried by putting the cooked rice in your freezer in a shallow pan.)

Combine dressing ingredients together and toss with salad ingredients; toss with rice and serve. You can use additional orange segments and pepper strips for garnish if you want. Divide entire tossed salad between four plates and serve.

Sweet Potato Stew

½ TB. margarine

2 cups fresh sweet potatoes, cooked and sliced

1 (8-oz.) can crushed pineapple in natural juice

¼ tsp. ground cinnamon

⅓ tsp. salt

Heat margarine in a large frying pan. Add sweet potato slices and pineapple. Sprinkle with cinnamon and salt. Simmer uncovered until most of the juice has evaporated (about 10–15 minutes), turning potato slices several times. Serve.

Serves six
Nutrition Information
(½ cup serving) Calories: 135 Protein: 1.3 grams Sodium: 78 mg Total fat: 1.6 grams Saturated fat: 0.3 gram Cholesterol: 0 mg Dietary Fiber: 2.3 grams

Papaya Sorbet

1 ripe papaya (1¼ lb.), diced

¼ cup plain low-fat yogurt

½ cup light corn syrup

1 tsp. fresh lime juice

Place papaya in a 9-inch square baking pan and freeze for about 1 hour. Place frozen papaya in food processor with yogurt, corn syrup, and lime juice. Process until smooth. Freeze at least 1 hour. Makes 2 cups.

Serves four
Nutrition Information
Calories: 160 Protein: 1.4 grams Sodium: 60 mg Total fat: 0 gram Saturated fat: 0 gram Cholesterol: 1 mg Dietary Fiber: 0.3 gram

Spicy Poached Pears

Serves four
Nutrition Information
Calories: 165
Protein: 1 gram
Sodium: 5 mg
Total fat: 0.7 gram
Saturated fat: 0.1 gram
Cholesterol: 0 mg
Dietary Fiber: 3.8 grams

Copyright © 1995, The American Dietetic Association. "Skim the Fat: A Practical and Up-to-Date Food Guide." Used with permission.

½ cup cranberry juice cocktail

⅓ cup water

¼ tsp. ground cloves

¼ tsp. cinnamon

⅛ tsp. ground ginger

4 ripe bosc pears, peeled

1 cup apple juice

1 TB. orange juice

Pour cranberry juice, water, and spices into a deep saucepan; cover and bring to a boil. Trim the bottom off pears, if necessary, so they stand up straight. Remove cores. Add pears to saucepan and simmer uncovered until tender (15–25 minutes, depending on how ripe the pears are). Remove pears and set aside. Cook remaining liquids over medium-high heat, stirring periodically, until mixture has reduced by half. Drizzle this juice-syrup over pears and serve while warm, or chill and serve later.

Nutrition and Health Directory

Nutrition Organizations

American Dietetic Association (ADA)
120 South Riverside Plaza
Suite 2000
Chicago, IL 60606-6995
312-899-0040
Consumer Nutrition Hotline
Tel: 1-800-366-1655
www.eatright.org

American Heart Association (AHA)
National Center
7272 Greenville Avenue
Dallas, TX 75231
Tel: 1-800-AHA-USA1 (242-8721)
www.americanheart.org

American Cancer Society
1599 Clifton Rd. NE
Atlanta, GA 30329
Tel: 1-800-227-2345
www.cancer.org

American Institute for Cancer Research (AICR)
1759 R St. NW
Washington, DC 20009
Tel: 1-800-843-8114
www.aicr.org

American Diabetes Association (ADA)
ATTN: Customer Service
1701 North Beauregard Street
Alexandria, VA 22311
Tel: 1-800-DIABETES (342-2383)
www.diabetes.org

Arthritis Foundation Information Line (AFIL)
PO Box 7669
Atlanta, GA 30357-0669
1-800-568-4045
www.arthritis.org

American College of Sports Medicine
PO Box 1440
Indianapolis, IN 46206-1440
Tel: 317-637-9200
www.acsm.org

National Eating Disorders Association
603 Stewart St.
Suite 803
Seattle, WA 98101
Tel: 206-382-3587
Help line and treatment referral line: 1-800-931-2237
www.nationaleatingdisorders.org

National Association of Anorexia Nervosa and Associated Disorders (ANAD)
PO Box 7
Highland Park, IL 60035
Tel: 847-831-3438
Fax: 847-433-4632
E-mail: anad20@aol.com
www.anad.org

Celiac Disease Foundation
13251 Ventura Blvd.
Suite #1
Studio City, CA 91604
Tel: 818-990-2354
Fax: 818-990-2379
E-mail: cdf@celiac.org
www.celiac.org

The Food Allergy and Anaphylaxis Network (FAAN)
11781 Lee Jackson Highway
Suite #160
Fairfax, VA 22033
Tel: 800-929-4040
Fax: 703-691-2713
E-mail: faan@foodallergy.org
www.foodallergy.org

Joy Bauer Nutrition
Individual Nutrition Counseling
116 East 63rd Street
New York, NY 10021
Tel: 212-759-6999
Fax: 212-759-7766
www.joybauernutrition.com

Vegetarian Resource Group
PO Box 1463
Baltimore, MD 21203
Tel: 410-366-VEGE
E-mail: vrg@vrg.org
www.vrg.org

American Botanical Council
PO Box 144345
Austin, TX 78714-4345
Tel: 1-800-373-7105
Tel: 512-926-4900
Fax: 512-926-2345
www.herbalgram.org

**Food and Drug Administration Center for Food Safety
and Applied Nutrition**
5100 Paint Branch Parkway
College Park, MD 20740-3835
Tel: 1-888-SAFEFOOD
www.cfsan.fda.gov

**National Center for Complementary and Alternative Medicine
NCCAM Clearinghouse**
PO Box 7923
Gaithersburg, MD 20898
Tel: 1-888-644-6226
Tel: 301-519-3153
E-mail: info@nccam.nih.gov
nccam.nih.gov

**Office of Dietary Supplements
National Institutes of Health**
6100 Executive Blvd.
Room 3801, MSC 7517
Bethesda, MD 20892-7517
Tel: 301-435-2920
Fax: 301-480-1845
E-mail: ods@nih.gov
ods.od.nih.gov

United States Pharmacopoeia
12601 Twinbrook Parkway
Rockville, MD 20852
Tel: 1-800-822-8772
Tel: 301-881-0666
www.usp.org

Monthly Newsletters

Consumer Reports on Health
101 Truman Avenue
Yonkers, NY 10703
Tel: 1-800-234-2188
www.consumerreports.org

Environmental Nutrition
PO Box 420235
Palm Coast, FL 32142-0451
Tel: 1-800-829-5384
www.environmentalnutrition.com

Nutrition Action Health Letter
Center for Science in the Public Interest
1875 Connecticut Ave. NW
Suite #300
Washington, DC 20009
Tel: 202-332-9110
Fax: 202-265-4954
www.cspinet.org

Tufts University Diet and Nutrition Letter
PO Box 57857
Boulder, CO 80322-7857
Tel: 1-800-274-7581
www.healthletter.tufts.edu

Your Body Mass Index (BMI)

Body Mass Index (BMI) has been replacing traditional height and weight tables as an index of healthy weight in relation to disease risk. The BMI formula is your weight in kilograms (1 kilogram = 2.2 pounds) divided by height in meters squared. However, every height and weight variance has already been calculated, so you don't have to bother with the math. Use the following BMI chart to determine if your weight poses health risks. The general rule is that a BMI of 24 or less is associated with the lowest risks of weight-related diseases. If your BMI is between 25 and 29 you are considered to be overweight, which increases your chances for several health complications, including heart disease, Type 2 diabetes, and certain cancers. If your BMI is 29 or higher, you are considered obese, with multiple health risks. Please understand that if you are very muscular, your BMI might not be accurate: muscle is denser than fat, and may throw the table off. Extra weight due to increased muscle mass has not been linked to health complications.

National Heart, Lung, and Blood Institute (NHLBI)
NHLBI Information Center
PO Box 30105
Bethesda, MD 20824-0105
301-592-8573 phone
301-592-8563 fax
Website: www.nhlbi.nih.gov
E-mail: NHLBIinfo@rover.nhlbi.nih.gov

Body Mass Index Table

Body Weight (pounds)

BMI (Height in inches)	Normal						Overweight					Obese										Extreme Obesity														
BMI	19	20	21	22	23	24	25	26	27	28	29	30	31	32	33	34	35	36	37	38	39	40	41	42	43	44	45	46	47	48	49	50	51	52	53	54
58	91	96	100	105	110	115	119	124	129	134	138	143	148	153	158	162	167	172	177	181	186	191	196	201	205	210	215	220	224	229	234	239	244	248	253	258
59	94	99	104	109	114	119	124	128	133	138	143	148	153	158	163	168	173	178	183	188	193	198	203	208	212	217	222	227	232	237	242	247	252	257	262	267
60	97	102	107	112	118	123	128	133	138	143	148	153	158	163	168	174	179	184	189	194	199	204	209	215	220	225	230	235	240	245	250	255	261	266	271	276
61	100	106	111	116	122	127	132	137	143	148	153	158	164	169	174	180	185	190	195	201	206	211	217	222	227	232	238	243	248	254	259	264	269	275	280	285
62	104	109	115	120	126	131	136	142	147	153	158	164	169	175	180	186	191	196	202	207	213	218	224	229	235	240	246	251	256	262	267	273	278	284	289	295
63	107	113	118	124	130	135	141	146	152	158	163	169	175	180	186	191	197	203	208	214	220	225	231	237	242	248	254	259	265	270	278	282	287	293	299	304
64	110	116	122	128	134	140	145	151	157	163	169	174	180	186	192	197	204	209	215	221	227	232	238	244	250	256	262	267	273	279	285	291	296	302	308	314
65	114	120	126	132	138	144	150	156	162	168	174	180	186	192	198	204	210	216	222	228	234	240	246	252	258	264	270	276	282	288	294	300	306	312	318	324
66	118	124	130	136	142	148	155	161	167	173	179	186	192	198	204	210	216	223	229	235	241	247	253	260	266	272	278	284	291	297	303	309	315	322	328	334
67	121	127	134	140	146	153	159	166	172	178	185	191	198	204	211	217	223	230	236	242	249	255	261	268	274	280	287	293	299	306	312	319	325	331	338	344
68	125	131	138	144	151	158	164	171	177	184	190	197	203	210	216	223	230	236	243	249	256	262	269	276	282	289	295	302	308	315	322	328	335	341	348	354
69	128	135	142	149	155	162	169	176	182	189	196	203	209	216	223	230	236	243	250	257	263	270	277	284	291	297	304	311	318	324	331	338	345	351	358	365
70	132	139	146	153	160	167	174	181	188	195	202	209	216	222	229	236	243	250	257	264	271	278	285	292	299	306	313	320	327	334	341	348	355	362	369	376
71	136	143	150	157	165	172	179	186	193	200	208	215	222	229	236	243	250	257	265	272	279	286	293	301	308	315	322	329	338	343	351	358	365	372	379	386
72	140	147	154	162	169	177	184	191	199	206	213	221	228	235	242	250	258	265	272	279	287	294	302	309	316	324	331	338	346	353	361	368	375	383	390	397
73	144	151	159	166	174	182	189	197	204	212	219	227	235	242	250	257	265	272	280	288	295	302	310	318	325	333	340	348	355	363	371	378	386	393	401	408
74	148	155	163	171	179	186	194	202	210	218	225	233	241	249	256	264	272	280	287	295	303	311	319	326	334	342	350	358	365	373	381	389	396	404	412	420
75	152	160	168	176	184	192	200	208	216	224	232	240	248	256	264	272	279	287	295	303	311	319	327	335	343	351	359	367	375	383	391	399	407	415	423	431
76	156	164	172	180	189	197	205	213	221	230	238	246	254	263	271	279	287	295	304	312	320	328	336	344	353	361	369	377	385	394	402	410	418	426	435	443

Source: Adapted from *Clinical Guidelines on the Identification, Evaluation, and Treatment of Overweight and Obesity in Adults: The Evidence Report.*

A Closer Look at the Foods We Eat

If you're looking for nutritional information on specific foods and beverages (calories, fat, calcium, iron, and so on), visit the following websites:

www.nutritiondata.com

www.nal.usda.gov/fnic/foodcomp/search/

For those of you interested in learning more about the popular alcoholic beverages, the following table shows you just how many calories are in a typical serving.

Alcoholic Beverage	Serving Size (Fluid Ounces)	Approximate Calories
Beer	12	150
Light beer	12	100
Bloody Mary	6.0	140
Gin and tonic	6.0	180
Daiquiri, frozen	6.5	350
Piña colada, frozen	6.5	360
Margarita, frozen	6.5	440
Margarita	3.5	236
Manhattan	4.0	255
Long Island iced tea	4.0	275
Cosmopolitan	4.0	150
Screwdriver	7	175
Tequila Sunrise	5.5	190
Tom Collins	7.5	120
Gin/rum/vodka/whiskey (100 proof)	1.5 (1 shot)	125
Gin/rum/vodka/whiskey (80 proof)	1.5 (1 shot)	100
Wine, red and white	6.0	120
Champagne	6.0	140
Wine, sweet dessert	6.0	270
Martini	3.0	175
White Russian	3.0	250
Whiskey Sour	4.0	175
Vodka Collins	8.0	175
Vodka and cranberry juice	5.5	172
Rum and Coke	6.0	185
Rum and Diet Coke	6.0	120

Index

F

G

Q-R

W

X-Y-Z

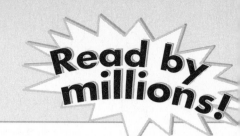
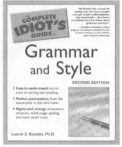
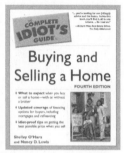
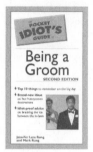
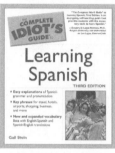
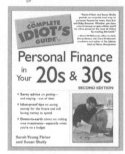
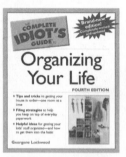
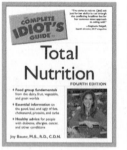
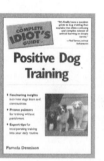
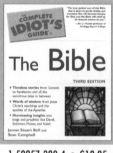
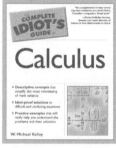
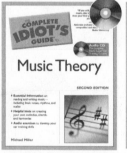
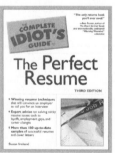
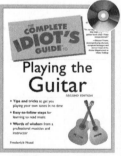
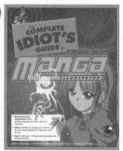
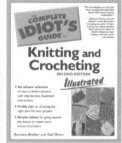